SEXUALITY AND CHRONIC ILLNESS

SEXUALITY AND CHRONIC ILLNESS
A Comprehensive Approach

LESLIE R. SCHOVER, PH.D.
SØREN BUUS JENSEN, M.D.

THE GUILFORD PRESS
New York　　　　*London*

© 1988 The Guilford Press
A Division of Guilford Publications, Inc.
72 Spring Street, New York, NY 10012

Printed in the United States of America

Last digit is print number: 9 8 7 6 5 4 3 2

Library of Congress Cataloging-in-Publication Data

Schover, Leslie R.
    Sexuality and chronic illness.

    Bibliography: p.
    Includes index.
    1. Chronically ill—Sexual behavior. 2. Sexual
disorders. I. Jensen, Søren Buus. II. Title.
[DNLM: 1. Chronic Disease. 2. Sex Behavior.
3. Sex Disorders. WT 500 S376s]
RC108.S38   1988   616.85′83   87-23640
ISBN 0-89862-715-X

Preface

We see sexual health as one important aspect of physical, social, and mental well-being. Sexuality is one of the most fundamental ways that humans share intimacy. Chronic illness, by interfering with a person's vitality, physical attractiveness, genital function, and social interactions, may create distance in relationships. Major diseases remind each of us that death is a solitary experience. To remain a sexual person, then, is to affirm life and one's connection with others.

Unfortunately, sexual health remains a neglected area of care in most medical settings. The information this book provides is relevant not only for physicians and mental health professionals but also for other members of the health care team, including nurses and occupational and physical therapists.

Part 1, "The Integrative Model of Sexuality Assessment and Treatment," is designed to teach the basic skills a clinician needs to comfortably discuss sexuality with patients, to assess sexual problems using both medical and psychological approaches, and to create a comprehensive treatment plan. In Part 2, "Specific Illnesses and Sexuality," we explore the special issues that apply to men and women who have the chronic illnesses most likely to impair sexual function: cardiovascular disease, diabetes, end-stage renal disease, chronic obstructive pulmonary disease, and cancer. We also look at several health problems that can profoundly affect sexuality: chronic pain, infertility, major psychiatric disorders, and alcoholism. Part 3, "Training and Ethical Issues," provides guidelines for training the primary health-care team and the sexuality specialist in sexual health care, and includes a discussion of ethical issues.

We would like to thank the individuals and organizations who made it practical for us to share our clinical and research knowledge across so many thousands of miles.

Seymour Weingarten, Editor-in-Chief of Guilford Press, suggested that Leslie Schover co-author this book with a physician after she presented a workshop on the topic at the American Psychological Association meeting in 1983. When we met in 1984, after several years of following each other's work, Søren Buus Jensen suggested collaborating on just such a volume and all the pieces fell into place.

We are also grateful for secretarial assistance on early drafts from Frances K. Gange of M. D. Anderson Hospital and Tumor Institute and Evalynne Laidman of the Cleveland Clinic Foundation.

The American Cancer Society has played an important role in Leslie Schover's research, funding a grant (PBR-15) on Sexual Function and Urologic Cancer Treatment as well as providing a public forum for discussion of sexual rehabilitation for cancer patients. The Danish Association for Cancer Patients and the Danish Research Council also have encouraged Søren Buus Jensen's work and provided funding for travel that allowed us to work on this and other projects. We owe our meeting to the International Academy of Sex Research, an organization that has fostered worldwide professional communication between workers in this field.

Leslie R. Schover
Søren Buus Jensen

Contents

THE INTEGRATIVE MODEL OF SEXUALITY ASSESSMENT AND TREATMENT

1

Sexuality and Chronic Illness: An Integrative Model

The physical effect of a chronic disease is often quite specific—damage to one organ or a subtle change in body chemistry. The psychological impact of an illness is broad, however, altering many aspects of a person's lifestyle. In the past 5 to 10 years, the relationship between illness and sexuality has received increasing attention. Now that behavioral medicine and sex therapy have come of age as specialties, an area of health care combining both approaches has emerged: the prevention and treatment of sexual problems in men and women who are chronically ill.

As clinicians, we tend to focus on sexual pathology, but we also need to have a concept of sexual health. Such a model provides a goal for our interventions and reminds us to assess individuals' or couples' strengths and resources, even in the midst of crisis counseling. The World Health Organization's definition of sexual health fits these requirements:

> Sexual health is the integration of the somatic, emotional, intellectual, and social aspects in ways that are positively enriching and that will enhance personality, communication, and love. (World Health Organization, 1975, p 2)

Sexual health care, then, is the process of facilitating sexual health through prevention and through intervention when problems occur. Perhaps the most important message we can convey is to maintain a balanced perspective when dealing with sexuality. Too much energy has been wasted on attempts to pigeonhole sexual problems as "organic" versus "psychogenic," especially when the patient is already labeled chronically ill. No matter what risk factors are present for sexual dysfunction, clinicians must identify the psychological, physiological, relationship, and societal threads that weave together to create the pattern we finally observe.

Perhaps a model of sexual health could not have been well defined until after World War II. Not only has sexuality become a less taboo topic, but the rising standards of living in industrialized countries, the loosening of bonds with the extended family, effective contraception, and the modern view that marriage is based on love rather than on economic concerns have also combined to focus tremendous emotional energy on

3

sexuality. Within this context, the risk that a major illness will impair sexual function becomes more threatening than it was in any previous historical period.

AN INTEGRATIVE MODEL OF SEXUAL HEALTH CARE

To help patients attain sexual health, the caregiver needs a way to integrate all aspects of functioning. Our model of sexual health care resembles the biopsychosocial model of medicine proposed by Engel (1977, 1980). The biopsychosocial model unites scientific and clinical approaches to patient care by viewing a disease as the outcome of interactions within a system. The system includes macroscopic components such as family and society as well as microscopic elements like cells and molecules. In contrast, the traditional medical model assumes that a specific disease agent acts in linear cause–effect fashion to produce a diseased person.

Figure 1-1 illustrates the integrative model using the example of a 45-year-old woman who could no longer reach orgasm after a hysterectomy and bilateral oophorectomy for benign fibroid tumors. Her sexual problem is depicted as a kind of "blob" to emphasize that the symptom looks different depending on the observer's orientation. A biological perspective, represented by the circle, reveals that the sudden decrease in circulating estrogen after surgery produced frequent hot flashes and severe vaginal dryness, interfering with the patient's desire for sex and enjoyment of intercourse.

A psychological viewpoint, denoted by the triangle, allows us to see that the patient feared her hysterectomy had left her "half a woman." She also had a history of phobic reactions, such as a fear of driving over bridges.

Social factors, represented by the rectangle, include the perceptions of her spouse, her family of origin, and society. The patient's husband believed the myth that hysterectomy impairs a woman's sexuality. The patient had also recently discovered that her husband was having an extramarital affair. She grew up in a family that valued women for their fertility, but was only able to bear one child. The hysterectomy was a reminder of her failure. Societal attitudes also contributed to the problem, since the media bombarded her with messages that sexuality is the province only of the young and beautiful.

Each of these factors is important in its own right, yet all interact to create the symptom picture. The arrows from factor to problem are bidirectional, since a sexual anxiety can in turn affect the biological, psychological, and social spheres of our patient's life.

To create a treatment plan for the problem we must also consider the influence of time. The patient's individual time is marked by her age, her sexual history, and the recent revelation of her husband's affair. Historical time also sets the scene, including society's sexual attitudes and the types of help currently available for a sexual dysfunction.

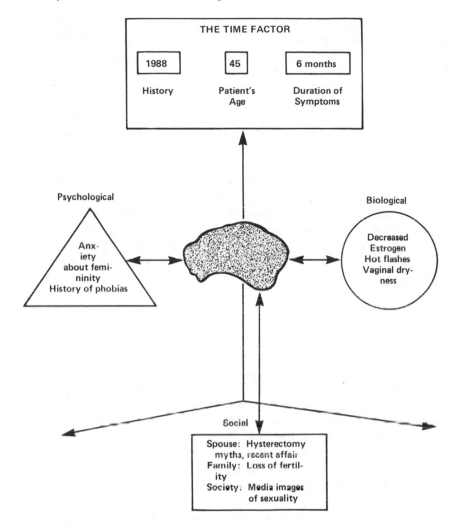

Figure 1-1. The integrative model applied to a problem of inorgasmia.

Although the integrative model seems as wholesome as apple pie, there is resistance to using it. Health care systems encourage specialization rather than integration. The result may be a strange kind of relay race. The medical specialist rushes to find a medical cause for a sexual problem, relegating psychosocial factors to a secondary, "wastebasket" role in diagnosis. The biologically oriented physician prefers to run the whole course alone, but if unsuccessful, passes the baton to the mental health clinician, instructing this colleague to complete the next lap. Since the patient expected a physiological cure, the "shrink" is not free to run at top speed, but must often drag an angry and confused patient across the course. We propose, instead, that teamwork is the essence of running an efficient and winning race. In a relay, each runner is equally important.

Mind-body dualities are not very helpful in assessing sexual problems. Yet physicians are trained to think in such terms, taking action to treat the symptom, in contrast to the mental health professional's process orientation (Brown & Zinberg, 1982; Hejl, 1984). The fast pace of work in many health-care settings produces staff overload and burnout, sapping the energy needed to cope with patients' emotions or to collaborate creatively with other clinicians. The medical physician wants a compliant patient who will follow instructions, while the mental health professional seeks to foster patient responsibility and autonomy in coping with illness. Although the field of sexology attempts to transcend interdisciplinary boundaries, it has not yet risen above these squabbles. This book is our effort to use our knowledge as psychiatrist and psychologist—Scandinavian and American— to create a more comprehensive system of assessment and treatment for sexual problems.

THEORETICAL ORIENTATIONS IN SEXOLOGY

Theories about the causes and treatment of sexual problems, like theories in other areas of medicine and psychology, have followed the vagaries of etiological fashion. Although there was a renaissance of anatomical studies in the 16th to 18th centuries, sexual problems were still commonly ascribed to witchcraft (Benedek & Kubinec, 1982). With the psychiatric enlightenment of the 19th century, dysfunctions began to be viewed as medical symptoms. The focus, however, remained on paraphilias and other examples of sexual "degeneracy" (Haeberle, 1983).

Americans are most familiar with the radical shift of Freudian theory to a belief that very early learning and family relationships determined later sexual problems. Sexual dysfunctions were regarded by the analysts as symptoms of more profound disturbance that could be cured only with full-scale psychoanalysis. In Europe, however, the period from 1900 to World War II marked the birth of the scientific study of sex. The German pioneers, including Bloch, Hirschfeld, and Marcuse began to integrate data not only from medicine and psychology, but also from anthropology, history, and philosophy into a more comprehensive view of sexuality. Their work was largely unknown in the United States until recent years (Haeberle, 1983). In Scandinavia, the focus during the 1930s and 1940s was on the fight for sexual freedom, including the right to abortion, to contraceptives, and to free expression for homosexuals (Hertoft, 1983).

In the United States, the psychoanalytic emphasis on psychogenic sexual dysfunction was superseded and made even more extreme by the work of Masters and Johnson. With the publication of *Human Sexual Response* (1966) and *Human Sexual Inadequacy* (1970), sexual problems were taken out of a medical context and put almost exclusively into a psychological one. Sexual dysfunction was the result of simple conditioning, and what was learned could be unlearned. Numerous journal articles and textbooks repeated a statement whose origins remain mysterious, that 90% of sexual problems are caused solely by psychological factors.

Such sweeping assertions are often based on naive enthusiasm or a desire to market a new treatment rather than on scientific evidence. When sex therapy came into vogue, it seemed to be *the* answer to the problem of sexual dysfunction. Clinicians rushed out to weekend workshops, eager to add this new technique to their repertoires. Sexual problems were no longer the province of physicians or even of mental health professionals. Legally, anyone could use the title "sex therapist."

The basic techniques of sex therapy have changed relatively little since Masters and Johnson's original publications. The most notable contribution has been the work of Helen S. Kaplan (1974, 1979), who combined systems and psychodynamic psychotherapy approaches with the series of behavioral exercises that constitute the treatment programs for various sexual dysfunctions. Most sex therapists of the 1980s use an eclectic range of interventions, recognizing that even Masters and Johnson drew on behavior therapy principles, particularly the work of Wolpe and Lazarus. There is also more variety in treatment format, with few centers utilizing the full co-therapy team, daily-session model developed in St. Louis.

Although the success rates of sex therapy have not matched the initial levels reported by Masters and Johnson (1970), when practiced by qualified clinicians, sex therapy continues to be one of the more effective psychotherapies (Arentewicz & Schmidt, 1983; De Amicis, Goldberg, LoPiccolo, Friedman, & Davies, 1985; Heiman & LoPiccolo, 1983; Winther, Jensen, & Hertoft, 1984; Zilbergeld & Kilmann, 1984). Success in reversing symptoms is reasonable, but long-term outcome looks brightest when measured in terms of patients' overall sexual satisfaction.

By the mid-1970s another faction began to clamor for attention—the neoorganicists. These researchers and clinicians have channeled most of their efforts into treating erection problems, but their influence is seen in articles about drug therapy for premature ejaculation (Cooper & Magnus, 1984; Girgis, El-Haggar, & El-Hermouzy, 1982) and neurological causes of inorgasmia in women (Brindley & Gillan, 1982). Whether the culprit is a neurological deficit, a hormonal abnormality, vascular disease, or something more exotic such as a shortage of a crucial neuropeptide, the treatment of choice is medication or surgery. Some of the innovations of the neoorganicists have been technically successful, notably the penile prosthesis. Tunnel vision, however, can limit both assessment and treatment so that the patient's ultimate goal of a satisfying relationship is not attained, despite the superficial "cure" of the sexual problem.

SEXUAL PROBLEMS IN MEDICAL PATIENTS: THE TIP OF THE ICEBERG

Although more attention has been paid in recent years to sexual problems in patients who are chronically ill, those who are referred for sexual counseling in fact represent the tip of the iceberg. We use diabetic men as an example from our own work, but we believe that the statistics are similar for patients with a variety of other illnesses.

Approximately 50,000 diabetic men live in Denmark, and according to several surveys, about half experience some type of sexual problem. Out of these potential 25,000 patients, how many receive any sexual counseling? Only 10% of men in a random sample of patients from a diabetes clinic had ever discussed sexuality with a physician (Jensen, 1986). Presumably, even fewer patients treated by a general practitioner would receive information about sexual function and diabetes. None of the patients with sexual problems had been referred to a sexuality specialist, although such services are well publicized in Denmark and 10% of the patients surveyed (i.e., a potential pool of 2,500 men nationwide) would welcome the opportunity to receive sex therapy.

Whether in Europe or the United States, standard practice is still to ignore sexual health. Neither physician nor patient brings up the topic, so that the great majority of problems remain untreated. Only by changing the attitudes of professionals at the primary care level will we reach the large group of patients that needs help rather than the small minority who take the risk of asking for sexual information and advice.

Sexual counseling for medical patients requires interdisciplinary cooperation. We advocate a system in which the primary health care team routinely assesses patients' sexuality, providing basic information on staying sexually active and satisfied in spite of a chronic illness. The great majority of medical patients can benefit from brief, educationally oriented counseling. Only a minority require referral to a mental health clinician who provides intensive sex and marital therapy or coordinates a treatment program combining medical and psychological approaches.

In organizing this book, we have tried to keep in mind both the needs of the primary care clinician who is not a specialist in sexuality and the mental health professional who sees the more complex cases. Although psychologists and psychiatrists may find some of the interviewing skills in Part 1 rather basic, the sexuality specialist reader can use the sections intended for the primary team when educating and supervising referral sources. The primary care clinician, in turn, needs to know enough about intensive assessment and treatment to make appropriate referrals. We carry this model through Part 2 by including three cases in each chapter illustrating a specific health problem—two cases that are routine and can be handled by the primary care team and one that is complex and should be referred to the sexuality specialist. In Part 3 we discuss training for the primary care clinician who wants to gain proficiency in sexual counseling and for the mental health professional learning to become a sexuality specialist. Ethical issues, of course, are relevant for everyone.

AN EXAMPLE OF THE INTEGRATIVE MODEL AT WORK

Our ideal of how the world should operate and our experience of reality are all too often at variance. To illustrate how we believe the integrative model can improve sexual health care, let us follow a hypothetical patient as he seeks treatment for a sexual problem in today's health care marketplace. To explore the diversity of opinions a patient might encounter, we set our story in a large eastern city in the United States.

Fred's diabetes was diagnosed when he was 59. He was treated with oral medication and a restricted diet for 4 years. Over the last 2 of these years, he gradually lost the ability to achieve full erections. He and his wife Angie had been married since their college graduation. Before the sexual problem began, they had had intercourse about twice a week. Both spouses had been satisfied with their sex life. When the erectile dysfunction became chronic, however, Angie asked her husband to stop initiating sex. "You just get frustrated," she said, "and then you take it out on me the next day. Besides, I don't like getting all excited and then having it go nowhere."

Fred, a civil engineer, believed in finding solutions to problems. He made an appointment with his internist and explained that he was having difficulty getting erections. The physician told Fred that diabetic men often become impotent. He suggested that, at age 63, Fred should be grateful not to have any more severe health problems. "You don't need to come back to see me until next year," he concluded.

Fred began to wonder if he really was crazy to be upset about a sexual problem. A friend of the family was seeing a psychologist because of a phobia about flying. Fred scheduled a visit with the therapist to discuss his own dysfunction. At the end of an assessment interview, the psychologist suggested a course of biofeedback. For 5 weeks, Fred learned to produce alpha brain waves. He felt more relaxed after the sessions, but with no discernible effect on his erections.

Angie, who had been skeptical all along about biofeedback, told her husband he should consult a "real doctor"—a psychiatrist. Fred called his county medical society and got the name of a reputable practitioner. The psychiatrist diagnosed a clinical depression and prescribed a tricyclic antidepressant. Fred's sleep improved and he did feel more energetic, but his erections were unchanged or maybe even a little worse.

At about this time, the newspaper ran an article about the inflatable penile prosthesis. The idea of a mechanical solution to his problem appealed to the engineer in Fred. A local urologist was mentioned in the newspaper, so Fred gave him a call. It was a month before an appointment could be scheduled. When the day finally arrived, the urologist took a quick history. "Diabetic, huh," he said with a wise look. "Do you ever have morning erections anymore?"

"I don't know," Fred replied. "I never seemed to have them too often in the past, and I really haven't noticed lately."

The urologist used a small Doppler stethoscope to assess Fred's penile blood pressure and pronounced it to be only 74% of the brachial pressure.* "You have pelvic arteriosclerosis," he said. "Take this kit home with you. For the next 2 nights, I want you to paste a ring of stamps around your penis. If you don't break the stamps, you need surgery. Call me next Monday and tell me the results."

Fred did not break the stamps either night. He returned to the urologist's office for a serious discussion of the risks and benefits of a penile prosthesis. The urologist was ready to schedule surgery for the following week, but Fred wanted time to think after hearing about the 15% chance of needing a revision later on, his greater risk, as a diabetic, of infection during healing, and the 2 weeks that he would need to take off from work after surgery. Angie was also not enthusiastic about the prosthesis. She asked her husband if it could cause long-term health problems, like cancer. She cautioned, "And what if the surgery damaged your heart?"

Fred was confused and discouraged. What kind of expert could really give him a definitive answer to his problem? He called the county medical society again. This time they referred him to the sexual dysfunction clinic of the city's most famous medical school. When Fred called to make an appointment, he was surprised by the requirement that Angie come with him, but his wife agreed to try it.

The couple was interviewed jointly by a psychiatry resident. She began by obtaining a picture of their relationship, both marital and sexual. Angie's problems with vaginal dryness, hot flashes, and difficulty reaching orgasm after stopping her estrogen therapy 2 years previously were explored in detail. The couple also talked about their fears that Fred's diabetes would

---

*The specialized medical tests mentioned in this narrative are explained in detail in Chapter 6.

lead to incapacitating side effects. Angie expressed her frustration with her husband's habit of sneaking sweet desserts. Fred complained that his wife never hugged him anymore and slept on the far side of the bed. Angie began to cry. The interviewer explained how common these patterns were with a chronically ill spouse. She promised the couple that the clinic would perform some special medical examinations, and then the staff would confer to arrive at a treatment plan for the erection problem.

This time Fred's medical assessment included a complete physical examination as well as specialized tests of erectile function. Penile blood flow was recorded, and penile blood pressures were taken before and after lower-extremity exercise. An electromyograph was used to record the latency of the bulbocavernosus reflex. Heart-rate beat-to-beat variation was monitored during deep breathing, and sensory thresholds were measured on Fred's penis. Finally, Fred slept for 2 nights in the clinic so that both his sleep and his nocturnal erections could be measured. Before scheduling the sleep studies, the physician had Fred stop his antidepressant medication since the drug inhibits the rapid eye movement (REM) sleep periods in which erections normally occur.

The resident met again with the couple to give them feedback. Fred's autonomic nervous system was not affected by his diabetes. He had a mild decrease in blood circulation to his penis, especially after exercise, but his nocturnal erections were really in the normal range for his age. The discrepancies from the urologist's earlier test results could be explained by the more extensive and sophisticated nature of this clinic's workup and the elimination of the antidepressant medication. The suggested treatment plan was to have Fred cut down on his cigarette smoking and to have the couple come in for 15 weekly sessions of sex therapy. The counseling would focus on improving couple communication and helping both partners express caring more easily. The clinicians felt that with a more relaxed and sensual sexual interaction, Fred's erections might become firmer. Quitting smoking might also improve the blood flow to his penis. They advised Fred not to consider a penile prosthesis unless this treatment left the couple dissatisfied.

Fred worried about the expense of the psychotherapy. His insurance policy would cover prosthesis surgery but did not pay for couple sessions. Since the clinic operated on a sliding fee scale, however, the couple decided they could afford the costs. The staff, in turn, agreed to try to limit the treatment to 10 sessions if possible.

Three months later Fred and Angie were much happier with their relationship. Fred was complying with his diet without pressure from his wife and had completely stopped smoking. The couple was setting aside 2 evenings a week for leisure time together. Each partner was far more aware of the other's needs for closeness and affection. Their sexual routine involved more extensive caressing, often ending in noncoital orgasm for each partner. About half the time, Fred was able to achieve an erection firm

Table 1-1. The Integrative Model Applied to the Case of Fred

	Psychological Factors	Physiological Factors	Relationship Factors	Social Factors
Assessment Results	• Poor compliance with diabetic diet • Anxiety about long-term diabetic complications • Clinical depression	• Mild pelvic vascular deficit • Heavy smoker • Antidepressant medication • Wife's postmenopausal vaginal atrophy	• Poor communication of affect and sexual preferences • Decrease in expressing affection since sexual problem began • Sexual routine performance-oriented; Focus on erections and intercourse • Wife overprotective of husband's health, encouraging him to take passive role	• Primary care physician disapproves of sexuality for older adults • Insurance does not cover couple therapy
Treatment Results	• Encourage more active role for Fred in controlling his diet and quitting smoking • Use cognitive behavioral techniques such as self-monitoring, positive thinking, and self-reinforcement • Try to eliminate antidepressant because of exacerbation of erectile difficulty; if depression persists, try other medications	• Quit smoking • Educate couple on water-based vaginal lubricants; use vaginal estrogen cream if conservative treatment fails	• Communication training • Negotiation on expressing caring more effectively in nonsexual contexts • Sensate focus and enrichment of sexual routine • Give wife insight into husband's need to actively control his health, enlist her support for his efforts in that direction	• With Fred's permission, send assessment report to his physician; follow with phone call to increase physician's knowledge of clinic services • Sliding fee scale; reduce planned sessions from 15 to 10

enough for satisfying intercourse. The use of a water-based lubricant made intercourse more comfortable for Angie, so that her ability to reach orgasm returned to its normal level. Both spouses felt they had met their goals and saw no need for further treatment.

Fred and Angie are not an actual couple, but rather a composite of patients we have seen. We can only guess how many Freds are discouraged by the attitudes of their primary health care team from ever getting help and how many others drop out of the treatment system somewhere along the way or go home with a penile prosthesis that cannot revitalize a flagging relationship.

Table 1-1 illustrates how the integrative model of sexual health care can be applied in assessing and treating Fred's erection problem. This book is designed to help the reader formulate similar treatment strategies. We would like to shorten the odysseys of the Freds of this world and to create more happy endings.

2

Couple Therapy and the Integrative Model

Sexual problems occur in relationships. Even when a person's only sexual outlet is masturbation, a fantasied partner is usually involved. Sex therapists have espoused the view that the "patient" is optimally the couple, although individuals or groups can be treated using a sex therapy format.

In medical settings, however, the patient is the patient. When assessing and treating a sexual problem in someone who is chronically ill, the clinician's first task is often to shift the focus from the individual to the dyad. In this chapter, we present a model of health care for couples that is relevant not only to sexual problems, but to the wider impact of chronic illness on an intimate relationship. We often use the term "spouse" for the sake of convenience, but what we have to say can apply to unmarried partners or to homosexual couples as well.

THE COUPLE MEETS THE MEDICAL MODEL

When a chronic illness develops in one partner, the anxiety and stress is shared by the other. Yet in most medical settings, little effort is made to involve the family in health care despite growing evidence of their important role in health maintenance and compliance with medical instructions (Doherty & Baird, 1983; Minuchin, Rosman, & Baker, 1978). Rather than giving medical information to a couple, the physician may tell the diagnosis only to the patient, or worse, inform the spouse but not the patient (Krant & Johnston, 1978). This latter pattern is particularly common when the patient is a woman, but we have also seen the opposite case.

Since couples do not expect to be seen jointly by the physician, the spouse often does not accompany a patient to the doctor's office or to the hospital. The physician who does wish to see the spouse must make a special effort to set up a couple appointment. Not only is the clinician breaking medical tradition, but the patient may have a hidden agenda for excluding the spouse, especially when sexual problems are at issue.

14

A 48-year-old engineer was referred to the Danish sexology center. He had previously been evaluated by his general practitioner and by a plastic surgeon who wished to implant a penile prosthesis. The surgeon wrote, "Hans is the most well-adjusted man I have seen in months. There must be an organic reason for his erection problem, although all of our laboratory evaluations were negative." Neither of the two physicians involved in the case had met Karen, Hans's wife.

When the couple appeared for their appointment, they presented an incongruous picture. Although the spouses were the same age, Karen looked 10 years older than her husband. Her face was caked with heavy make-up and her lacy, outmoded dress looked like it had been pulled out of an attic storage chest.

Each day, Karen laid in bed until an hour before Hans was to arrive home from work. At that time she dressed, put on her make-up, and prepared dinner. Evening cocktails were followed by a candle-lit meal. As soon as the dishes were done, Karen was ready for sex. If foreplay did not quickly result in an erection, she got out of bed and took her sleeping pills, returning to lie as far away from Hans as possible, with her back turned. Karen rarely left the house or saw anyone except her husband.

In an individual session, Hans said that coming home was like stepping into a padded cell in which he was the inmate's only contact with the outside world. Karen refused to participate in couple therapy, but Hans came in for several sessions. He despaired of changing his marital relationship, but did acknowledge that a penile prosthesis would not solve his problems.

Physicians and nurses rarely are taught techniques of couple therapy. When contemplating a joint visit, the clinician may fear being overwhelmed by the couple's conflicts. It takes practice to maintain a neutral position that gives the message, "I am here to coach both of you to work as a team in coping with this illness." The clinician who tries to enlist a spouse's support in helping the patient remain on a diet, quit smoking, or follow a medication schedule may end up feeling like a ping-pong ball, slammed alternately by husband and wife, who shout:

Wife: See! I told you the pills were important!

Husband: Then why did you forget to pack them when we went away for the weekend?

Wife: They're your pills! Why didn't you pack them?

Health care professionals need more training in interviewing couples and families. An experienced clinician might interrupt the above dialogue, saying, "Let's forget what happened last week, and see if we can plan how to make things go smoothly this week. What can your wife do tomorrow to help you remember to take your pills? And how would you feel about your husband's suggestion? Do you have some other ideas?"

Taking a couple approach to chronic illness can be rewarding for clinicians. Many diseases can only be controlled by lifestyle changes that affect the whole family. Giving the spouse an active role in health care increases the chance that a patient will comply with treatment. The majority of spouses seen in medical settings are supportive and loving. Getting to know a couple gives the physician, nurse, or other health care provider an enhanced sense of involvement in the family's intimate ties and in their efforts to maintain a high quality of life. The clinician also learns to recognize quickly the distressed couple that will need extra help to meet the challenge of illness. Early intervention with a disturbed family can often prevent turmoil that would otherwise interfere with medical care.

We advocate scheduling periodic couple visits routinely when treating chronically ill patients (see Chapter 6). If the health-care team sees a cross-section of couples, clinicians are less likely to dread that each interaction will be a struggle. The clinician who schedules couple visits only after family problems have disrupted medical care risks burnout. Crisis sessions reveal families' weaknesses, but do not teach us about their strengths.

THE IMPORTANCE OF THE PARTNER
IN HEALTH MAINTENANCE

A couple's relationship can affect the development and management of a chronic illness in a variety of ways. Simply being married is correlated with better physical and mental health for both men and women (Verbrugge, 1979). Divorced or separated people have the poorest health, followed by the widowed. Although the data are not absolutely clear, it appears that men's health is more adversely affected than women's by being unmarried (Stroebe & Stroebe, 1983; Verbrugge, 1979).

Perhaps married people are healthier because of a selection bias, that is, the healthiest and most competent people are the most likely to marry. Selection effects do not seem powerful enough to account for the strong relationship between marital status and health, however (Stroebe & Stroebe, 1983; Verbrugge, 1979). Another hypothesis is that marriage provides a buffer against stressful life events that could damage health.

We need more research on how marital status influences the quality of life of the chronically ill. Spouses often play a role in getting a patient to seek medical attention. The American Cancer Society has a poster that reads, "A nagging wife may save your life." After a disease is diagnosed, the spouse's support becomes even more crucial in helping the patient adjust to medical regimes. Behavior therapists are just beginning to tap the potential of the spouse as a "cotherapist" in treating obesity (Brownell & Stunkard, 1981) or in helping patients quit smoking. While some protective effects of marriage are relatively nonspecific, such as the benefits of intimacy, social support, or touching, the spouse also can play a concrete role in helping a chronically ill patient to comply with medical treatment or to reduce high-risk behaviors like substance abuse. Some of the causes of excess mortality in bereaved spouses, especially widowers, suggest poor self-care: auto accidents, cirrhosis of the liver, homicide, and suicide (Stroebe & Stroebe, 1983).

Certainly not all aspects of a marriage relationship promote health. If one spouse is stressed at work and brings frustrations home, the other partner's health may be adversely affected. That is one interpretation of the finding in the Framingham heart study that men married to college-educated working women developed more coronary disease (Haynes, Eaker, & Feinleib, 1983). Recently, another large epidemiological study also found an association between wives' educational levels and Type A husbands' heart disease, especially when wives were active and dominant (Carmelli, Swan, & Rosenman, 1985).

At least for mental health, the quality of the marital relationship is a predictor of better adjustment (Gove, Hughes, & Style, 1983). Marital unhappiness or a lack of intimacy is correlated with the severity of depression within samples of married psychiatric patients (Crowther, 1985; Waring & Patton, 1984). Assortive mating may explain this finding, however. A number of studies suggest that men and women with major psychiatric disorders choose spouses who have similar psychopathology (Merikangas, 1982). Of course, some couples meet in psychiatric treatment settings or because they live in similarly disadvantaged neighborhoods as a result of their limited coping skills. The evidence is weaker that partners select each other on the basis of similar personality styles. Type A behavior, for example, does not show high concordance between husbands and wives (Haynes et al., 1983).

Studies of couples with a diabetic spouse illustrate that the ability of both partners to cope with illness is also predictive of sexual function (Jensen, 1985a, 1985b). One of us (SBJ) interviewed 51 couples, rating their "disease acceptance" as good, moderate, or poor. The rating was based on both partners' success in meeting the crisis of the diagnosis, complying with medical instructions, maintaining a supportive social network, and achieving good self-esteem. Emotional reactions to illness, including depression, anxiety, and denial, were also included in the judgment. Only 15% of couples with good disease acceptance reported a sexual dysfunction, in contrast to 57% of those with moderate or poor disease acceptance.

Corroborating evidence came from a standardized questionnaire filled out separately by each partner. Respondents were asked whether they agreed completely, agreed somewhat, disagreed somewhat, or disagreed completely that they had experienced 15 negative emotional reactions to diabetes. The number of problems reported by both partners correlated significantly with sexual function. In future studies, this approach could be expanded to study the relationship between couples' coping styles and their ability to stay sexually active despite an illness (see Chapter 6).

COUPLES' STRENGTHS IN COPING WITH ILLNESS

Since general coping skills and sexual function are linked in the chronically ill, the clinician treating sexual problems should identify and foster strengths in the relationship that can mitigate the stress of illness. Of course there is no formula for marital happiness; anyone who discovers the magic equation will be a strong contender for the Nobel Peace Prize. We can, however, provide guidelines for evaluating partners' joint resources.

Health care professionals should become aware of four varieties of tasks that partners in a well-functioning relationship have mastered: allocating marital roles, respecting each others' boundaries, achieving a good level of communication, and agreeing on relationship rules. These couple skills interact to foster a supportive relationship. We describe each type of task in more detail, illustrating theoretical concepts with case examples, visual schemata, and brief exercises that can be used as part of couple assessment.

Allocating Marital Roles

As a relationship develops, each partner is assigned roles to play. Some roles center around everyday chores, such as child care, earning wages, cooking, cleaning, and balancing the checkbook. Others are less concrete: nurturer, initiator of contacts with friends, liaison with the extended family, or financial decision-maker. When allocating roles, partners must retain some flexibility in sharing daily tasks, avoid functioning in a parent–child model, and set aside private time for "adult" activities together.

Role Flexibility

Some couples allocate tasks according to traditional gender roles. Such relationships may be termed *complementary*. Other couples create *symmetrical* relationships, sharing tasks so that each partner invests an equal effort across the board. Most relationships, in fact, blend the two styles, with some tasks divided along gender lines while others are assigned by preference: "Let's take turns giving the kids their baths, but since I like cooking and you're the gardener, we'll each take responsibility for our favorite jobs."

Of course the assignment of roles is rarely so overt and permanent, even in couples who reject sex-role stereotyping. Not only does division of labor shift over time, but partners often have different perceptions of who does what. An interesting exercise, shown in Figure 2-1, is to have a husband and wife generate a list of roles and then each draw a graph representing the man's and woman's responsibilities. Each partner can chart roles first as they were before illness interfered with the family life, and then for the present situation.

When a couple has a very complementary relationship, they may have difficulty altering role responsibilities during an illness. The classic example is the traditional wife who has no idea of how to keep track of family finances and so feels helpless when her husband is hospitalized.

Avoiding a Parent–Child Interactive Style

One common pattern when the husband in a traditional marriage becomes ill is for the wife to act parentally while he regresses into childishness. Many wives do in effect become mother, not just to their children but to their husbands as well. When the husband shows symptoms of illness, the wife nags him to see the doctor. Once a disease has been diagnosed, she limits her husband's activities; monitors his eating, drinking, and bowel habits; and discourages him from independence, even in simple tasks like making his own breakfast or remembering to take his medications. The husband also relinquishes his role as a sexual adult, or perhaps the partners fear that sexual activity will be harmful to his health. The role of invalid is not compatible with the role of lover, especially when a man believes the "macho" doctrine that he must be the initiator and leader in sexual matters. Loss of sexual function and wage-earning capacity are very difficult issues for men who become ill.

Of course this parent–child pattern may also be seen when a wife becomes ill. Again, rigid sex-role expectations contribute to the interaction; since women are fragile, illogical, and ineffectual, a strong and clear-headed man must direct the wife's medical care and hold the family together. A decrease in sexual activity may stem from the man's overprotectiveness and the wife's concept of herself as impaired and chronically ill. Women who have traditional sex-role attitudes also are especially vulnerable to loss of self-esteem if illness affects their physical attractiveness or impairs their ability to take care of family tasks.

Scheduling Adult Time

A couple needs time to relax and enjoy togetherness after outside work and household chores are finished. During child-raising years, some couple time must be held separate from leisure time that includes the whole family. Privacy not only fosters sexual interactions, but allows emotional sharing and provides an opportunity to resolve conflicts. When couples have a sexual dysfunction, an absence of adult time is often observed (Jensen, 1985b). Sometimes the lack of privacy contributes to a sexual problem, but in other

Step 1. Partners make a list of roles important to their family life. Examples might include child care, wage earning, cooking, being the social secretary, nurturing, long-range planning, initiating sex.

Step 2. Each partner separately completes the chart below.

Write your list of roles on the lines of this chart. Think about the 6 months *before* illness affected your family life. For each role, color in the percent of the line that best describes how much of the work *you* did. The remaining white space will represent your partner's percent of responsibility. For example, if you did 80% of the cooking, the first line would look like this:

	10%	20%	30%	40%	50%	60%	70%	80%	90%	100%
Role:										
Cooking										

Step 3. Each partner fills in the chart again, but now estimates role responsibilities since the illness, over the past 3 months.

Step 4. With the therapist, the partners compare their charts and try to arrive at a joint estimate of their role responsibilities before and then after the illness. In a complementary relationship, each partner's chart would look like this:

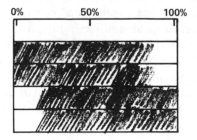

In a symmetrical relationship, Both charts would look like this:

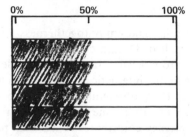

Figure 2-1. An exercise evaluating the impact of illness on marital roles.

cases the low priority given adult time represents an avoidance of sexuality in reaction to the dysfunction.

When one partner becomes ill, adult time is often sacrificed. The healthy partner scrambles frantically to complete the work of two, especially in young couples who have children.

Tim and Pat were in their mid-30s. After an auto accident left Tim paraplegic, he was hospitalized for 5 months in a rehabilitation facility. Pat continued to teach school and take care of the couple's daughters, aged 5 and 7. She visited her husband several times a week, but the children only saw him for an hour on Sundays.

Tim's homecoming was less joyful than he expected. Adjusting to life in a wheelchair was difficult, in spite of changes made in the house and car to help him become independent. The children had grown used to Pat's meeting all their needs and reacted negatively whenever Tim tried to replace his wife as bedtime storyteller or lunch giver. If Tim tried to initiate sexual activity, Pat often said she was too tired. She also became irritated with her husband if she felt he wanted to be babied, for example, calling her from the next room and asking her to bring him a coke. After these incidents, Pat would feel guilty and try to apologize, but Tim would turn on the television and refuse to talk.

Couple therapy focused on balancing marital roles, encouraging Tim to take over his old tasks and to plan positive interactions with his children and private time with Pat. The couple's sexual relationship improved markedly when Pat no longer saw lovemaking as another marital obligation, but as a chance to feel close to her husband and to give and receive pleasure.

Figure 2-2 presents a couple evaluation sheet for assessing the partners' skills in scheduling adult time together. Each partner uses a time line to describe how a typical day was spent before a chronic illness began and currently. The amount of adult time is highlighted and compared in the past versus the present. To increase the amount of adult time available, each partner offers to make several schedule changes and also suggests concessions that the other could make. A space is provided for final solutions, arrived at mutually with the therapist's help.

Respecting Each Other's Boundaries

When two people build a relationship, they must find a comfortable degree of intimacy, agreeing on how deeply to share feelings, how much time to spend together, and how openly to express affection. We observe a continuum of degrees of intimacy in relationships. Intimacy is not a static concept, so that a couple can travel through different stages of closeness over time.

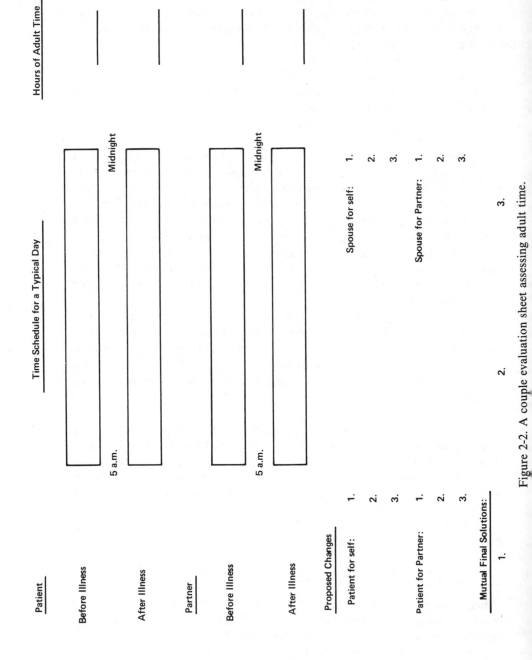

Figure 2-2. A couple evaluation sheet assessing adult time.

22

When a couple has the optimal balance between intimacy and autonomy, their boundaries touch yet remain distinct. They are aware of each other's needs and emotions. An illness can upset the balance achieved, evoking fear and anger. A couple's previous success in resolving intimacy issues will determine how well they cope with an illness. Disease can prevent one partner from enjoying the couple's favorite leisure pursuits, force the spouses to spend far more time in each other's company than usual, reduce the amount of adult time, or, conversely, exert pressure on the partners to prove their love by being more affectionate than usual.

During the crisis period of an illness, couples have a tendency to oscillate between the more extreme points of the intimacy range. In their attempts to support each other, the partners may begin to violate each other's autonomy. The result can be a switch into withdrawal or even flight.

Lisa was regarded by family and friends as the perfect spouse during the first few months of her 28-year-old husband's treatment for Hodgkin's disease. She worked from 8 a.m. to 3 p.m. each day and then, if Steve was hospitalized, spent the evening in his room. When he was at home, she cooked his lunches for the week on Sunday, freezing them in microwave trays so that he could heat them by pushing a button. She spoke of the illness as "our" cancer, illustrating that the couple had moved from closeness to fusion.

During Steve's most intensive chemotherapy, Lisa stopped working and sat with him all day in the hospital. She felt guilty if she read a magazine instead of distracting her husband from his illness with conversation. She refused friends' invitations to take off an afternoon and go shopping, but did cheerfully attend her sister's baby shower, never revealing her grief at having to put off motherhood, perhaps forever, because of her husband's cancer treatment. No matter how ill Steve became, he maintained a stoic calm and was never irritable with his wife. The couple had attained a kind of symbiosis.

As Steve finished his chemotherapy, however, and began to recover, the young couple's relationship showed the effects of this unnatural degree of closeness. Steve wanted to resume sexual activity, but his wife felt no sexual desire. Lisa was bewildered by her feelings, but thought perhaps she had become tired out by the stress she was under. The couple was now in withdrawal. Steve had become friendly with one of his nurses and confided his sexual frustration to her. She reacted with sympathy, and made a date to meet Steve at a local pub. Although they did not have intercourse, they spent some time kissing in Steve's car. The next time that Lisa refused his sexual advances, Steve told her about this encounter. Lisa left and went to her mother's for the night. The couple had reached the flight stage of their intimacy conflict.

The oscillation cycle can also begin with withdrawal. If an illness is life threatening, both partners must cope with the fear of death. The healthy partner risks being left behind. The ill partner fears being replaced by someone new. Reactions to this separation anxiety often depend on a person's past experiences with loss. The crisis may reactivate unresolved mourning for a parent or a previous spouse. When one partner stops communicating feelings, touching, or reaching out sexually, the other may try to regain intimacy by initiating sex, smothering the withdrawn spouse with affectionate gestures, or making anxious inquiries as to what the partner is thinking or feeling. Other spouses fear being perceived as demanding, so they wait silently for intimacy to return to normal. For the clinician, these latter couples with each partner locked in their twin cells of fear and loneliness are the most poignant. Fortunately, brief couple therapy can often help the partners see that their confinement is voluntary.

Couples in relatively new relationships are more likely to react to an illness with a decrease in intimacy. Withdrawal does not have to lead to flight, however, if the partners can develop a sense of trust over time.

Although Harry was 68 and his wife was 60, they had only been married for 2 years when he had a myocardial infarction (MI) that left him with heart failure. Harry was not a candidate for cardiac bypass surgery, and his physicians warned the couple that his lifespan was limited. Harry and Cynthia's marriage had been stormy from the beginning. They had begun an affair while Harry was still married to his first wife, a fact that became known in their small and religious southern town. Harry's children refused to visit his house, and Cynthia's daughter snubbed her in public. The couple switched church congregations but still felt rejected by many old friends.

Cynthia was also bitter because Harry proved different as a husband than he had been as a lover. He rarely showed affection or gave her compliments, and their sex life became increasingly perfunctory. In subtle ways, especially after his heart attack, Harry let his wife know that he shared his children's suspicions that she had married him for his money. Cynthia was indignant but at the same time was angered when she discovered that she would benefit very little from her husband's will. Harry also felt guilty about involving a younger, healthy woman in caring for him and was depressed by his difficulty in achieving erections or even in comfortably enjoying mutual caressing. He suggested to his wife numerous times that she leave him and find a man who could satisfy her sexually. Cynthia would respond with reassurances of her fidelity and commitment.

Although the couple never resumed a satisfying sex life, Harry's behavior changed radically after his wife supported him through a respiratory arrest and hospitalization. He became very open in avowing his love for her and wanted her in close proximity, preferably in physical contact, as much as possible. Cynthia continued to be wary, but stood by her husband until his death 8 months later.

Achieving Good Communication

A couple's ability to allocate marital roles and to arrive at a comfortable level of intimacy depends on good communication skills. Clinicians who work with couples learn to recognize effective communication and spot maladaptive patterns that interfere with partners' ability to negotiate compromises. Because communication is such a complex process, professionals who are new to couple counseling need a model that alerts them to different communication styles and helps them to recognize hidden messages.

A model that we have found helpful in teaching and clinical supervision is based on the concept that each person's defense mechanisms, or habitual ways of processing information from inner experience and from the outer world, also shape communication with the partner. Most people use a variety of communication styles, but one or two may be more typical of them, particularly when under stress. Table 2-1 illustrates this schema.

As an example, suppose you were counseling Jeff, a 46-year-old multiple sclerosis patient, and his wife Jane. Jeff primarily uses denial as a communicative style, while Jane is apt to react to the world by withdrawal. When Jeff's neurological symptoms are diagnosed as multiple sclerosis, he ignores the situation as much as possible. He cannot tell his physician how often he feels unusual sensations in his lower limbs and, indeed, did not seek medical attention until he had fallen several times and finally twisted his

Table 2-1. Communicative Styles that Affect Couples' Abilities to Cope with Illness

	Definition	Example
Denial	Refusal to hear one's own feelings or the partner's concerns	"So I had a little tumor. It's gone now and I don't see why you're nagging me to go in for a check-up."
Projection	Failing to realize that the other's feelings are separate from one's own.	"I know that you would feel better if we just stayed home tonight and rested."
Passive Acceptance	Swallowing the other's feelings rather than being aware of one's own	"You're right. We shouldn't marry now that I'm infertile. I want you to be happy with someone else."
Withdrawal	Focusing on one's own fantasies but failing to test them against reality	"I don't bother to date anymore. I know a man wouldn't be attracted to a woman who has a colostomy."

ankle. When asked whether he is frightened by his prognosis, he says that doctors make mistakes and perhaps his illness has been misdiagnosed.

Jane's response to the family crisis is to appear depressed and apathetic. Household chores go unfinished. She spends a large proportion of the day worrying about the future, but does not share any of her concerns with Jeff.

This couple avoids overt conflict because Jeff is unaware of his feelings or his wife's, while she lives in her own inner world, rarely trying to understand her husband. Unfortunately, their mutual pact of uninvolvement, while it minimizes pain, leaves them unprepared for Jeff's worsening health.

Sexually, Jeff and Jane silently agree to be celibate. Jeff does not want to initiate sex, because his occasional erectile dysfunction reminds him of his disease. He does not wonder if Jane is sexually frustrated and she, in turn, feels no desire for erotic contact.

When interacting with a health professional, Jeff is willing to talk but expresses little affect. Jane is usually silent, unless asked a direct question. The partners do not make eye contact with each other or turn to one another spontaneously during the consultation. The clinician must evaluate their communication by asking how each typically expresses caring and anger and how one partner knows when the other is frightened, annoyed, or sad.

Nonverbal Cues

Clinicians should remain alert to discrepancies in a couple's verbal and nonverbal communication. Primary care physicians and nurses can regard body language as a diagnostic sign, just like shortness of breath, pallor, or ankle edema. Do the partners look at each other when they talk? Does one sit with folded arms, turned slightly away from the other? Does the wife smile sweetly as she tells her husband how ineffectual he is? During the counseling process, such observations can be used to help the couple understand their own communication.

Communicative Styles and the Therapeutic Relationship

The same patterns that interfere with couple communication also distort the interaction between the clinician and the couple. Clinicians will recognize the couple who simply forgot that the physician, when eliciting informed consent before surgery, warned of erection problems (denial); who assume that the doctor is just as anxious as they are to have a long conversation at midnight about the causes of constipation (projection); who feel compelled to agree with the nurse who said that older pople should not be interested in sex (passive acceptance); or who thought the hospital would call if the prescription was to be refilled when the bottle was empty (withdrawal). Clinicians must take care to communicate clearly themselves and to identify communication patterns that may interfere with good care.

Agreeing on Relationship Rules

As Sager (1976) has pointed out, every relationship develops a set of contracts that governs its daily functioning. These rules are usually unspoken and each partner may interpret them somewhat differently. When a couple faces a chronic illness in one partner, their flexibility in rewriting the marital contract determines their success in coping with the crisis. Of course some relationship rules are more adaptive than others. The following are some "contracts" that promote good coping in the midst of a health crisis.

A basic commitment exists so that if conflict occurs, the relationship is not threatened. In stable relationships, partners tolerate conflict without expecting it to escalate to divorce. Partners have a sense of themselves as "we" and can picture themselves growing old together. The sexual revolution in the 1960s led couples to question whether commitment included lifelong sexual fidelity. Currently, however, a return to monogamy seems to be in progress, perhaps spurred on by epidemics of sexually transmitted diseases like herpes and acquired immune deficiency syndrome (AIDS).

Partners share power equally and openly. At first impression, many couples appear unbalanced in terms of power. One partner speaks for both or seems to make all decisions. On deeper acquaintance, however, the clinician finds that an apparently powerless spouse actually wields a great deal of covert authority. Two of the issues most often used in a passive-aggressive manner to control a relationship are illness and sex.

Alice, aged 38 and on renal dialysis, complained of loss of sexual desire. She and her husband, Ralph, were interviewed together. They agreed that he preferred to have sex daily while she would be satisfied if intercourse took place only once a month.

Alice: My husband really calls the shots about sex in our house. He's always pressuring me, and I always feel guilty.

Ralph: *She's* the one in charge. I could stand on my head and beg for sex, but it wouldn't do any good. Sex only happens when she's ready. And I'll tell you, when your wife only wants sex once a month, you'd better be in the mood all the time or else you'll miss your chance. Talk about pressure!

Each partner contributes his or her unique strengths to the relationship. Well-functioning couples can tolerate diversity. In fact, relationships often develop because one partner supplies what the other lacks.

Jill: When we met I thought you were such a warm, gentle person. Just watching you sit there, smoking your pipe, I felt you would be my roots.
Walter: And you were so bubbly, always with something exciting to report. I guess I felt you made life more vivid.

Yet, the same qualities that draw partners together may subsequently become a source of conflict.

Jill: You never have anything to say. I'm so sick of sitting there while you hide behind the newspaper and the pipe smoke!
Walter: You just want to talk, talk, talk! Can't I relax in peace and quiet for a few minutes after a busy day?

When one spouse becomes ill, the partners' diverse ways of handling stress are often exaggerated. The reserved partner sits in a corner while the other calls all their friends and discusses the latest treatment plan. The result is an increase in bickering and a decrease in intimacy.

When conflict occurs, it will be resolved. In a well-adjusted couple, disagreements lead to compromise and new solutions for daily life problems. Even though sharp words may be exchanged, or one or both partners may sulk for a while, negotiation ensues. For some couples, however, compromise is difficult. Perhaps an issue is so sensitive that neither partner dares to approach it, and an undercurrent of tensions disturbs daily interactions.

Each partner is accepted by the other unconditionally. Unconditional love is an essential element of trust in relationships. When each partner feels valued as a person, the couple can weather traumas such as a disability in one partner. Indeed that is the meaning of the marriage vow, "for richer or for poorer, in sickness and in health, until death do us part."

Unconditional acceptance also lays the groundwork for constructive criticism. A husband can ask his wife to work fewer evenings because he wants to change what she *does*, not what she *is*. She can listen, knowing that the request comes out of a desire for a better partnership. If such trust is not an integral part of a relationship, a chronically ill partner is likely to fear that the marriage will fall apart.

The most important time is here and now. Couples who can focus on the present have an easier time handling the stress of an illness. Diseases bring uncertainty about future health and lifespan, often disrupting a family's future plans. A good solution is to enjoy each day as much as possible and to limit plans to the immediate future. Many couples have difficulty forgetting "the good old days before I got sick," or giving up the illusion of control over the future.

It takes work to keep a relationship going. It has often been said that rising divorce rates reflect our unrealistic attitudes about relationships. We think that romantic love should strike like a thunderbolt and then last forever. Although passionate love brings partners together and helps them stay bonded in spite of conflict, the real glue of relationships is each partner's willingness to change, to allow the other to grow, and to make time for togetherness.

Even during an illness, relationships should not be neglected. As we mentioned earlier, couples often sacrifice their adult time to keep up with daily life tasks. Yet disease makes each partner vulnerable to fear of loss and to loneliness. Taking time to communicate and to reduce the impact of the illness on intimacy is the key to maintaining marital happiness despite health problems. One part of that intimacy is sexuality. There too, a couple's unspoken agreements can help or hurt them as they undergo the stress of an illness.

Couple Skills and Sexual Health

The same skills that shape a couple's general relationship, allocating roles, respecting boundaries, communicating effectively, and agreeing on relationship rules, also promote a satisfying sex life. We review each of these areas of sexual adaptation, noting how mastery promotes continued sexual activity during an illness.

Allocating Sexual Roles

Many couples give all the responsibility for initiating sex to one partner, usually the husband. Such a pattern may work well until one spouse becomes ill.

Bill's emphysema became so severe that he had to retire from his job as a construction foreman. He kept busy with household chores but felt depressed. He and Joan did not discuss the change in their lives. They spent their evenings watching television.

Bill also had developed erectile dysfunction. During sex he often became breathless and then lost his erection. Joan noticed that her husband came to bed later and later and avoided touching her. She missed the intimacy and pleasure of their sex life, but she had never felt comfortable asking for lovemaking. Now she feared that her husband would see any sexual advance as a demand and would feel more inadequate than he already did.

When men become ill, they often stop initiating sex. Wives, however, may not know how to take over the role of seducer and keep sexual feelings alive. Even when a sexual dysfunction develops, men continue to take responsibility for sexual initiation, but the frequency often drops radically (Jensen, Meidahl, & Sjögren, 1984). The influence of traditional male sex roles on a couple's sex life becomes even more crucial when we realize that many chronic illnesses physiologically impair men's sexual function more than women's.

We have already discussed the incompatibility of a parent–child relationship with continued sexual activity. Diseases that limit mobility or disturb bowel or bladder function lead to role confusion when the healthy spouse must switch from caretaker to lover, helping with catheter care at one moment and caressing the next. Some couples delegate as little physical caretaking as possible to the healthy spouse. When roles must be mixed, however, sexual attraction and mutual respect can help both partners transcend the embarrassment.

Sexual Communication

An illness often interrupts a couple's sexual routine. For 20 or 30 years they have made love the same way. Communication has become almost superfluous. Now the ability to share emotions and preferences, verbally and nonverbally, becomes crucial. No two partners will always be in the mood for sex at the same time or always prefer the same types of sexual stimulation. Asking for a new caress, however, means risking rejection. In the optimal relationship, each partner can communicate a sexual desire but does not always expect it to be granted. Perhaps a man with emphysema finds the missionary position for intercourse too fatiguing, but his wife has never volunteered to try a position that would give her the active role in movement. The husband needs to be able to verbalize his desires, at the same time knowing that his wife will not accede out of pity or guilt if she finds the idea repugnant.

Many couples believe that the only normal way to reach orgasm is through intercourse. Yet our experience with cancer patients clearly shows that partners who have occasionally helped each other reach orgasm with noncoital stimulation before cancer treatment are far more likely to resume sex after the illness (Schover, Evans, & von Eschenbach, 1986). Couples who relegate all noncoital caressing to the category of "foreplay" are not as adaptable as those who see sex as "loveplay." Changing such practices calls for good communication.

Sexual communication can also be taken to extremes. Sexual variety is pleasant, but each partner must respect the other's boundaries so that sex is never frightening or painful. Not every sexual wish needs to be spoken or acted out, and a session of lovemaking does not have to end with an "instant replay" analysis.

Respecting Sexual Boundaries

When couples disagree about the variety of frequency of sexual activity they must arrive at some compromise. What feels like comfortable intimacy to one partner may be overwhelming to the other. Although conflicts about sexuality in a couple often involve each partner playing a fixed role, that is, the pursuer versus the distancer, in reality each feels that boundaries are being transgressed.

Especially for inexpressive patients, sexuality becomes one of the only ways to experience intimacy. Yet, couples function best when they regard sex as one but not the only way of being close. Otherwise, an illness that interferes with sexual function can precipitate a panic. If the wife is ill, the husband may continue to demand sex as a way of maintaining a sense of contact with her. She complies, feeling it is her duty as a wife, but in fact is passive and distant, making her husband feel more desperate. Conversely, a man who conforms to traditional sex-role expectations may withdraw emotionally from his wife if he becomes sexually dysfunctional. Such patients benefit from counseling on substituting other ways of being close for some of the missing sexual interactions, such as cuddling, sharing a hobby, or having a quiet talk.

Couples also get into trouble when one partner regards sex as an ideal way to make up after a fight, but the other is still turned off and angry. Overtures of apology may need to precede sexual advances.

Agreement on Sexual Rules

Our society's emphasis on sexual performance has been a negative influence for many couples. Their sex lives have become overly rule-bound by maxims such as:

• Sex is a failure unless both partners reach orgasm.
• Sex is a serious business.
• Sexuality belongs to the young and the beautiful.

When confronted by an illness, couples must reexamine their sexual rules and take a less performance-oriented attitude towards lovemaking, exploring new ways of pleasuring each other. Sexuality can also assume too much importance in life. A sense of humor belongs in the bedroom just as it does in the rest of the house. Playfulness can ease the tension in accommodating lovemaking to the limitations imposed by an illness. Couples can focus on each partner's attractive points rather than striving to match a glossy magazine fantasy of perfection.

Although couple issues are inextricable from a discussion of sexuality, not every patient has a traditional, heterosexual relationship. To conclude this chapter we discuss two common types of patients seen in medical settings; the patient involved in an extramarital affair and the single patient.

THE EXTRAMARITAL AFFAIR

One of the situations that makes clinicians most apprehensive about tackling sexual issues is the extramarital affair. It is easy for physicians or other professionals to get caught in the triangle of patient, spouse, and lover. If an affair predates the diagnosis of a chronic illness, the patient's confrontation with mortality may either provoke termination of the extramarital relationship or cause the patient to disclose its existence to the spouse.

When Paul, the wealthy 54-year-old owner of an importing business, found out that he had end-stage renal disease, he brought his 36-year-old girlfriend rather than his wife to the hospital. The couple requested a consultation to discuss sexual function and dialysis. Paul said that his greatest fear was to be critically ill and lose touch with his girlfriend. She would have no legitimate way of keeping in contact with him or even of knowing his medical status. Paul and his girlfriend described his wife Ginger as a very prim and proper woman who had always disliked sex. She kept busy with her children and her many volunteer projects. Although Paul and his girlfriend were discreet, they believed that a less disinterested wife would have discovered their affair long ago. Paul did not want to leave his marriage. He needed Ginger's help in running their large establishment and in entertaining business clients. Ginger had asked to accompany her husband to the hospital, but he told her that her job was at home, taking care of house and children.

Ginger entered the scene, however, and the girlfriend had to leave when the physicians decided to teach Paul and his family to use home dialysis equipment. After a few days, Paul sent his wife to the psychologist. Believing that his time on earth was limited, Paul told Ginger about his affair. He suggested to her that she and his girlfriend ought to be able to cooperate like "sisters" in supporting Paul and satisfying his needs. Since Paul had assured Ginger that he would never divorce her, he was shocked when she reacted to his disclosure with tears and angry scenes.

Ginger did not match her husband's description of a frigid socialite. A softly pretty woman, she told a story of years of loneliness and resentment at being excluded from her husband's emotional life. She felt more like an employee than a wife, and was especially angry at her husband's lack of attention to their three children. Ginger was needy enough to overcome feeling betrayed because the psychologist had counseled Paul with his girlfriend. She did actively try to enlist the psychologist's support against the girlfriend, pointing out that the girlfriend had repeatedly been a guest in the couple's home and asking how any woman could be so callous.

The psychologist had to walk a thin line, trying to support Ginger, meeting with the couple to help them decide how to proceed, and talking on the phone to the girlfriend, who had no other way to find out the progress of Paul's health. The situation was only tenable because it was clearly a short-term crisis and because all the protagonists were appealing and fairly insightful people. Even Paul had a boyish charm, although he was basically narcissistic. The poignancy of his illness overshadowed the cruelty of his manipulations.

The upshot of the story was ironic, however. Paul had a successful renal transplant and, restored to good health, was left to manage an angry wife and a newly assertive girlfriend.

Any illness may also stimulate one partner to begin an affair. The patient may feel it is his or her last chance to find happiness or sexual pleasure. The partner may have an affair to deny grief over a spouse's impending death, or even to act out resentment at the spouse for becoming ill.

Sam was dying of cancer at age 40. He and Amy, age 25, had been married for 5 years and had a 3-year-old daughter. Both spouses had stormy relationships with their own families and had been isolated and miserable before finding each other. Their marriage was bonded by their view of outsiders as the enemy. When Sam's cancer was diagnosed, he was ready to seek any form of treatment, including nontraditional therapies. His rage and his conviction that the cancer resulted from occupational exposure to chemicals soon alternated with periods of delirium and severe pain from bone metastases.

One day Amy asked to see the psychiatrist, who had met with the couple earlier. Tearfully, she confessed that in her loneliness she had gone out drinking with her husband's best friend and they had ended up having sex together. The clinician was supportive but tried to help Amy gain some insight into her feelings. They discussed her needs for nurturance, her anger at the friend who had taken advantage of her vulnerability, and her even greater rage at the husband who was leaving her to fight the world alone. The therapist focused on Amy's temptation to tell her husband about the affair. By the end of the session, Amy said she saw why she had had a sexual encounter and was resolved not to cause Sam needless pain by telling him about it. The next day, however, Amy recounted the incident in detail to her husband. Her need to act out her anger was stronger than her ability to control her impulses in the face of great stress.

Clinicians must be aware of their own attitudes about extramarital affairs and try to remain as neutral and nonjudgmental as possible. Our role is as consultant to the couple, not as arbiter of morality.

SEX AND THE SINGLE PATIENT

We have focused on couples in this chapter because the medical model is built around the individual patient. In fact, single patients may need special attention from the health-care team. Patients who live alone lack social support when a chronic illness develops. Often they hesitate to ask friends or relatives for the kind of intensive help usually provided by a spouse. Such men and women may benefit from finding a peer network, such as the support provided by a self-help group or other community services like visiting nurses or transportation for senior citizens. The elderly often benefit from the companionship found in senior citizen's centers. For older men, such programs are a ready source of dating partners as well, since most participants are women

Dating relationships are more vulnerable than marriages to the stress of illness. When a full commitment has not been made, it is easy for healthy partners to decide they would prefer someone who is not infertile, disfigured, or in danger of dying in the next few years. Sometimes the patient pushes the dating partner away to avoid risking rejection.

Irma, a handsome woman of 66, had been dating a man 9 years younger when she had to have a mastectomy. He lived 100 miles away, so the couple only met about once a month. Irma told her boyfriend that she was going to be hospitalized for surgery but did not give him any clue as to the type of operation. Afterward, she stayed for several weeks with her brother, but did not contact her boyfriend, despite having received several calls from him during her hospitalization. Irma believed that her boyfriend would find a healthy woman his own age once he knew about her cancer. She did not want to face the pain of what she imagined his reaction would be to her mastectomy.

Some illnesses leave a public disfigurement that alienates potential dating partners at the moment of meeting. Single men and women who have facial scars, have lost a limb, or have obvious neurologic impairment are often reluctant to meet new people. It takes courage and a solid sense of self-esteem to face rejection with equanimity.

Other consequences of illness are private, but nevertheless affect developing love relationships. When does one tell a date about a mastectomy, an ostomy, infertility, or a sexual dysfunction? If divulged too early in a relationship, such information may prevent the partner from coming to value the patient enough to overlook imperfection. If left until too late, however, the disclosure may be such a shock that it provokes anger and a sense of betrayal. No easy answer exists.

The single patient is also less likely to request help for these sexual concerns. A man or woman may fear that the health care team disapproves of sex before marriage or sees the patient as asexual. Patients who are homosexual may be even more private about their sex lives, especially with the recent resurgence of homophobia because of AIDS. Thus the sensitive clinician must make an extra effort to assess sexual concerns in unmarried patients.

3

The Matrix of Normal Sexuality

Clinicians who treat sexual problems need a thorough knowledge of sexual behavior and function. This chapter provides an overview of the normal range of sexual behavior, the sexual response cycle, sexuality across the life cycle, and a system for diagnosing sexual dysfunction. Since each of these topics could fill several chapters, we focus on information essential for evaluating and treating the chronically ill patient. The references we cite provide a starting point for readers who want further knowledge.

DEFINING NORMALCY IN HUMAN SEXUAL BEHAVIOR

Although we need some reference points, sexual "normalcy" is difficult to define. One way to identify what is normal is quantitatively, that is, what the average person does. If we use such criteria, extramarital affairs are normal in the United States (L. J. Sarrel & Sarrel, 1984). Another way to look at normalcy is qualitatively. Is a sexual act morally and legally acceptable? Whose standards should then be used to judge? Sexuality is a biological process but is also inseparable from culture; each society and era has its own mores (J. LoPiccolo & Heiman, 1978).

If we view sexual normalcy from the perspective of the World Health Organization's definition of sexual health and the integrative model of sexual health care described in Chapter 1, we can identify biological, psychological, social, and temporal aspects.

The biological facets of sexual normalcy include the usual sequence of sexual development from prenatal months, through childhood, adolescence, adulthood, and old age. In adulthood, normalcy can also be defined as the capacity to experience the physiological sexual response cycle of desire, arousal, orgasm, and resolution (H. S. Kaplan, 1979; Masters & Johnson, 1966).

Psychological normalcy consists of optimal psychosexual development, so that an individual masters the sexual tasks of each developmental phase. Personality and communicative style allow satisfying sexual relationships to take place. Each phase of the sexual response cycle brings pleasure and intimacy.

Regarding sexual normalcy from a social perspective, the individual accepts societal norms for choice of sexual object and activities. Within a given society, sexual norms may differ according to a subgroup's religion, education, political beliefs, or socioeconomic status. Each family also develops a code of sexual ethics that is superimposed on societal norms. Within a couple, a standard of sexual normalcy also develops. If the partners' beliefs about sexuality are incongruent, severe relationship conflict can result.

An example is the woman who marries a transvestite and then cannot accept her husband's sexual preferences (Wise, 1985). Which partner should be asked to change when such a couple seeks help? More commonly, partners disagree on sexual variety, having different values and thus opinions about the types of sexual caressing that are pleasurable. One partner wants to try anal intercourse or to vary positions for sex while the other believes that only vaginal intercourse in the missionary position is normal. Couples may disagree on who should take the initiative in starting a session of lovemaking or about the optimal time of day for sexual activity. One partner may be angered or shocked to discover that the other masturbates occasionally. The issue is the poor matching between partners. Yet, one spouse will often try to enlist a therapist's aid, asking the expert to confirm that indeed it is "normal" for a husband to want daily sex and "sick" for a wife to experience desire only once a week. Although societies have often sought to regulate sexual behavior, we take the position that between consenting adults, any sexual behavior is normal unless it causes physical or psychological damage.

Time is important in defining sexual normalcy both in terms of a society's and an individual's history. Sexual mores have probably changed more rapidly in the last century than at any other time in history (Haeberle, 1983; Hertoft, 1983), creating a great deal of confusion about what is normal. For the individual, sexual time is measured not only in years, as when we focus on life stages, but also in the fluctuations of sexual desire over such short periods as weeks, days, or minutes.

Because sexual normalcy is so complex, we cannot take a linear, cause-and-effect view of sexual problems. Usually a problem results from an interaction of "abnormalities" in several facets of sexuality. Although it is tempting to focus on biological abnormalities when a patient is chronically ill, we must struggle to maintain an integrative point of view. Let us begin, however, by taking a closer look at the biological underpinnings of sexuality, the sexual response cycle.

THE SEXUAL RESPONSE CYCLE

Although sexual behavior varies tremendously, the physiological process of the sexual response is relatively fixed. The concept of a multiphasic sexual response cycle was first used by Masters and Johnson (1966) and has become an organizing principle for sex research and sex therapy (H. S. Kaplan, 1979, 1983). Most specialists divide the sexual response cycle into the phases of desire, arousal, orgasm, and resolution. Each phase can be characterized in terms of a person's subjective experience and by observable physiological events.

The Desire Phase

Sexual desire is difficult to define or to measure. Many authorities on sexuality use the terms "sex drive" or "libido," comparing desire with the appetite for food or the need for sleep. Sexual desire is certainly necessary for the survival of a species, but sexual behavior can be shaped by cultural evolution far more radically than can eating, sleeping, and other physiological processes. Thus it is more accurate to regard desire as a motivation or interest in sex.

Desire is intangible, but we can infer its presence from people's subjective experiences. We assess the frequency of their sexual thoughts and fantasies and how often they notice sexually arousing stimuli in their environment. We also ask about frustration when a partner is unavailable and about efforts to initiate sexual activity. In defining sexual desire, we must carefully separate subjective experience from the choice to engage in sexual activity. Masturbation and sexual activity with a partner are only indirect evidence of sexual desire.

Physiological Factors and Sexual Desire

Given our vague definition of sexual desire, it is not surprising that we only dimly understand its physiological substrates. Certainly the experience of sexual desire depends on hormones and central nervous system processes, but the question is which hormones and neurotransmitters and which areas of the brain are crucial.

Researchers agree that the androgens are the hormones most important in stimulating sexual desire for both men and women (Bancroft, 1984). For readers who are not familiar with the sex hormones, a more complete description is given in Chapter 5.

In men, as long as testosterone levels are within the normal range, significant correlations between the amount of circulating hormone and the frequency of sexual desire or activity are rarely observed (Tsitouras, Martin, & Harman, 1982). Testosterone may operate according to a threshold model (Bancroft, 1984). As long as a man produces a minimum level of hormone, his sexual desire will be normal. Excess androgens have little or no additional effect.

In women the situation is complicated by the menstrual cycle (Bancroft, 1984). Because most mammals show a peak in sexual activity at the time of female ovulation, researchers have searched for an upsurge in women's sexual desire at midcycle (Sanders & Bancroft, 1982). The data currently available suggest that women's sexual desire peaks slightly just before and after menstruation (Bancroft, 1984) but not at midcycle.

Androgen levels vary only somewhat across the menstrual cycle. In general, studies of sexual desire and arousal in the laboratory and in real life suggest that baseline androgen levels do correlate with women's interest in sex (Persky *et al.*, 1982; Schreiner-Engel, Schiavi, Smith, & White, 1981). Estrogen and progesterone have few discernible effects on women's sexual desire, however (Bancroft, 1984).

Sexual desire is also influenced by the pituitary hormone prolactin, definitely in men (Schwartz, Bauman, & Masters, 1982) and probably in women (Lundberg, Hulter, & Wide, 1985; Weizman *et al.*, 1983). High prolactin levels suppress sexual interest and pleasure, probably by means of a central nervous system mechanism. The neurotransmitter dopamine inhibits prolactin release by the pituitary gland. Dopamine is also thought to facilitate sexual desire and arousal. Perhaps abnormally high prolactin levels are associated with low sexual desire because brain dopamine is simultaneously reduced. One final puzzle piece is the relationship between prolactin and beta-endorphin. Beta-endorphin may stimulate prolactin release as well as modulating other aspects of hypothalamic control of pituitary hormones (Frantz *et al.*, 1982). It has long been known that opiate addiction produces a state of sexual apathy (Mirin, Meyer, Mendelson, & Ellingboe, 1980). Endogenous opiate peptides seem to have a similar effect on sexual desire (Mendelson, Ellingboe, Kcuhnle, & Mello, 1979).

Clinicians also like to refer to "sex centers" in the brain (H. S. Kaplan, 1979, p. 79). We can confidently state that the limbic system is involved in humans' sexuality, but we really know very little about the cortical localization of sexual desire. In fact, the study of neurological deficits and human sexuality is still in its infancy. We can only conclude at present that sexual desire is the necessary, initial phase in the response cycle, but it remains the most mysterious aspect of sexuality.

The Arousal Phase

Sexual arousal, like desire, has a private, subjective component—the experience of sexual "excitement" and the sensations of sexual pleasure that result from genital stimulation. The ability to focus on pleasurable genital feelings or on an exciting mental erotic image is crucial to sexual arousal. An aroused person can dismiss distracting thoughts about daily cares or anxieties about sexual performance.

Sexual arousal is easier than desire to measure physiologically. Both men and women show signs of generalized arousal similar to that observed with other strong emotions. Changes include increases in heart rate, blood pressure, respiration rate, and overall muscle tension (Masters & Johnson, 1966). The hallmark of sexual arousal is genital vasocongestion. Increased blood flow to the penis causes erection. In women the breasts and external genitals become engorged while the vagina expands in width and depth and produces lubrication.

Physiological Mechanisms of Erection

Recently, scientists have made strides in unraveling the mechanisms of genital vasocongestion. The great majority of studies have focused on men. Erection is not simply a parasympathetic reflex, as was once thought. A nerve plexus surrounding the back and sides of the prostate (Figure 3-1) is crucial in producing erection (Lepor, Gregerman, Crosby, Mostofi, & Walsh, 1985; Lue, Zeineh, Schmidt, & Tanagho, 1984). Composed of both parasympathetic fibers and sympathetic nerves, the prostatic plexus presumably controls the dilation of the arteries that bring blood to the penis. In a young man with normal erections, the amount of blood flow during erection increases 25 to 60 times over baseline levels (Wagner & Green, 1981, p. 29). Within the shaft of the penis, blood fills up the spaces in the spongy tissue of the twin cavernous bodies. The cavernous bodies are surrounded by a tough capsule of tissue, the tunica albuginea. As blood pressure builds within, the penis swells and then becomes stiff. The corpus spongiosum, which surrounds the urethra and widens to become the glans of the penis, also fills with blood but does not grow rigid. The glans then cushions the penis during intercourse.

The corpora cavernosa contain smooth muscle cells as well as a rich supply of capillaries and nerve fibers. Although parasympathetic (cholinergic) nerves are present, the sympathetic (adrenergic) nerves are the most abundant (Benson & McConnell, 1983) and play a crucial role in erection (Melman, 1983; Wein, Van Arsdalen, & Levin, 1983; Zorgniotti & Lefleur, 1985). The "resting state" of the penis may actually involve an active sympathetic nerve process that keeps the spongy tissue empty of blood. Vasoactive intestinal polypeptide (VIP), a powerful vasodilator, is also present in large quantities in the corpora cavernosa. VIP seems to act directly to relax smooth muscle fibers (Gu *et al.*, 1983; Willis, Ottesen, Wagner, Sundler, & Fahrenkrug, 1983), allowing the spongy tissue to fill with blood. Decreased venous drainage also helps maintain an erection (Wagner, 1982).

Physiological Mechanisms of Female Arousal

The mechanisms of genital vasocongestion and vaginal expansion and lubrication in women are not nearly as well understood as the arousal phase processes in men. The lack of focus on female arousal mechanisms is

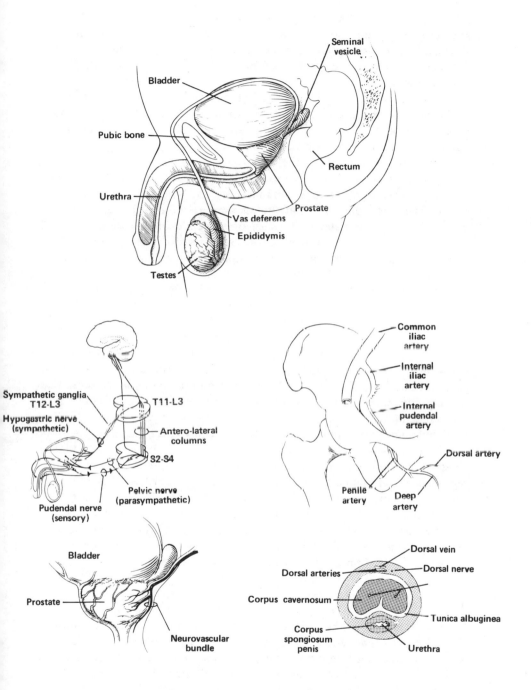

Figure 3-1. The male internal genital organs.

reflected as well in the paucity of illustrations and precise descriptions available. We do not include a parallel figure because such is not helpful to the understanding of these mechanisms. Masters and Johnson's (1966) description is still the most detailed set of observations of female genital changes during the arousal phase. Blood pools in the tissue of the labia majora, labia, minora, and clitoris. The labia swell, and, with high levels of excitement, the labia minora turn red. In some women, the clitoral glans expands visibly. At higher levels of arousal, the clitoris retracts against the pubic bone and disappears beneath its hood of skin.

The upper two thirds of the vagina deepens and widens in a series of muscular contractions and relaxations. Within 30 seconds of the onset of arousing stimulation, the vaginal lining (mucosa) "sweats" droplets of lubrication. The cervix does not contribute to vaginal lubrication, and Bartholin's glands near the vaginal entrance only secrete one to three drops of moisture. At high levels of arousal, the outer third of the vagina swells to form the "orgasmic platform." This area provides increased friction against the penis, adding to both partners' sensory pleasure.

We know that arterial flow to the vaginal walls increases with sexual arousal (Wagner & Levin, 1978) leading to the secretion of vaginal lubrication. A series of studies in Denmark suggests that VIP is an important neurotransmitter in the female genital tract, promoting vasodilation and smooth muscle relaxation just as in the penis (Ottesen, 1983). The nerves containing VIP and the adrenergic nerves cluster together in the female genital tract, again similar to the penis. It would certainly make sense that the mechanisms underlying female genital changes during arousal resemble those causing penile erection.

One point to remember is that arousal is controlled by several systems of nerves that function independently and thus can be selectively damaged by an illness. Although genital blood flow and smooth muscle contractions are regulated by autonomic and peptidergic nerves, the sensation of genital pleasure is transmitted through the sensory nervous system. In both men and women, the pudendal nerve and its terminal branches carry sensory messages from the genital, perineal, and anal areas to the spinal cord and brain (Wagner & Green, 1981). The pudendal nerve also controls striated muscle contractions crucial to the next phase of the response cycle—orgasm.

The Orgasm Phase

Orgasm, like arousal, has an experiential component and is a measurable physiological event. Orgasmic pleasure seems to be similar for men and women. Both genders report that orgasm begins with an exquisite sensation of inevitability, the "point of no return" (Bohlen, Held, Sanderson, & Ahlgren, 1982a). The orgasm then is described as "waves" of pleasure, often centered in the genital area. In both men and women, the striated muscles of the genital and anal area contract a variable number of times. The time between contractions gradually increases during an orgasm. Psychological processes important in orgasm include a sense of trust in the partner and tolerance for some loss of control. Although orgasm feels similar to men and women, some important physiological aspects of their orgasms differ.

Physiological Mechanisms of Male Orgasm

In men, the feeling of orgasmic inevitability corresponds to the emission phase of orgasm (Lipschultz, McConnell, & Benson, 1981; Newman, Reiss, & Northup, 1982). The smooth muscles of the genital area are activated, controlled by short adrenergic neurons that are part of the sympathetic nervous system. The vasa deferens, prostate, and seminal vesicles contract (Figure 3-1). The mature sperm cells, which had been stored in the epididymis (tubules capping each testicle), travel up the vasa deferens and mingle with the other components of semen. About 80% of seminal fluid is produced by the seminal vesicles and the rest by the prostate. The semen is deposited in the part of the urethra that runs through the prostate gland. At the same moment, the opening of the bladder into the urethra shuts tightly.

When the contractions of orgasm begin, the semen is ejaculated in the only free direction, outward through the urethra. The striated muscles at the base of the penis that pump during ejaculation are controlled by the pudendal nerve.

Physiological Aspects of Female Orgasm

No evidence exists for an emission stage in female orgasm despite the fact that women experience a sensation of orgasmic inevitability (Bohlen et al., 1982a). Ladas, Whipple, and Perry (1982) created a furor several years ago by announcing that some women ejaculate a fluid from the urethra during orgasmic contractions. They said the fluid was chemically distinct from urine (Belzer, Whipple, & Moger, 1984) and was produced by Skene's glands, a network of glands emptying into the urethra and thought to be a vestige of the prostate (Tepper, Jagirdar, Heath, & Geller, 1984). Bohlen (1982) has pointed out that the amount of fluid observed at "female ejaculation" is far greater than that produced in men by the prostate and seminal vesicles. He believes it is more likely to be urine. Another research team, indeed, found that fluid expelled by women during orgasm was chemically identical to urine (Goldberg et al., 1983).

Ladas and colleagues (1982) also suggested that female ejaculation, and indeed most coital orgasms in women, result from stimulation of an area on the lower to middle anterior vaginal wall, corresponding to Skene's glands. They named this area the *Grafenberg Spot* (*G spot*, for short). A few other researchers have reported that women experience the greatest pleasure from stimulation of the anterior vaginal wall, but no else has observed such a clearly defined area of sensitivity. In fact, many women prefer stimulation of the upper anterior vagina or of the posterior vaginal wall (Alzate, 1985; Goldberg et al., 1983; Hoch, 1983). A woman's orgasm can theoretically be produced by stimulating any area innervated by the pudendal nerve, including the clitoris, perineum, anus, and vagina.

Another gender difference in orgasm is that women can have multiple orgasms, that is, more than one orgasm within a single episode of sexual stimulation (Bohlen, Held, Sanderson, & Boyer, 1982b; Masters & Johnson, 1966). Men are subject to a refractory period—an interval after ejaculation in which they cannot reach orgasm again (Masters & Johnson, 1966), a period that women do not experience.

Some clinicians believe that both men and women can learn to experience multiple orgasms by performing Kegel exercises to increase the strength of the pubococcygeal (PC) muscles (Graber & Kline-Graber, 1979; Hartman & Fithian, 1984). Controlled studies of the relationship between Kegel exercises and orgasm have not demonstrated a significant effect of PC muscle strength, however (Chambless et al., 1982; Roughan & Kunst, 1981; Trudel & Saint-Laurent, 1983).

The Resolution Phase

The resolution phase of the sexual response has received little attention since it was first described by Masters and Johnson (1966). Researchers are more interested in understanding desire, excitement, and orgasm than in studying their aftermath. During resolution, physiological measures return to their baseline, prearousal levels. Subjectively, orgasm is followed by a sense of relaxation and that nebulous feeling, satisfaction.

If sexual arousal does not lead to orgasm, resolution still takes place, but more gradually. Muscle tension decreases, heart rate and respiration slow, and genital vasocongestion ebbs. Some men and women experience an unpleasant sensation of tension or fullness because of prolonged vasocongestion. Men usually locate this feeling in the scrotum, while women complain of pelvic cramping. Great variability exists, however, in the experience of resolution without orgasm. On some occasions, satisfaction and relaxation are felt regardless of the lack of sexual release.

One unsolved mystery is why men have a refractory period, and what prevents them from reaching a second orgasm immediately. With our current emphasis on improving sexual performance, "remedies" for the refractory period would be quite marketable. Most mammals do have a refractory period, and its length is fairly constant within each species (McIntosh & Barfield, 1984a). While it is always dangerous to extrapolate from rats to humans, a series of animal studies (McIntosh & Barfield, 1984a, 1984b, 1984c) suggests that areas of the brain sensitive to dopamine and norepinephrine affect the length of the refractory period in a complex interaction with serotonin. Perhaps studies of medication effects in humans will shed more light on the central nervous system control of the refractory phase.

SEXUALITY AND THE LIFE CYCLE

Human beings are sexual from birth. Infants and young children are capable of having erections, vaginal lubrication, or orgasms. In Western societies, where childhood sexual play and even masturbation are still regarded as taboo (L. J. Sarrel & Sarrel, 1984, pp. 7 27), adolescence is defined as the beginning of true sexual feelings. Certainly an upsurge of erotic awareness accompanies the physical and hormonal changes of puberty. Most teenagers experience anxiety about secondary sex characteristics. They worry if they develop earlier or later than peers or if breasts or penis size seems inadequate. All too often they are inadequately prepared for their first menstruation or ejaculation.

Each individual's sexual development is shaped by his or her unique history. Not only must the physiological developmental sequence unfold according to nature's rhythms, but psychological and social development must be nurtured as well. Psychology and psychiatry have created several alternate models of psychosexual development. The biological theorists believe hormones and neurons to be the most powerful determinants of adult sexuality. The psychoanalysts focus on early interactions between child and parents. Behaviorists are somewhat less deterministic, seeing sexuality as a complex of learned habits that can be changed during adulthood by new life experiences.

Clearly, we cannot review these controversies adequately in a book on sexuality and illness. We can, however, list psychosexual factors that often shape adult sexuality to guide the clinician in evaluating a patient's sexual history. These include:

- Family attitudes about emotional expressiveness, physical affection, and sexuality;
- Parents' ability to foster a child's sense of autonomy and self-esteem;
- The child's self-image as physically attractive and able to move gracefully and competently;
- Experiences of childhood sex play and masturbation;
- Emotional reactions to puberty;
- Experiences of separation and loss in close relationships;
- Sexual traumas such as incest, molestation, or rape;
- Comfort with choice of sexual objects as an adolescent and adult;
- Initial sexual interactions with a partner.

Children or adolescents who have chronic illnesses confront special crises in sexual development. As they are poked and prodded by medical personnel, they may learn that their privacy can be invaded with impunity and that touch is impersonal and painful. Such children are especially vulnerable to sexual abuse or exploitation. Children with medical problems may also have an image of their bodies as defective. They need support to see puberty as a normal part of growth and to feel sexually healthy and desirable.

SEXUALITY ACROSS ADULTHOOD

Much of our knowledge about sexual practices is derived from large survey studies of sexual behavior, beginning with the Kinsey reports in the 1940s (Kinsey, Pomeroy, & Martin, 1948; Kinsey, Pomeroy, Martin, & Gebhard, 1953) and including more recent efforts by Hunt (1974), Hite (1976, 1981), and Blumstein and Schwartz (1983). Most surveys focus on young to middle-aged adults, aged 18 to 45. All survey research shares the problem of sample bias. Most subjects are gathered from the readership of a certain magazine or by networking. Even when researchers try to collect data from a random sample of adults, many of those contacted refuse to participate in a study about sexuality.

Since surveys are our major source of information on people's actual sexual behavior, it is worth taking a more detailed look at one project that used careful methodology to generate a random sample of women representative of marital status and social class in the population. Table 3-1 lists major findings from cohorts of Danish women 22, 40, and 70 years of age (Garde & Lunde, 1982; Nielsen *et al.*, 1986a; Nielsen *et al.*, 1986b). Women were recruited from national health registries. Because the research focused on a general physical examination for preventive purposes, and on an interview about life history and social conditions, few women refused to participate. Sexual information was gathered by a female physician in an additional, structured interview.

Although survey studies may never provide accurate estimates of the number of people who engage in oral sex or extramarital sex or the mean frequency of intercourse for couples, they do give us a useful picture of the extreme variability in people's sexual practices. The message for a clinician who treats sexual problems is to dispense with stereotypes and judgments as much as possible when evaluating a patient.

When couples are in their 20s or 30s, their sex lives are often affected by the tasks of establishing a family. Both spouses work hard to meet career goals and raise children. Time and energy for intimacy between husband and wife may be limited. For many couples, the advent of middle age brings a renaissance of interest in sex. Career goals have largely been achieved, the children are leaving the nest, and it is time to reevaluate life priorities as a clearer sense of mortality sets in. Some men and women negotiate middle

Table 3-1. Sexual Experience in Three Cohorts of Danish Women

Age at Time of Survey	22	40	70
Number of Subjects	221	225	179
Age at first coitus	16	18	21
Age at first orgasm	16	21	23
Women with coital experience	98%	99%	96%
Women who have masturbated	81	47	38
Women currently sexually active	83	94	22
Women who have felt sexual desire at least once	98	67	88
Women who have reached orgasm at least once	91	96	95
Women who have had a homosexual experience	0	1	0
Women who have had an extramarital affair	38	14	7
Women with a current sexual problem	22	36	11
Women wanting sexual counseling	11	11	5

age easily, whereas others leave their long-term relationships and explore new ways of finding sexual and emotional gratification.

The majority of chronically ill patients are age 50 or older, a time when aging brings both physical and emotional changes. Aging is a lifelong process, but we will concentrate our attention on the years beginning with the 6th decade of life. Clinicians who treat sexual problems in the chronically ill need to be familiar with the impact of normal aging on the sexual response cycle (Schover, 1984, 1986b).

SEXUALITY AND AGING

Aging may play a role in a person's sexual function, self-image, and frequency of sexual activity. Although aging is a biological process, psychological and social factors are important determinants of sexual change versus stability during the later years of the life cycle.

The Frequency of Sexual Activity Across Adulthood

The conventional wisdom has been that sexual frequency and function automatically decline with age in both men and women. In the past 10 years, however, researchers have found new evidence of stability in levels of sexual activity and capacity from perhaps age 40 onward to the end of life. The keys to sexual stability are good health and a cooperative partner.

Early studies of aging and sexuality were cross-sectional in design, including the Kinsey surveys and a series of studies performed at Duke

University in the 1960s (George & Weiler, 1981). A consistent decline in the frequency of intercourse was observed with age. Within each age group studied, women lagged behind men in both sexual desire and activity levels. As George and Weiler (1981) pointed out, however, cross-sectional studies confound aging and cohort effects. A man born in 1900 was probably raised with sexual attitudes quite different from those of one born in 1920, since the latter would thus come of age in the tumultuous times that accompanied the Second World War. Since sexual mores have changed so rapidly in our century, we cannot expect people in different age groups to share the same sexual expectations or practices. Indeed, when George and Weiler followed one of the Duke samples of elderly people for 6 years, studying only those men and women whose partnerships remained stable, they found the most common individual pattern to be stability of desire and activity.

A number of other research studies suggest that the most important predictors of sexual motivation and activity in a person's later years are the importance and frequency of sex in earlier life (Giambra & Martin, 1977; Martin 1981; White, 1982).

Research on aging and sexuality has also suffered from other methodological flaws (George & Weiler, 1981; Robinson, 1983), including vague definitions of sexual function; failure to assess a range of sexual activities, including masturbation or noncoital activity with a partner as well as intercourse; biased sampling procedures; and a lack of attention to the tendency for subjects to report socially desirable sexual attitudes.

One recent large study (Brecher, 1984) exhibits each of these flaws. The publishers of *Consumer Reports* undertook a survey of older readers' sexuality. Over 4,000 men and women at least 50 years old filled out a sexuality questionnaire distributed by the magazine. Older respondents clearly had more conservative sexual attitudes. Brecher, however, believes the data show that sexual activity declines as a result of aging and never mentions the influence of cohort effects. The questionnaire did not distinguish clearly between coital and noncoital activities when measuring sexual frequency, although masturbation was assessed separately. Questions on erectile function were poorly constructed so that the actual incidence of problems is unclear. The respondents were better educated and more affluent than an average group of older Americans, and presumably more interested in sex, since they took the time to fill out a lengthy questionnaire. The findings, though, are touted as representative of all older Americans. The most positive aspect of the study is its message that older men and women can remain sexually active and satisfied

When older couples do cease sexual activity, the choice usually rests with the male partner (George & Weiler, 1981; White, 1982). Men become sexually inactive because of lack of desire, ill health, or erectile dysfunction. Women, however, report that sex ceases because of loss of a partner or at the husband's wishes. Women are also at a disadvantage because they tend to marry older men. The shorter male life expectancy combines with this custom to generate a ratio of four single women for every single man over age 65 (Corby & Zarit, 1983).

The Lack of a Male Menopause

Research before the 1970s also suggested that there is a male menopause. Hormone levels were believed to decline in elderly men, causing dysfunctions of sexual desire and arousal (Schover, 1984, pp. 8–23). More recent studies of healthy older men, however, have found only mild changes in the levels of testosterone and other hormones important in the hypothalamic–pituitary–testicular feedback cycle (Harman & Tsitouras, 1980; Purifoy, Koopmans, & Mayes, 1981; Winters, Sherins, & Troen, 1984). Only a small percentage of men over 50 have abnormal hormone levels that could impair sexual function. Because levels of testosterone vary widely, small decreases have little measurable effect on sexual desire, erections, or the ability to reach orgasm. Only one research group has observed even modest correlations between levels of testosterone and the frequency of sex in men over 60 (Tsitouras, Martin, & Harman, 1982).

Men also continue to have fairly stable amounts of nocturnal penile tumescence (NPT) with aging. Several nightly reflex erections occur during periods of REM sleep in males of all ages, from infancy to the 9th decade of life. NPT does not depend on an erotic stimulus such as a sexual dream or even on the sensations evoked by bladder fullness or friction against the penis. The erections are one aspect of autonomic nervous system activation during REM sleep.

The amount of NPT each night does decline in healthy men between the ages of 20 and 50, but then remains constant through age 80 (Kahn & Fisher, 1969; Karacan, Williams, Thornby, & Salis, 1975). Men over 50 have an average of 90 minutes per night of NPT, comprising two or three separate episodes. After age 70, NPT episodes are less perfectly synchronized with REM sleep and more of the erections are only partially firm. The striking finding, however, is that erectile capacity is retained unless the reflex is impaired by a medical problem such as a hormonal abnormality, decreased penile blood flow, or neurological damage.

The Impact of Menopause on Female Sexuality

Menopause is an undebated aspect of aging in women. The effects of menopause on sexual function, like so many other aspects of sexual physiology, are only now being clarified. As with male aging, the expert consensus had been that menopause signaled a decline in sexual desire and arousability. Adequate levels of estrogen were believed necessary for women's sexual pleasure (Morrell, Dixen, Carter, & Davidson, 1984).

Recent studies suggest that estrogen certainly enhances vaginal blood flow and lubrication and maintains a normal vaginal pH (Semmens, Tsai, Semmens, & Loadholt, 1985). Without estrogen, the mucosa become thin and fragile, and the vaginal walls lose elasticity. Hormonal replacement therapy takes 18 to 24 months to fully restore normal vaginal function in postmenopausal women. The researchers cited above and others (Bachmann et al., 1984) have observed that women who remain sexually active after menopause have less vaginal atrophy, although the differences are small.

Estrogen deficiency also brings annoying hot flashes and formication, or crawling skin sensations, which may disturb women's sleep and cause discomfort during daily activities. The loss of physical well-being and dyspareunia at menopause may reduce some women's sexual desire (McCoy, Cutler, & Davidson, 1985), although other women note few sexual problems with menopause. In studies of postmenopausal women, about one third report coital pain (Bachmann et al., 1984; Morrell et al., 1984). Sarrel (1984) examined 185 women who attended a climacteric clinic in London. Not only did 37% report dyspareunia, but 39% had low sexual desire, 23% had difficulty reaching orgasm, 10% experienced stress incontinence during intercourse, and 17% believed their clitoral sensitivity to be reduced. Because these women sought medical help, the incidence of problems in this group may be higher than that in postmenopausal women at large, but the findings indicate a need for better education and brief sexual counseling.

Reductions in circulating estrogen, progesterone, and androgens do not seem to affect postmenopausal women's sexual desire or ability to experience pleasure with touch. Hormonal levels do not predict postmenopausal women's daily sexual desire and function (Bachmann et al., 1984; Bachmann et al., 1985; Persky et al., 1982) or their responses to erotic stimuli (fantasy and film) in the laboratory (Morrell et al., 1984). In general, postmenopausal women have reduced serum androgen levels because so little estrogen is available to be converted to androgens. Nevertheless, levels of adrenal androgens and hormones produced by the ovarian stroma appear to be sufficient to maintain normal sexual function.

Sherwin (Sherwin, 1985; Sherwin, Gelfand, & Brender, 1985) did find that adding androgens to a regimen of replacement hormones increased women's sexual desire, arousability, and fantasies after bilateral oophorectomy. Women who lose their ovaries may have more profound hormonal deficits than those undergoing a natural menopause, however.

Aging and the Sexual Response Cycle

The normal process of aging does have some minor effects on the sexual response cycle. The changes that occur should not be considered sexual dysfunctions; rather, they represent a general slowing and decrease in intensity in the arousal and orgasm phases. The subjective experience of sexual pleasure alters very little.

Desire. Since sexual desire is mediated by androgens, the discussion earlier in this chapter of hormonal changes with aging is relevant. Androgen levels seem to remain above the threshold for normal sexuality in men and women from midlife onward. Aging does not produce an abrupt loss of sexual desire, but life events such as losing a partner or becoming ill can disrupt the motivation to stay sexually active.

Arousal. Even though 20 years have passed since Masters and Johnson (1966) published their laboratory observations of sexual arousal in aging men and women, their work remains the standard in the field. Their sample was not large (39 men and 34 women over age 50), but no comparable study using more modern technology has yet been published.

Masters and Johnson found that older men took a longer time and needed more penile stimulation to achieve erections. Their maximal erections were not as firm as those of younger men and detumesced more readily and rapidly. Older men were not always able to regain an erection if they lost it. Women over 50 similarly needed prolonged genital stimulation to produce vaginal lubrication. The amount of lubrication was decreased. Other measures of genital vasocongestion and breast engorgement, including vaginal expansion, also showed mild decreases with age. For both men and women, the changes in sexual arousal were not of a magnitude to cause sexual dysfunction.

Orgasm. Masters and Johnson (1966) are also still the source of the best data on aging and orgasm. Older men were better able to delay ejaculation and felt less frustration than formerly if sexual arousal did not lead to orgasm. Some no longer experienced the sensation of ejaculatory inevitability, and the pleasure of orgasm itself was more prolonged but less intense. The force of semen expulsion and the number of muscular contractions during ejaculation also decreased.

Older women noticed less change in the sensation of orgasm but did have fewer and weaker muscle contractions. A few postmenopausal women reported a cramping pelvic pain at orgasm. Older women could still have multiple orgasms, however, even though both older women and men exhibited a faster return to baseline levels of vasocongestion after orgasm. In men, a well-known effect of aging is the increase in the length of the refractory phase, sometimes to the extent that men in their 70s and 80s need several days between orgasms.

Myths about Sexuality and Aging

Western society has more pessimistic attitudes and beliefs about sexuality and aging than most other cultures in the world (Winn & Newton, 1982). Our media images of sexual attractiveness focus almost exclusively on the young, healthy, and physically perfect (Schover, 1986b). Our expectation that older men and women will become asexual is undoubtedly responsible for more sexual problems than all the physiological changes described in this chapter.

Besides the myth that aging is the end of sexuality, older adults must deal with exhortations to "use it or lose it." They have been authoritatively told that long periods of inactivity cause permanent sexual dysfunction (Masters & Johnson, 1981). The dread of celibacy is especially destructive when one spouse's chronic illness interferes with a couple's sexual activity. The healthy spouse is not only left frustrated and lonely, but may also feel doomed to permanent sexual inadequacy.

The evidence that sexual inactivity leads to vaginal atrophy is very tenuous. There is even less reason to believe that celibacy causes organic erectile dysfunction. The phenomenon of NPT indeed assures that the erection reflex occurs several times each 24-hour period (Schover, 1984, pp. 38–39). In the absence of research findings documenting the "use it or lose it" hypothesis, we should not publicize it further.

One final "myth" about sexuality and aging is the belief that sexual acting out, especially pedophilia and exhibitionism, is a common symptom of senile dementia. We have been unable to find documentation of the incidence of inappropriate sexual behavior in demented men or women, although Wise (1983) suggests that elderly people who act out sexually have damage to the frontal lobes of their brains. A very impressionistic survey of the staff of a nursing home for elderly men in Canada suggested that 25% of residents had annoyed staff by sexual comments, masturbating in public, or making sexual overtures (Szasz, 1983). Such behavior, however, must be put into context. The lack of touch, affection, privacy, and personal autonomy experienced in nursing home environments encourages residents to feel angry and sexually frustrated. The lack of an appropriate sexual outlet may lead to actions that the staff labels disruptive and dismisses as symptoms of dementia (Wasow & Loeb, 1977).

SEXUAL PROBLEMS

Having examined the elements of normal sexuality, we are ready to consider the types of sexual problems that people experience. Two major categories of sexual disorders are the deviations and the dysfunctions. In chronically ill patients, sexual dysfunctions such as premature ejaculation or low desire are far more common than deviations. The course of a chronic illness would have a negligible effect on a patient's preferred sexual object, although it might limit opportunities to engage in deviant behavior.

We thus will not discuss sexual deviation in any detail. Sexual arousal in response to children, like the other paraphilias, is defined as abnormal in American medical and legal systems. The potential for exploiting and harming a child sets such behavior apart. A homosexual orientation, however, is no longer regarded as a disease. Clinicians who treat sexual problems must be aware of their own attitudes and feelings about homosexuality. Particularly in medical settings, a health professional sees a cross-section of the population. Since homosexual men and women experience sexual anxieties and dysfunctions just as heterosexuals do (Paff, 1985), a homophobic clinician limits his or her usefulness and may actually add to the stress of illness for the homosexual patient.

Acquired Immune Deficiency Syndrome and Safe Sex

The epidemic of AIDS and its continued grim prognosis call for all health care professionals working with sexual issues to educate patients on guidelines for safe sex. Unless a vaccine is developed, the HIV virus will change the face of "normal" sexuality for all of us. The stress of being an AIDS patient in our health care system has been vividly underlined by mental health professionals counseling this group (Forstein, 1984). The panic of health care professionals and the emotional isolation of the AIDS patient is far more intense than is warranted even by the discovery of the deadly HIV virus. Clinicians who are attuned to sexual issues can help moderate their colleagues' fears and promote better health care for the AIDS patient (Morin, Charles, & Malyon, 1984).

Patients and their sexual partners who are in a high-risk category (having sexual contact with gay men or with intravenous drug users, or sharing needles during intravenous drug use) should be given guidelines for safe sex. People are advised to get to know potential partners and to reduce their number of partners (H. S. Kaplan, 1987). Showering together before sex is a way of combining foreplay with a check for sores or swollen lymph glands. Both partners should avoid contact between the mouth and anal area and should not swallow semen, urine, or feces. Wearing a condom may reduce, although not eliminate, the risk of sexually transmitted diseases from oral sex or vaginal or anal intercourse. Washing any body part that has touched the anal area before touching it with the mouth and urinating after sex are also important. Individuals with positive antibody tests for the virus should avoid street drugs and maintain good health habits to keep their immune systems functioning as effectively as possible (Gay Men's Health Crisis, 1985).

DIAGNOSING SEXUAL DYSFUNCTIONS

We begin our discussion of diagnosing sexual dysfunctions with a caveat. Sexual dysfunction categories are the most popular ways to describe sexual problems, but they are lin ·ting as well. When a researcher reports that 50%

of men have erectile dysfunction after coronary bypass surgery, what do we really know? We do not know whether all men had willing sexual partners available, whether they continued to enjoy noncoital sexual activity in spite of the lack of erections, or if the erection problem occurred on a quarter, a half, or all of the occasions.

Diagnostic systems for the sexual dysfunctions draw on our knowledge of the sexual response cycle. In subtle ways, however, our diagnostic categories are shaped by Western society's definitions of "functional" sex. For example, we assume that both partners should desire a sexual encounter and feel sexually aroused. The man's arousal should be evident in an erection firm enough to allow vaginal penetration, even if the lovemaking does not culminate in intercourse. The woman should experience vaginal lubrication and expansion. Each partner should be able to reach orgasm by means of his or her preferred type of sexual stimulation. The timing and intensity of orgasm should also be satisfactory.

It is difficult to step outside of the sexual definitions of one's culture, yet not all individuals judge a sexual experience by the above criteria. Working in a sex therapy clinic tends to reinforce a clinician's adherence to cultural definitions of "good sex," since in many patients dysfunctions developed because of their rigid or narrow sexual expectations, such as the belief that a woman should reach orgasm through coitus alone without clitoral stimulation or that a man should achieve and maintain erections without any direct caressing of his penis. It is rare that a couple seeking sex therapy is unconcerned about the man's degree of erection or thinks it is fine for one partner to participate a bit unenthusiastically in sex for the other's sake. In medical settings, however, patients referred for evaluation and counseling might never have sought treatment on their own initiative. The clinician needs to be judicious about "diagnosing" a sexual dysfunction and recommending treatment if the couple sees their sexual routine as normal and satisfying.

Another limitation of current diagnostic systems is our focus on the individual patient. We have a vocabulary to describe a woman's problems reaching orgasm or the severity of a man's erectile dysfunction. It is more difficult, however, to "label" a couple in which one partner wants sex twice a week and the other prefers it twice a day. Who gets a diagnosis? How do we describe a couple's deficits in balancing intimacy with autonomy? What is the diagnostic label for a couple in which one partner wakes at 6 A.M. and wants to make love while the other is a "night owl"?

With these caveats, we present the diagnostic system we find most useful for clinical and research purposes. The multiaxial problem-oriented diagnostic system for sexual dysfunction is the product of a number of years of experience in a sex therapy program (Schover, Friedman, Weiler, Heiman, & LoPiccolo, 1982) and has been translated and modified for use in Scandinavia (Jensen & Hertoft, 1984).

The multiaxial system recognizes that patients often have more than one sexual problem. Sexual function has multiple dimensions, or axes, each contributing an important part to the whole picture. The axes include the first three phases of the sexual response cycle: desire, arousal, and orgasm. Since no clearly defined sexual dysfunctions are observed in the resolution phase, it was not included in the diagnostic system. The other three axes include coital pain, dissatisfaction with the frequency or variety of sexual activity, and qualifying information that might be helpful in planning treatment for sexual problems.

Table 3-2 lists the diagnostic categories as we currently use them. If the patient is in a committed relationship, a complete diagnosis includes assessment of both partners. The system is designed to be used with a couple interview and a multiple-choice self-report questionnaire completed by each partner (see Chapter 6). A manual outlines the criteria for each diagnosis.* Whenever a diagnosis is made, the clinician codes the problem as *lifelong versus not lifelong* (i.e., some period of normal function has occurred), *global versus occurring only in some sexual situations*, and as a *presenting problem defined by the patient versus a problem identified by the clinician during the assessment*. Diagnostic categories are intended as descriptions of behavior, affect, and cognition. A diagnosis does not imply knowledge about the cause of the problem.

Desire Axis

Low sexual desire is diagnosed not only when the frequency of various sexual activities is low but also when the patient lacks interest in and attention to sexual stimuli. We must be careful not to overlook the patient with low desire who says, "Yes, I want sex," but really means "I want to want sex." We have set a somewhat arbitrary standard of "low" frequency as less than once every 2 weeks, drawing from our clinical experience and the survey literature. The lack of desire may be global or it may be a situational response, for example, to one particular partner. An aversion to sex is distinguished from low desire because it involves an actively negative emotional reaction to sexual situations. Aversion to sex is not uncommon in women seeking help in a sex therapy clinic, but is rare in men (Schover & LoPiccolo, 1982).

The desire phase axis does not include a diagnostic category of excess sexual desire. Although compulsive sexual behavior is a fashionable new "problem" (Quadland, 1985), we see it as a difficulty with the function of sexual relationships in daily life rather than as a surfeit of desire. When both partners could be termed "normal" in their individual levels of desire, conflicts about sexual frequency are coded in the dissatisfaction axis rather than as a desire-phase dysfunction.

*Copies of the manual for the multiaxial diagnostic system may be obtained from Joseph LoPiccolo, Ph.D., Department of Psychology, University of Missouri, Columbia, MO, 65201.

Table 3-2. Multiaxial problem-Oriented Descriptive System
for Sexual Dysfunction: Revised Version

Desire Phase
  Low sexual desire
  Aversion to sex
Arousal Phase
  Decreased subjective arousal
  Difficulty achieving erections
  Difficulty maintaining erections
  Difficulty achieving and maintaining erections
  Decreased physiological arousal, female
Orgasm Phase
  Anhedonic orgasm
  Decreased intensity of orgasm
  Premature ejaculation before entry
  Premature ejaculation, less than 1 minute
  Premature ejaculation, 1 to 3 minutes
  Premature ejaculation, 4 to 7 minutes
  Inorgasmic (male or female)
  Inorgasmic except for vibrator or other mechanical stimulation
  Inorgasmic except for masturbation
  Inorgasmic except for partner manipulation
  Coitally inorgasmic
  Infrequent coital orgasms
  Dry ejaculation
  Orgasm with flaccid penis
  Ejaculation with seepage of semen
Coital Pain
  Vaginismus
  Dyspareunia (male or female)
  Pain during or after ejaculation
  Other pain exacerbated by sexual activity
  Decreased genital sensation

Arousal Axis

In the arousal phase, a patient may have a subjective lack of arousal, an absence of physiologic arousal, or both. A problem with lack of subjective arousal usually includes a failure to experience pleasure from genital touch as well as an absence of mental excitement. Often the patient is unaware of the cues of generalized physiological arousal, such as increased pulse, deepened breathing, or muscle tension.

Problems with physiological arousal include difficulty achieving and/or maintaining erections for men and vaginal dryness and tightness in women. Genital arousal and subjective arousal are not always linked. For example, a man may have a full erection without feeling excitement. Conversely, a man may feel aroused but not achieve erection, especially if medical factors are interfering with genital vasocongestion.

Table 3-2. Continued

Sexual Dissatisfaction
  Desired frequency lower than activity level
  Desired frequency higher than activity level
  Desires wider variety of sexual activities
  Objects to partner's desire for sexual variety

Qualifying Information
  Prefers gender opposite to partner's
  Bisexual
  Transvestism
  Fetishism
  Voyeurism
  Exhibitionism
  Sexual pleasure from inflicting pain
  Sexual pleasure from experiencing pain
  Sexual assaultiveness
  Assault survivor
  Sexually abused child
  Sexual abuser of children
  Unconsummated marriage
  No current sexual activity
  Sexual pleasure from humiliating partner
  Sexual pleasure from being humiliated by partner
  History of severe psychopathology
  Current severe psychopathology
  Severe marital distress
  History of substance abuse
  Current substance abuse
  History of spouse abuse
  Current spouse abuse
  Active extramarital affair

Modifiers for Each Descriptive Category
  Lifelong vs. not lifelong
  Global vs. situational
  Presenting complaint

Orgasm Axis

Orgasm may be disturbed in a number of ways. Some men and women have no orgasms at all or can only reach orgasm with certain intense types of stimulation such as the regular friction of a vibrator. In men the most common problem of this type is inability to reach orgasm during vaginal intercourse. Perhaps a third of American women cannot reach orgasm through intercourse alone without concurrent clitoral stimulation. Since infrequent coital orgasm is so common, many sex therapists do not label it as a dysfunction in women (H. S. Kaplan, 1974, pp. 377–383). We include it in the descriptive system, however, because many couples seek help to improve the woman's ability to be coitally orgasmic. Thus, it is important to know whether the pattern is one of the patient's presenting complaints.

Other patients have problems with the quality of orgasm. Some men ejaculate with no sensation of pleasure, which we call anhedonic orgasm.

More common is the complaint that orgasm occurs, but the intensity of pleasure is no longer as strong and satisfying as in the past. Women are less likely than men to report problems with orgasmic intensity.

Men may also experience abnormal orgasms often (but not always) associated with organic impairment. These include "dry" ejaculation in which no semen emerges from the penis but the sensation of orgasm and the striated muscle contractions still occur; reaching orgasms with a flaccid penis, often with reduced orgasmic pleasure; and orgasm with just a seepage of semen instead of a pulsing expulsion as in normal ejaculation.

Finally, premature ejaculation is a problem in the timing of male orgasm. Our system classifies premature ejaculation in terms of the time from penetration to orgasm because knowledge about the severity of the dysfunction has been useful in planning treatment (Schover *et al.*, 1982). Normative data suggest that the average duration of intercourse is 7 to 10 minutes.

Coital Pain Axis

The coital pain axis includes categories describing genital and nongenital pain that could interfere with sexual pleasure. Vaginismus is included here because the involuntary spasm of the pubococcygeal muscles causes pain when the man attempts to penetrate for intercourse. Vaginismus in its less severe forms often exacerbates dyspareunia (Fordney, 1978) because a woman tenses her circumvaginal muscles in anticipation of painful intercourse. We also classify reduced genital sensation on this axis. Even though it is not a true pain syndrome, it is a distortion of normal sexual pleasure.

Dissatisfaction Axis

Sexual dissatisfaction is the axis that codes couple disagreements on how often to have sex or about the types of caressing to include. Many couples are dissatisfied with both sexual frequency and variety. Often one partner is labeled sexually inhibited or uninterested, but is in fact, well within the normal range. It is the mismatching between partners that creates a problem. If one partner truly lacks sexual desire, he or she receives a desire phase diagnosis, and the dissatisfaction with frequency category is used only for the frustrated partner whose level of desire is normal.

Qualifying Information Axis

The qualifying information categories listed are ones we have found useful in planning treatment. Others can certainly be added, depending on the clinical setting. The purpose of these codes is to "red flag" problem areas that can affect the outcome of any type of therapy for a sexual dysfunction.

THE INCIDENCE OF SEXUAL DYSFUNCTIONS

Research on the incidence of sexual dysfunctions suffers from the same flaws as other survey research. Samples are rarely gathered randomly, and standard criteria have not been used in diagnosing sexual problems. Researchers who use a detailed, structured interview to gather data may arrive at different definitions of a sexual problem from researchers who depend on self-report questionnaire data. Whether data collection preserves anonymity can also affect a subject's willingness to disclose a problem.

Many small surveys of sexual problems in groups of healthy and ill people have been published. The wide range of rates of dysfunctions reported reflects varying methods of subject recruitment, the different ages and health histories of populations surveyed, and different ways of eliciting information. Table 3-3 compares five such studies.

Two surveys were based on data gathered from volunteers who responded to an advertisement to participate in research on couples. The Sex History Form data, detailed further in Chapter 6, Table 6-2, were gathered from 92 couples who answered a newspaper advertisement for people in stable relationships to participate in a questionnaire study. All couples filled out a detailed questionnaire designed to correspond to the multiaxial diag-

Table 3-3. Rates of Sexual Dysfunction in Four Surveys of American Adults

Dysfunction	Schover (1981)[a]	Jensen et al. (1980)[b]	Frank et al. (1978)[c]	Schover et al. (1987)[d]	Schein et al. (1986)[e]
Male low desire	0%	3%	16%	11%	14%
Female low desire	10	23	35	10	18
Erectile dysfunction	3	0	9	21	27
Female low arousal	14	24	48	10	50
Premature Ejaculation	23	7	36	8	41
Male difficulty reaching orgasm	1	0	4	4	3
Male decreased orgasmic pleasure	4	3	—	2	—
Female difficulty reaching orgasm:					
Global	9	7	15	4	—
Situational	18	30	33	26	—
Total	27	37	48	30	18
Male dyspareunia	2	0	—	6	2
Female dyspareunia	8	8	—	10	21

[a] $n = 92$ men, $m = 32$ years; $n = 92$ women, $m = 30$ years.
[b] $n = 40$ men, $m = 38$ years; $n = 40$ women, $m = 38$ years.
[c] $n = 100$ men, $m = 37$ years; $n = 100$ women, $m = 35$ years.
[d] $n = 300$ men, $m = 55$ years; $n = 76$ women, $m = 41$ years.
[e] $n = 64$ men, $m = 35$ years; $n = 148$ women, $m = 35$ years.

nostic system. Rates of sexual dysfunction were quite a bit lower than those observed by Frank, Anderson, and Rubenstein (1978) who studied 100 couples who responded to calls from local community groups for volunteers to participate in a study of couples "whose marriages were working." Questions in the latter study were less detailed, however, asking only whether a problem existed rather than using criteria for identifying dysfunctions by the frequency or severity of symptoms.

In two other studies, researchers surveyed patients visiting their general practitioner. Jensen and colleagues (Jensen, 1982; Jensen, Olsen, & Rønne, 1980) asked a random sample of Danish patients aged 26 to 45 to fill out a sexuality questionnaire (modified from the Sex History Form) and to participate in a structured interview. The response rate was 90%. Results were similar to American norms for the Sex History Form. Compared with a study of reports by 36 general practitioners of patients' sexual problems, however, this careful study of consecutive patients found a tenfold higher incidence of dysfunction (Jensen, 1982).

Schein *et al.* (1986) asked patients visiting a family practitioner for routine care to fill out a sexuality questionnaire. Their data resemble Frank *et al.*'s (1978) findings more than the Sex History Form norms, again perhaps because their questionnaire asked only whether a problem existed rather than using standardized criteria to assess dysfunctions.

Schover, Evans, & von Eschenbach (1987) used the same criteria embodied in the Sex History Form in a structured interview, assessing sexual function in cancer patients for the period before cancer symptoms interfered. Although the cancer patients were older than the groups studied by other researchers, in most respects, rates of sexual dysfunction are similar to the Sex History Form norms. Higher rates of erectile dysfunction and lower rates of premature ejaculation in male cancer patients probably reflect their greater average age.

Recognizing sexual dysfunctions is more crucial than knowing their exact incidence in the general population. It is helpful, however, to have some idea of norms of sexual function for young, healthy couples to provide a context for evaluating groups of chronically ill patients. These five surveys underscore the need to use clearly defined diagnostic categories in conducting survey research so that one is not comparing apples to oranges.

SEXUAL DYSFUNCTIONS IN OLDER ADULTS

Since many chronically ill patients are over age 50, data on the incidence of sexual problems in the elderly would be of particular value to the clinician working in a medical setting. Unfortunately, accurate information about sexual problems in older people is even scarcer than the facts about young men and women.

Few older adults seek help for sexual problems in sexual dysfunction clinics. At the Johns Hopkins clinic, only 3% of couples seen over a 10-year period included a partner over age 60, and no patient was older than 70 (Wise, 1983). When the records of all couples including a partner over 50 were reviewed, the most common diagnosis was erectile dysfunction (70%). A majority of men (59%) and many women (40%) had a major medical illness. Psychiatric disorders, including depression, anxiety reaction, or personality disorder, were diagnosed in 64% of men and 69% of women (Wise, Rabins, & Gahnsley, 1984). This group of elderly couples undoubtedly had more physical and mental problems than those who do not seek counseling.

Kinsey *et al.* (1948) reported that in the general population erection problems were present in 2% of men in their 40s, 7% of men in their 50s, 18% of men in their 70s, and 80% of men in their 80s. Kinsey's sample, however, of 5,000 men included only 126 subjects over age 60. It is frustrating that the recent Consumers Union survey (Brecher, 1983) merely notes that 44% of men over 50 report less firm erections than in their younger days and 32% lose erections more frequently during sexual activity. No rates of true erectile dysfunction are reported. If we estimate male sexual dysfunction indirectly by examining sexual inactivity, abstinence increased in that survey from 2% of married men in their 50s to 7% of men in their 60s and 19% of those 70 and older.

Although clinical experience suggests that low sexual desire is one of the more common sexual problems in older men and women (Wise *et al.*, 1984), we do not know its incidence in large community samples.

Kinsey's study of female sexuality (Kinsey *et al.*, 1953) suggested that women actually have an easier time reaching orgasm as their sexual experience increases with age. In the Consumers Union survey, 19% of women in their 50s, 22% of women in their 60s, and 28% of those over 70 were seldom or never orgasmic during sexual activity with a partner (Brecher, 1984). If one interprets the statistics on partner sexual activity to represent orgasmic capacity during intercourse, the above data are quite similar to rates of orgasmic dysfunction in younger women (Morokoff, 1978). The minor changes with aging are probably cohort effects.

CONCLUSION

The matrix of normal sexuality is the background against which we highlight the facts in the rest of this book. Having reviewed our knowledge about illness and relationships, sexual normalcy, the sexual response cycle, and the diagnosis of sexual dysfunctions, we are ready to examine the impact of illness on sexual function, activity, and satisfaction.

4

Emotional Factors and Sexuality in Chronic Illness

To meet the crisis of an illness, patients must mobilize their resources. We have already discussed ways in which the quality of a couple's relationship affects the partners' ability to cope with illness. We have described the matrix of normal sexuality and a typology of sexual dysfunction. Now we focus on the individual. Why do some men and women remain sexually active and functional in spite of chronic disease while others develop problems? Part of the answer rests on physiological factors and will be taken up in Chapter 5. For now, we examine how emotional factors influence sexual function after a chronic illness is diagnosed.

We believe that sexual function is linked to general emotional health. An entire literature has developed on coping skills in medical patients (Coyne & Holroyd, 1982; Lazarus & Folkman, 1984). We are beginning to understand the role of factors such as locus of control, self-efficacy, hardiness, and Type A behavior in mediating patients' responses to disease. Researchers in behavioral medicine have largely ignored sexuality as an area of coping, however. How do the illness and the patient's ability to cope influence continued sexual function and satisfaction?

THEORIES FROM BEHAVIORAL MEDICINE APPLIED TO SEXUALITY AND CHRONIC ILLNESS

The diagnosis of a chronic disease can be viewed as a crisis. Crisis theory has guided psychotherapists since the early work of Lindemann (1944), Erikson (1963), and Caplan (1964). The initial diagnosis is just one type of crisis associated with illness. If an illness worsens or complications develop, such as blindness or limb amputation in a diabetic, the sense of crisis is renewed. Chronic diseases also intensify normal developmental life crises such as puberty, marriage, or birth of a child.

As an example, a woman learning that she must have a mastectomy passes through several stages in reacting to her health crisis (Horowitz, 1982). At first there is the outcry: "Why me? Will my husband still want me?

Will I die of my cancer?" Next comes denial, for example, shopping for a revealing bathing suit the week before surgery or telling friends she is just having a biopsy. After the operation come the intrusive thoughts. Every billboard and TV commercial seems to picture a large-breasted model wearing low-cut clothes. A woman friend is being cruel by ostentatiously wearing a tight sweater. A hug from the husband is a reminder of the breast prosthesis. If the woman has adequate social support and inner resources, she will work through her preoccupation with her lost breast and complete the crisis period with a return to normal life activities, including a joyful sex life.

Moos (1982) suggests that, to negotiate a health crisis successfully, the person needs to have an accurate cognitive appraisal of the situation and to be able to perform adaptive tasks using appropriate coping skills.

Cognitive appraisal is the patient's perception of harm, the damage already done by an illness; threat, the potential for further harm; and challenge, the chance that the crisis could lead to a higher level of adaptation (Lazarus, 1966). A man recovering from a myocardial infarction and worrying about sexuality wonders whether he will be able to have adequate erections now that he is taking cardiac medication (harm). Will having intercourse increase the risk of another heart attack (threat)? Perhaps the illness will present an opportunity for him and his wife to discuss sexuality with the physician, improving their rather poor sexual communication (challenge).

The patient is faced with a number of adaptive tasks (Moos, 1982). He must adjust to temporary immobility, to the drowsiness that his medication causes, and to the pain of occasional episodes of angina. He needs to develop a trusting relationship with his medical team and to maintain good communication with family and friends. His ability to adapt depends not only on his state of health but also on his social and physical environment (Shontz, 1982). His likelihood of resuming sex is increased by his ability to return to a good job that will promote a sense of self-efficacy in resuming other daily life tasks. His economic success ensures that he has the best medical care available, including a cardiac rehabilitation program that promotes a healthy diet and regular aerobic exercise, and includes seminars for couples on family life topics such as sex after heart attack.

Shontz (1982) believes that good adaptation involves the same process, whether in healthy individuals or in those who are chronically ill. We agree, but believe that to adapt completely to an illness requires that the disease no longer dominate the person's inner world or daily activities. Thus, an illness presents a special challenge to coping skills.

Coping has been defined by Lazarus and Folkman (1984) as "the process of managing demands (external or internal) that are appraised as taxing or exceeding the resouces of the person" (p. 283). Coping may be problem focused, as when efforts center on taking action to remedy harm, reduce threat, or meet a challenge; or it may be emotion focused, as when coping skills are used to reduce psychological distress, whether through regulating inner states or changing behavior.

A woman suffering from multiple sclerosis can use problem-focused coping to adapt sexually to the illness. She may buy several extra pillows to use as props during caressing so that she can stay in a comfortable position in spite of reduced mobility. She can use an anesthetic gel on her vulva during times when her disease causes unpleasant genital paresthesias that distract from sexual arousal. For emotional coping, she may need to practice focusing on erotic fantasies to combat distracting sexual anxieties related to her illness. She can make special efforts to look attractive and to do all she can to fulfill her husband's sexual and emotional needs, reducing her sense of inadequacy and her fear that she is failing him as a wife.

A crisis is, by definition, a transitional period. Within a few days or weeks, some equilibrium will be reached. The clinician can assist patients in working through a health crisis, encouraging them to use their strengths to return to a more normal state. One area in which coping affects medical care is compliance, the patient's ability to follow medical advice and take responsibility for his or her own health care.

As society has put increasing value on sexual pleasure, the fear of sexual disability has become a more common motive for noncompliance with important preventive health measures and medical therapies. Women fail to examine their breasts because they fear mastectomy, even though finding a tumor as early as possible could not only save their lives but might also help them avoid radical surgery. Men often refuse to take antihypertensive medications that interfere with erectile function, even if they realize that untreated hypertension increases their risk of stroke or heart attack. Better information for the public is needed on the role of good health habits not only in preventing major illnesses, but ultimately in preserving sexual function or at least allowing sexual rehabilitation to take place. Sometimes we remind patients that as far as we know, in order to have a good sex life one has to remain in the land of the living.

A patient's ability to adapt depends on inner resources. Each individual acquires psychological strengths and weaknesses in the course of development. We believe that coping skills, a term that focuses on psychological health, and defense mechanisms, a way of classifying pathological reactions to stress, are two faces of the same coin. When a person lacks good coping skills, defense mechanisms will become evident. Then we see somatopsychological symptoms (Cullberg, 1984), such as denial, anxiety, anger, and depressed mood.

The four defense mechanisms that influence communication (Chapter 2) also help categorize individuals' ability to stay sexually active after the crisis of an illness. Each defense can be used adaptively or maladaptively (Table 4-1). Denial can be a way of ignoring pain and going on to have as normal a sex life as possible, but it can also lead to denial of important

Table 4-1. Defense Mechanisms and Their Impact on Sexuality and Illness

	Adaptive Use	Maladaptive Use
Denial	I will stay sexually active. I'll feel better soon, even if intercourse is a little painful now.	I'll just ignore this bleeding after intercourse. Maybe I'm having an early menopause.
Withdrawal	I need time to look at this ostomy and get used to its being a part of me. Then I'll be ready to let my partner see it.	Oh, she would probably faint or throw up if she saw a man with one testicle. I'll never have sex again.
Projection	My wife left me because of my diabetes, but she never treated me right anyway. I'll find someone better.	I never had premature ejaculation until my vasectomy. What have they done to me? I'm getting a lawyer.
Passive Acceptance	I don't like having sex without erections, but I needed the surgery and now I must accept the results.	Of course he broke our engagement. Nobody will ever marry a woman who has had cancer.

physical symptoms. Withdrawal can help a patient integrate a change in body image or can entail so much obsessional thinking that the person never takes action to try a new solution. Projection can free a patient from unproductive guilt about the cause of sexual problem but can also prevent a person from taking responsibility to get help when a problem can be remedied. Passive acceptance is helpful when the patient acknowledges that a sexual disability exists but goes on to enjoy lovemaking in spite of it. Acceptance, however, can also lead to inaction when solutions are available.

SEXUAL FUNCTION AND EMOTIONAL DISTRESS

Within groups of chronically ill patients, sexual problems occur more often in individuals who evince somatopsychological symptoms, suggesting that their coping skills have not been sufficient for adaptation, that is for achieving peaceful coexistence with the disease. Although sexual dysfunction and psychological distress have rarely been studied systematically in groups of chronically ill people, measures of both have been included in several studies. Jensen (1986) found that, even when peripheral neuropathy was taken into account, sexual dysfunction was more common in diabetic men who coped poorly in emotional terms with their illness. Similarly, Buvat *et al.* (1985b) found that Minnesota Multiphasic Personality Inventory (MMPI) profiles were significantly elevated in diabetic men with erectile dysfunction compared to diabetic men with good sexual function. A significant correlation between psychological distress on the Brief Symptom Inventory (BSI) and global sexual satisfaction was observed in a group of women about to receive treatment for early-stage cervical cancer (Schover, Fife, & Gershenson, 1985).

Of course, none of these studies can demonstrate a causal relationship between the emotional pain and the sexual problem. Even if sexual dysfunction is more common in medical patients who are emotionally distressed, the correlation may result from the sexual problem's influence on mood and self-esteem. In fact, psychological testing has been notoriously unsuccessful at distinguishing between organically caused and psychogenic erectile dysfunction for just that reason (Schover & von Eschenbach, 1985a).

Even without the influence of a chronic illness, psychological distress seems common in patients seeking help for a sexual dysfunction. Derogatis, Meyer, and King (1981) evaluated the psychological health of 325 men and women seen at the Johns Hopkins sexuality clinic. Based on a structured interview, a third of the men and half of the women received psychiatric diagnoses. The SCL-90, a questionnaire rating psychological distress, also revealed that clinic patients had mean levels of distress one to two standard deviations above the mean for a nonpatient population. Of course we do not know whether a strong association exists between psychopathology and sexual dysfunction in nonclinical samples. Perhaps sexually dysfunctional people who also suffer from other life problems are apt to seek help, and then are referred to a university-based sexuality clinic. Men and women with better coping skills may solve their own sexual problems rather than seek psychotherapy.

If we are to untangle the relationships among chronic illness, emotional distress, and sexual function, we need carefully designed longitudinal studies that use behavioral measures of psychological coping as well as inventories assessing psychopathology and a comprehensive assessment of sexual anxieties and problems.

Although our current knowledge is limited, the rest of this chapter takes a more detailed look at emotional factors and their impact on sexual function in the chronically ill. We discuss sexual problems as reactive to the stress of illness and then focus on the role of anxiety, anger, and depression in sexual dysfunction. We look in detail at defense mechanisms and sexuality, proceeding to a consideration of the patient's beliefs about sexuality and illness and of her or his self-image.

THE STRESS OF ILLNESS AND SEXUALITY

A life-threatening illness can rearrange life priorities literally overnight. Instead of worrying about a job promotion or this year's taxes, the patient wonders whether life will continue and at what price in terms of painful and debilitating medical treatment. When an illness is in the acute phase and the patient is in crisis, sexual function or attractiveness may have low priority compared with survival. For example, when cancer surgery is necessary to halt the spread of disease, most patients will submit to it, even if it means removal of a breast, the vulva, or even the penis. Similarly, in the first days after a myocardial infarction, fears about future sexual adequacy are rarely as disturbing as anxiety about the degree of cardiac damage or eventual ability to return to work.

The crises of illness are times of denial and of intrusive thoughts about the disease. Such mental states make it difficult to provide effective sexual counseling or education, even though for some patients sexual side effects of treatment are an important concern.

Leon, a 51-year-old actuary, was hospitalized for a radical cystectomy only 2 weeks after his bladder cancer was diagnosed. He was very concerned about having an ostomy and losing erectile function and had a 2-hour preoperative session with the hospital's sexual counselor. When she returned to see Leon a week after surgery, however, she discovered that he had retained little of the information provided. He had forgotten that he would have normal penile sensation; had only a vague idea of what a penile prosthesis was like, despite having seen pictures and samples of several types; and was convinced that he would no longer be able to feel any sexual pleasure.

The stress of illness, and its impact on sexuality, does not end with diagnosis and initial treatment. Medical care may disrupt a couple's daily routines, as discussed in Chapter 2. The patient may be chronically in pain or fatigued, so that sexual activity feels effortful. Some patients begin to view sex as something they give to their spouses to keep the peace, rather than as a well-deserved pleasure. Older women who grew up with very conservative sexual attitudes seem particularly vulnerable to such feelings, since, for many, sex was always a wifely duty but rarely a source of much gratification.

Violet, aged 76, asked her doctor to have a talk with her husband. She wanted him to tell the husband that she was too debilitated by her osteoporosis to continue sexual activity. Violet was upset when her physician suggested that sexuality was a normal part of life and offered to give her a pamphlet on comfortable positions for intercourse. She wanted permission to refuse sex, not advice on how to improve it.

Emotional responses to stress include anxiety, anger, and depression. The next three sections examine these somatopsychological symptoms and their relationship to sexuality.

ANXIETY AND SEXUALITY

Anxiety is certainly a prime etiological candidate for sexual dysfunctions in the chronically ill, but what kind of anxiety? Beck and Barlow (1984) point out that the literature on sexual dysfunction has invoked an old-fashioned, unitary concept of anxiety as a cause of sexual problems. They suggest, instead, that the type of anxiety responsible for sexual dysfunction is quite specific. During sexual activity, individuals with dysfunction are distracted by thoughts about failing to perform instead of focusing on arousing fantasies or on pleasurable sensations. Beck and Barlow have devised and carried out a series of ingenious experiments suggesting that cognitive distraction during sex decreases arousal, whereas the type of generalized physiological arousal associated with fear actually increases sexual arousal.

If we adopt their model of sexual anxiety, it seems self-evident that having an illness could provoke distracting fears about performance during sex. Medical patients often worry that a treatment will impair sexual function or that sexual activity is unhealthy. Each sexual encounter then becomes a test: Will it still work this time? Physical pain occurring during sex is a distraction in itself and also may elicit fears about health. Although sexual arousal can also direct a patient's attention away from pain (Whipple & Komisaruk, 1985), some patients interpret even innocuous, novel sensations during sex as a physical symptom, setting off a whole chain of anxious thoughts.

Doris, a 43-year-old homemaker, had been treated successfully with radiotherapy for cervical cancer 3 years previously. She told her gynecologist that she had recently lost all desire for sex and could rarely reach orgasm. Doris was taking replacement estrogens. On physical examination her vagina appeared moist and adequate in size. In fact she did not experience any pain with intercourse.

When the gynecologist moved the speculum in Doris' vagina, however, she exclaimed, "That's it! That's the feeling!" She explained that the thrusting of intercourse produced a sensation that reminded her of the pelvic fullness she experienced at the time of her cancer diagnosis. Each time she had intercourse, she worried for a day or two that she was having a recurrence of her cervical malignancy.

ANGER AND SEXUALITY

Anger is a common emotional response to an illness. The patient may wonder, "Why me?" or feel enraged by the interruption of life plans and loss of autonomy. Anger can interfere with sexuality, no matter whether the anger is directed at fate, at oneself, or at one's partner.

Battling with fate is a lost cause, since revenge or constructive action is impossible. Frustration may surface as a generalized irritability that interferes with a couple's relationship. Sex becomes one more way the healthy spouse feels obligated to nurture a crotchety, uncooperative partner. When a patient is angry, even lovemaking can take on an aggressive, tense aspect. Having sex may be a way of figuratively shaking one's fist at fate.

Often the spouse is the safest target for a patient's anger. Physicians or nurses may desert an abusive patient, but spouses are usually more understanding. Sometimes the ill partner envies the other's good health. Bitter remarks are common, such as, "How would you know what it's like? You don't have cancer." Resentment may also be evoked when the family gets along too smoothly. It is frightening to feel superfluous. A patient may react by trying to prove that the spouse still needs sex, or conversely by withdrawing from sexual intimacy.

When lifestyle has played a role in causing an illness, the healthy spouse may feel justified in being angry at the patient. Such patterns are common in couples where one partner is alcoholic or is a smoker with lung cancer. Anger becomes an even more divisive force when a disease is sexually transmitted.

Curtis was a truck driver with a waitress at every stop. Annie knew of his affairs, but loved her husband and did not want her four young children to grow up in a broken home. When Annie's pap smear showed cervical dysplasia, her gynecologist diagnosed genital condyloma. Untreated, cervical condyloma may develop into a cervical cancer. He warned Annie that her husband should be checked for the warts because, although she could be treated with laser surgery, a partner could reinfect her. Curtis refused to see a doctor, so Annie hoped for the best.

The next year, her pap smear revealed carcinoma *in situ*, and she had to have a vaginal hysterectomy. When Curtis came to visit her in the hospital, he was drunk. After accusing her of sleeping with other men and spending all of his money, he finally had to be taken away by the hospital's security guard. This episode was the last straw for Annie. After she was discharged, she got a job as a typist and moved out of the couple's apartment, taking the children with her.

DEPRESSION AND SEXUALITY

In samples of adults unselected for health or age, the incidence of depressive symptoms ranges from 9% to 20%. Surveys of medical patients, however, suggest that 20% to 30% are depressed in mood (Bukberg, Penman, & Holland, 1984; Derogatis et al., 1983). Only a smaller group would be diagnosed as having a major affective disorder by DSM-III criteria. Research with cancer patients, as well as with men and women suffering from other illnesses, reveals that depression is more prevalent in more debilitated populations. Depression in medical patients may be related to the disruption of their control over life events, interruption of pleasurable activities, loss of social support, effects of medications, or even metabolic or endocrine abnormalities.

In our experience, patients referred for evaluation of a sexual dysfunction in a medical setting are often depressed in mood. The sexual problem may be only one aspect of a generalized loss of the ability to experience pleasure. Sometimes patients will seek help for a sexual problem because they regard it as a medical symptom but consider depression to be a sign of weakness. Such men and women often feel relieved when the clinician helps them see the pervasive influence of their depression on their daily life. The labeling process is particularly helpful because with the effective treatments available for depression, we can give patients a renewed sense of hope.

Diagnosing depression is a difficult task when patients are medically ill. Inexperienced clinicians may mistake the denial or intrusive thoughts of an acute crisis for depressive cognitions. We must also be cautious in labeling the normal sadness or dysphoria that accompanies a serious illness as depression. Although careful evaluation for affective disorder is crucial when a medical patient is distressed, antidepressant medication is often overprescribed in this group, especially given the risks of cardiac arrhythmia, orthostatic hypotension, and even of sexual dysfunction. Nonpsychiatric physicians sometimes feel overwhelmed by the patient's misery and see medication as a way of taking action. The more sophisticated mental health clinician knows that short-term psychotherapies have also had good success in ameliorating unipolar affective disorders (Rush, 1982) and thus considers psychological treatment or a combination of medication and psychotherapy as a good alternative.

We advocate reserving medication for the patient with severe vegetative symptoms such as insomnia, early morning awakenings, fatigue, changes in appetite for food, depressed mood, inability to concentrate or make decisions, feelings of guilt or worthlessness, decreased sexual desire, and verbal or psychomotor slowing.

Besides the usual approaches to treating depression, we can use couple therapy to work simultaneously on alleviating depression and a sexual problem (Coyne, 1986).

Neal was a successful 33-year-old attorney when a seizure led to the diagnosis of a tumor in his frontal lobes. The tumor was successfully treated with surgery, but Neal continued to take high doses of phenytoin, and still had seizures occasionally. Although he was not supposed to drive a car, he sometimes did. Limited by subtle deficits in his short-term memory, he gave up his private law practice and joined a law firm as a junior employee.

Neal's wife of 2 years, Barbara, had great difficulty adjusting to his illness. She wanted to forget that surgery ever took place and became furious if she overheard Neal discussing his tumor with a friend. Neal's interest in sex had decreased greatly. It took long periods of intense penile caressing before he could achieve a full erection. Believing that the sexual problem was under her husband's control, Barbara accused him of withholding sex out of anger at his new dependence on her.

Neal's levels of testosterone and pituitary hormones were in the normal range. He had all the classic symptoms of a major affective disorder, however, including early morning awakenings, a recent weight loss of 10 pounds, social withdrawal, ruminations about his cognitive deficits and lost job skills, irritability, and anhedonia.

Because of his severe problems with sleep, appetite, and mood, a tricyclic antidepressant was prescribed for Neal, with careful monitoring to make sure it did not stimulate seizures. At the same time, couple therapy was offered to help Neal and Barbara adjust to the effects of his disability on their relationship.

Not only emotional responses to illness, but also the patient's habitual style of responding to emotional pain will influence sexuality. The next four sections take a closer look at the role of the defense mechanisms described in Table 4-1.

DENIAL AND SEXUALITY

Denial, as mentioned earlier in this chapter, can be adaptive or maladaptive in coping with an illness (Krantz & Glass, 1984). In the early stages of diagnosis and treatment, denial protects the patient against anxiety that might otherwise be overwhelming. Using denial, the patient can mobilize his or her resources to stay calm and endure uncertainty. Later on, however, denial interferes with treatment. Patients who deny the severity of their illness may fail to comply with a physician's instructions. Denial can also halt the healthy process of mourning, whether for a lost organ, lost health, or a lost spouse.

Denial may be evident in patients' sexual attitudes. Some ignore the impact of an illness on sexual function until confronted with a problem. A common example is the alcoholic who refuses to believe that his drinking could permanently impair erections. Others avoid situations that remind them of their health problem, such as the woman who after a mastectomy never undresses in front of her husband and makes love wearing a nightgown and breast prosthesis. Another type of denial is a refusal to think about sex at all. Patients who have been sexually active and functional until an illness often claim afterward to have no further interest in sex. Men are particularly likely to deny all sexual desire when a disease impairs erections. Women seem more vulnerable to illnesses that affect their physical appearance.

When sex is at issue, denial can be adaptive if it helps a patient overlook a disability and remain sexually active. Denial is not helpful if the patient rejects all sexual pleasure to avoid confronting the effects of illness.

WITHDRAWAL AND SEXUALITY

When a patient is unwilling to adapt to an illness, all aspects of rehabilitation are hampered. If a previously functional man or woman retreats into the invalid role, the spouse often reacts by becoming parental, as discussed in Chapter 2. A whole lifestyle develops around the patient's position in the family as "sick person." If the healthy spouse believes the patient's helplessness to be unjustified by physical limitations, great resentment can develop.

For some patients, sexual rehabilitation is the beginning of a fuller recovery. Treating a sexual dysfunction can boost a man's or woman's self-esteem, stimulating efforts to take control of other areas of life again, too.

Mack, a 63-year-old farmer, had a triple coronary artery bypass. Before surgery, angina limited Mack's activities, and he had delegated the management of his land to his son. After the bypass, Mack joined the community hospital's cardiac rehabilitation exercise class but made little effort to befriend the other participants. Pam called the program director to express concern over her husband's lack of progress. He no longer drove into town for his morning ritual of breakfast with his old cronies. At home Mack spent most of his time watching television or walking aimlessly around the fields. He would not reply to his wife's questions about what was bothering him, but every once in a while would make a comment that implied he was expecting to die in the near future. Since Mack's second heart attack, the couple had not tried to have any sexual activity. When Pam reminded her husband that the doctor had given them permission to resume intercourse after surgery, he replied that he was not yet ready.

An interview with the couple revealed that Mack had been experiencing erectile dysfunction for many months. He refused his wife's advances because he feared being unable to achieve penetration for intercourse. He no longer had erections on waking or when he tried self-stimulation. To Mack, this was the final blow to his sense of manhood and autonomy. Pam had not realized the extent of her husband's sexual dysfunction.

An extensive medical evaluation revealed some pelvic arteriosclerosis, which could be contributing to the erection problem. With counseling, the couple was able to resume noncoital caressing. Although both partners could reach orgasm, Mack's erections were not rigid and the couple missed having intercourse.

Mack decided to have a semirigid penile prosthesis implanted. After surgery, both partners were more satisfied with their lovemaking, and the frequency of sexual activity stabilized at about once a week. Mack also began going into town again, where he cheerfully endured a great deal of teasing from his friends who knew about his latest operation. Although he continued to allow his son to run the farm, he became more active in community affairs, acting as an agricultural advisor for younger men.

PROJECTION AND SEXUALITY

When an illness is diagnosed, a person's perspective narrows to a self-centered mode. As one patient with arthritis commented, "Nobody can join me on my island of pain." The person who is ill may use so much emotional energy to stay in control that capacity for empathy is reduced. The world shrinks as future plans, job, and family life are all threatened by possible disability or death. An increased tendency to project one's own feelings onto others or to blame the illness for unrelated problems may result.

Projection can be a detrimental coping strategy where sexuality is concerned. Instead of seeking help for sexual problems, patients may blame them on the illness, accepting them as inevitable. Even the break-up of a relationship may be attributed to the disease, although the clinician will almost always find that conflict predated the diagnosis.

Sexual problems also occur when a patient projects his or her own feelings onto the spouse.

Albert refused to try any sexual activity after his laryngectomy. When a therapist met with Albert and his wife, Bonnie, together, he asked Albert why he no longer was interested in sex. Albert replied that he would like sex, but knew his wife was only offering to make love out of pity and could not possibly still feel attracted to him. "I won't put her through that," he said. Even in the metallic tones of Albert's speech device, his resolve was plain.

"But honey, if I had a laryngectomy, would you think I was repulsive?" asked Bonnie.

Her husband shook his head. "Of course not!"

"Then why can't you see that I still want you?"

"It's different," was Albert's only answer.

PASSIVE ACCEPTANCE AND SEXUALITY

Passive acceptance of an illness can lead to the attitude that nothing can be done. This type of helplessness is a common reason that couples discontinue sexual activity after a medical treatment, even though sexual pleasure could be attained again with some effort and creativity.

Gretchen was an attractive 62-year-old woman who had an abdominal hysterectomy followed by radiotherapy for cancer of the endometrium. She had been married to Harold for 41 years, and they had continued to have mutually satisfying sexual activity once to twice weekly until her cancer was diagnosed. Gretchen had taken estrogen replacement pills after menopause, but had to discontinue them after her cancer treatment.

At her 3-month check-up, Gretchen told her gynecologist that she was having severe hot flashes and had not resumed intercourse because she feared it would be painful. Harold was asked to come in, and the gynecologist performed a gentle pelvic examination, pointing out to both partners that although Gretchen's vagina was somewhat shallower than before, with added lubrication, intercourse should be comfortable. If Gretchen found that her vagina did not stretch sufficiently with sexual arousal, her vagina could be expanded with a skin graft in a reconstructive operation.

The couple tried having intercourse after their appointment, but penetration was painful. Harold was frightened and turned off by his wife's dyspareunia and lost his erection on subsequent attempts. The gynecologist did not follow up on the sexual situation in future visits, but the couple was seen 4 years later as a part of a research project. They still helped each other reach orgasm through noncoital stimulation, but rarely had successful coitus. The researcher suggested that the couple try a series of sensate focus exercises. Gretchen was also sent back to her gynecologist to ask whether she would be a good candidate for vaginal reconstruction. A minor operation was indeed performed, and, over the next several months, the couple regained their prior degree of sexual pleasure and increased their frequency of sexual activity to twice weekly.

Two final psychological factors influencing sexuality during an illness are cognitions reflecting the patient's inner model of the world. Believing myths about illness and sexuality can prevent a man or woman from resuming a satisfying sex life. An impaired body image has the same effect, no matter what the physical reality to an outside observer.

MYTHS ABOUT DISEASE AND SEXUALITY

Out society promulgates a number of false beliefs about illness and sexuality. If a patient incorporates such myths into his or her inner cognitive world, the beliefs interfere with the motivation to adapt sexually by mastering new skills or even trying old tricks.

Some of the most common myths about sex and disease include the following:

- Sex saps one's strength and thus is harmful to anyone not in the best of health.
- Too much sex is unhealthy and causes illness.
- Having sex weakens the potency of medical treatments like medication or radiation therapy.
- Older people should not be sexually active or even feel sexual desire.

If one or both partners in a couple believe such myths, an illness often heralds an abrupt drop in sexual activity. A few authoritative words from the medical team can debunk the myths, but clinicians rarely remember to discuss such issues with patients and partners. Physicians usually take care to prohibit sexual activity when it might be harmful, for example during postsurgical recovery or when an illness can be sexually transmitted. They are often less scrupulous about encouraging couples to resume sexual activity, however.

Many chronic illnesses are associated with specific myths about sexuality. Although the impact of these beliefs will be discussed in more detail in the chapters of Part 2, they are listed here for illustration:

- Strokes and heart attacks are very common during sexual intercourse.
- Diabetic men always develop erection problems.
- Cancer is contagious through sexual activity.
- Transurethral prostatectomy or chronic prostatitis damage the erection reflex.
- Alcohol, marijuana, or cocaine improve sexual performance.
- Psychiatric patients are oversexed.

No scientific evidence exists to support any of these beliefs, yet we still hear them voiced by patients and even by some clinicians. As sex education improves worldwide, these myths may come to be historical oddities, objects of amusement, like turn-of-the-century treatises on the dangers of masturbation. Until that time, clinicians must remain alert for these beliefs and play the role of sex educator when necessary.

IMPAIRED BODY IMAGE AND SEXUALITY

Each person needs to feel desirable as a sexual partner. A man's or woman's sexual self-image is a blend of feeling physically attractive, skilled as a lover, and able to satisfy a partner's emotional needs for warmth, tenderness, passion, or playfulness. A chronic illness can be devastating to these areas of self-confidence.

Our standards of physical attractiveness are based on youth and vitality. In the United States, even the patients portrayed in television dramas or movies with a medical theme languish glamorously in their hospital beds, perfectly made up and clad in fashionable pajamas. The hero is never a pale, paunchy man in his 50s, staring glumly at his new surgical scar or carting his urine bag around on an IV pole. Almost all illnesses temporarily decrease physical attractiveness by their effect on the patient's energy level and appearance. Some diseases, however, also cause long-term disfigurement and physical disability.

Changes in a person's body image are not always directly proportional to physical changes in appearance. Of course one dimension is whether a change is visible at all. Sometimes the diagnosis of a chronic illness leaves a patient feeling stigmatized, even though little physical evidence of disease can be seen. Other changes are publicly visible, such as hair loss during chemotherapy or a facial disfigurement. Alterations in the breasts, abdominal, or genital area more more private, yet are devastating because they will be obvious to the sexual partner.

The degree of impairment in a person's body image depends on beliefs and feelings. How much emphasis does the patient place on physical beauty? Does the patient view an illness as stigmatizing? The diabetic whose daily insulin injections remind her of her disease, the man who knows that his cerebral hemorrhage has impaired his memory, the patient who must take medication daily to control seizures—all are vulnerable to feeling rejected or undesirable.

The partner's reaction to the disease also affects the patient's self-esteem. Can a husband stroke his wife's mastectomy scar? Is a wife willing to help her husband change his ostomy appliance? Does the spouse continue to initiate sex and reach out with an affectionate touch? The final piece of the puzzle is the reaction of others in the social environment. If the patient no longer feels accepted as a fully functioning person, if gazes are averted or full of pity, if friends and family become too kind and treat the patient like a fragile doll, the patient will have difficulty feeling sexually attractive.

Arlene, a handsome 34-year-old woman, became quadriplegic after an auto accident. Although she made an effort to be well-groomed and socially outgoing, she felt anxious and self-conscious in public. It was especially hard for her, a tall woman, to look up at the world. She noticed that people often failed to make eye contact with her. She also regretted her inability to help her 2-year-old daughter with normal daily activities such as bathing or dressing.

Michael loved his wife very much, but 6 months after her injury he still had not initiated any sexual activity. When Arlene asked him why, he said he feared that she would be unable to feel anything. Arlene told her husband that feeling close and sharing his excitement would give her pleasure, too. She was afraid that Michael was no longer attracted to her. When the couple began to experiment with sexual touching, each partner mourned for what they had lost, but they were also able to regain a sense of intimacy.

Some illnesses interfere with lovemaking skills. Diseases that actually disrupt physiological genital function will be discussed in Chapter 5. Here we are concerned with chronic limitations in mobility, such as those caused by amputations, spinal cord damage, or arthritis, or even by the chest and arm pain common after radical mastectomy. Often a couple's preferred intercourse positions are no longer comfortable. The partners must sometimes adjust to awkward preparations for sexual activity, including performing bowel or bladder care, arranging supporting pillows on the bed, or timing lovemaking to take place during a period of maximal pain relief.

A number of guides are available for patients with illnesses that necessitate special sexual preparations. Helpful publications include *Sexual Options for Paraplegics and Quadraplegics* (Mooney, Cole, & Chilgren, 1975), *Toward Intimacy* (Task Force on Concerns of Physically Disabled Women, 1980), and *Arthritis: Living and Loving* (Arthritis Foundation, 1982). Catalogues of sexual aids for the disabled can also be obtained.*

It takes time and effort to achieve a state in which lovemaking can feel playful and spontaneous in spite of the need for some preparation. Ultimately, it is the emotional quality of a sexual experience, however, that makes a relationship truly satisfying.

---

*One such catalogue is available through the Xandria Collection (Special Edition Catalogue for Disabled People), Lawrence Research Group, 1245 16th Street, San Francisco, CA, 94107.

5

Physiological Factors and
Sexual Problems in Chronic Illness

Clinicians who treat sexual problems in medical patients need a thorough knowledge of the physiological effects of illness on sexual function. We present a schema for evaluating medical risk factors as a part of the integrative model. The goal is to identify any need for medical treatment or any limitations on a man's or woman's ability to regain good sexual function through counseling or sex therapy. We are not interested in classifying sexual problems as organic versus psychogenic, however, since either/or distinctions interfere with comprehensive treatment planning.

When evaluating a patient, it is crucial to carefully review the medical history, a recent physical examination, and current medications (including abused substances). The following questions are important to keep in mind:

- Does the patient have a history of illness or take a medication that can affect hormone levels?
- Does the patient's history reveal risk factors for pelvic vascular insufficiency?
- Has the patient had an illness or medical treatment that can damage the central nervous system or the pelvic sensory nerves?
- Has the patient had an illness or medical treatment that can damage pelvic autonomic nerves? Is the patient taking medications that affect the autonomic nervous system?
- Has the patient had a medical problem that involved removing or damaging areas of the genitals?
- Has the patient had an illness or medical treatment that could cause pain during sexual activity?

This chapter addresses each of the questions in turn. When a patient is at risk in one of the above areas, the clinician can suggest specialized examinations, described in Chapter 6, to further investigate the problem.

HORMONAL FACTORS IN SEXUAL DYSFUNCTION

Although hormonal abnormalities are some of the rarest medical causes of sexual dysfunction, clinicians need a basic knowledge of behavioral endocrinology. The hormonal systems are so different in men and women that we will discuss hormonal mechanisms of sexual dysfunction separately by gender.

Sexuality, Fertility, and Hormones in Men

Testosterone is a steroid hormone produced by the Leydig cells of the testes. The hypothalamus (a part of the brain's limbic system) controls production of testosterone (Figure 5-1) by secreting a peptide called *gonadotropin-releasing hormone* (GnRH), into the blood that circulates to the pituitary gland (the "master gland" at the base of the brain). The anterior area of the pituitary, in turn, releases bursts of luteinizing hormone (LH) into the bloodstream (Vigersky, 1983). LH stimulates the Leydig cells of the testes to produce testosterone. Circulating LH peaks 4 hours after the onset of sleep (Schiavi, Fisher, White, Beers, & Szechter, 1984), accounting for the fact that men's serum testosterone levels are highest in early morning.

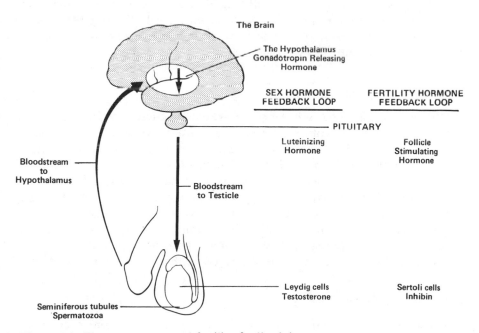

Figure 5-1. The testosterone and fertility feedback loops.

Once testosterone has been released into the bloodstream, most is bound to sex-hormone-binding globulin (SHBG). The bound hormone molecules are inactive and cannot enter target cells in the body. Free testosterone (about 3% of the total in the bloodstream) (Semmens, Rouse, Beilin, & Masarei, 1983) can be used by target cells, however. It enters the cells by way of special receptor sites and then is usually converted either to dihydrotestosterone (DHT) or estradiol (E$_2$), hormones that affect sexual desire, arousability, erections, and the ease of reaching orgasm. The hypothalamus senses the circulating levels of DHT and E$_2$ and responds by regulating further production of GnRH. Thus, the sex hormone system is a feedback loop.

Fertility depends on a feedback loop that is related to testosterone production, but also has some independence from it. GnRH also commands the pituitary gland to produce the follicle-stimulating hormone (FSH) (Vigersky, 1983; Figure 5-1), which acts in the Sertoli cells of the testicles to regulate the production of sperm cells. Both testosterone and FSH levels must be normal for spermatogenesis to take place. The testicles regulate the production of FSH by releasing a protein called *inhibin* into the bloodstream. Inhibin probably does its work in the pituitary gland.

Effects of Illness on Sexuality and Fertility in Men

It is important for clinicians to distinguish between hormonal effects on sexuality and changes in fertility. Both patients and health care professionals may confuse sexuality with fertility, assuming that one cannot be impaired independently of the other.

Damage to Spermatogenesis

Although testosterone is involved in sexual function and fertility, many illnesses or medical treatments impair the delicate process of spermatogenesis, leaving the Leydig cells in the testicles intact. During sperm cell production, stem cells within the seminiferous tubules (long cylindrical structures in the testicle) divide a number of times, taking 16 days to develop into mature sperm cells (Huckins, 1983). During cell division, genetic control mechanisms are especially vulnerable to "insults" such as radiation, cancer chemotherapy agents, or damage from infections like mumps orchitis. Such events can interrupt spermatogenesis, sometimes for a number of years. If the damage is severe, all the stem cells may be destroyed so that infertility is permanent.

Health and Testosterone

Leydig cells are not perpetually dividing, and thus testosterone production is harder than spermatogenesis to damage. Men who have cerebral accidents, myocardial infarctions, or major surgery do experience a temporary decline in testosterone that is probably caused by the hypothalamus responding to stress (Woolf, Hamill, McDonald, Lee, & Kelly, 1985). Evidence is growing that testosterone levels also vary with general health or vigor. In young men, testosterone levels increase with aerobic fitness (Remes, Kuoppasalmi, & Adlercreutz, 1979; Young & Ismail, 1978). Thus one would expect to find more men with abnormally low testosterone in chronically ill populations than in healthy, fit groups.

Testosterone and Male Sexual Function

Because testosterone plays a basic role in male sexual function, let us take a closer look at the mechanisms involved.

Serum testosterone levels vary widely in men. The normal range is between 300 and 1200 ng./dl. (or 10.4–41.6 nmol./L.), though the endpoints differ somewhat from laboratory to laboratory. When a man's testosterone level is abnormally low, sexual problems are common but by no means universal. Many reports exist in the literature of men with prepubertal levels of serum testosterone who continue to have normal sexual function (Davidson, Camargo, Smith, & Kwan, 1983; Heim, 1981; Salmimies, Kockott, Pirke, Vogt, & Schill, 1982). The sexual symptoms commonly associated with testosterone deficiency are similar, no matter what interruption in the feedback loop has caused the abnormality. Usually the man complains of reduced sexual desire, difficulty in achieving full erections, and difficulty in reaching orgasm. Some men report that the pleasure they achieve from penile caressing is reduced. The sexual dysfunction is rarely absolute. A man may still feel some interest in sex, but getting aroused is an effortful, prolonged process. On some occasions, successful intercourse may take place, with a rigid erection and a normal sensation of orgasm, although semen volume is lessened.

How does testosterone impair the sexual response cycle? The mechanisms remain mysterious. Testosterone probably acts in the human brain to promote sexual desire, but we do not know which areas of the brain are hormonally responsive or even which metabolite of testosterone is active in the brain. The interaction between testosterone levels and erectile function is even more mysterious. Prepubescent boys, and even infants, can get erections and reach orgasm. Why do some hypogonadal men maintain erectile function in spite of low testosterone levels while many others, especially older men (Heim, 1981), have erection problems? Is it just that the men lack sexual desire and thus cannot get aroused? Double-blind studies of testosterone replacement in hypogonadal men have found clear, dose-related increases in the frequency of spontaneous erections, orgasm, and sexual activity (Davidson, Camargo, & Smith, 1979; Salmimies *et al.*, 1982). Research has also demonstrated that NPT is depressed in men with low testosterone (O'Carroll, Shapiro, & Bancroft, 1985; Wincze, Bansal, & Malamud, 1986). Perhaps testosterone has a direct effect on the central or peripheral nerves that control the erection reflex.

Prolactin and Men's Sexual Function

One controversial hormone that can produce sexual dysfunction is *prolactin*, produced by the pituitary. Severe elevations in prolactin are rare and usually caused by a benign, hormone-producing tumor of the pituitary. Prolactin may be hundreds of times higher than normal in these patients. If the tumor is large enough, it may also cause vision problems and headaches and can be life threatening. Sometimes, however, the only symptoms of a tumor are sexual problems. A clinician evaluating sexual dysfunction must therefore remain alert for this small group of patients.

Not all hyperprolactinemic men have sexual problems, but low sexual desire, erectile dysfunction, and difficulty reaching orgasm are quite frequent (Buvat *et al.*, 1985b; Grunstein *et al.*, 1984; Rocco, Falaschi, Pompei, D'Urso, & Frajese, 1983; Schwartz *et al.*, 1982). Even if dysfunction is situational, a clinician should remain alert for indications of this hormonal abnormality. As Schwartz *et al.* (1982) and Buvat and colleagues (1985a) point out, sexual dysfunctions in severely hyperprolactinemic men may occur intermittently or only with certain partners or types of sexual stimulation. Some patients can even reach orgasm through masturbation but not during intercourse.

The sexual dysfunction associated with severe hyperprolactinemia is quite similar to that seen in men with low testosterone. Indeed, when prolactin is quite elevated, the level of total serum testosterone is often below normal (Buvat *et al.*, 1985b). The amount of free testosterone, however, remains adequate (Vermeulen, Ando, & Verdonck, 1982). Thus, testosterone levels do not tell the whole story. Merely giving replacement testosterone will not improve sexual function in severely hyperprolactinemic men. The prolactin level needs to be decreased, for example, by surgically removing a pituitary tumor or by giving the dopamine agonist medication, bromocriptine (Parlodel). Researchers believe that hyperprolactinemia may decrease sexual desire because of concurrent depletion of brain dopamine or interference with the conversion of testosterone to dihydrotestosterone (Drago, 1984).

The real controversy is about the impact of mild elevations of prolactin on sexual function. Medications that deplete brain dopamine, like the phenothiazines, butyrophenones, or sulpirides used to treat psychosis or the antihypertensives reserpine and methyldopa, can cause mild hyperprolactinemia (De La Fuente & Rosenbaum, 1981). Opiates also stimulate prolactin secretion (Judd *et al.*, 1982). For an unknown reason, hyperprolactinemia is common in men and women on chronic dialysis for end-stage renal disease. Some researchers have observed sexual dysfunction in mildly hyperprolactinemic patients, which improves when prolactin levels are normalized (Ermolenko *et al.*, 1986; Muir *et al.*, 1983; Ruilope *et al.*, 1985; Weizman *et al.*, 1983). Buvat *et al.* (1985a), however, do not believe that mild hyperprolactinemia causes sexual problems.

Prolactin apparently can affect mood as well as sexual function. Hyperprolactinemic women are often depressed and hostile, although dysphoria is not as well documented in men (De La Fuente & Rosenbaum, 1981; Fava, 1984; Kellner, Buckman, Fava, & Pathak, 1984). Perhaps the sexual dysfunction is just one aspect of a more general syndrome of psychological distress. Certainly erectile dysfunction and difficulty achieving orgasm may be secondary to a lack of sexual interest and subjective arousal.

The Incidence of Hormonal Abnormalities in Men

Table 5-1 lists base rates of low testosterone and hyperprolactinemia found in several series of men consecutively referred for treatment of sexual dysfunction. The treatment setting clearly influences the incidence of hormone abnormalities. Men sent to an endocrinologist are more likely to have endocrinopathy, as are men followed in a VA clinic, a setting in which patients are often elderly and have histories of alcoholism or other chronic illnesses. Hormone abnormalities are uncommon, yet are frequent enough to justify routine screening (see Chapter 6) since appropriate therapy can often restore normal sexual function.

Table 5-1. Rates of Low Testosterone (T) and Hyperprolactinemia (PRL) in Men with Sexual Dysfunction

Study Setting	N	Low T(%)	High PRL(%)	Total abnormal (%)
Endocrine clinic (Spark, White & Connolly, 1980)	105	28	8	36
VA outpatient medical clinic (Slag *et al.*, 1983)	188	19	4	23
Sex clinic (Masters & Johnson) (Schwartz *et al.*, 1982)	136	15	8	23
Sex clinic (psychiatry) (Jensen, Colstrup, Wagner, Nystrup, & Hertoft, 1983)	50	4	2	6
Sex clinic (multidisciplinary) (Segraves, Schoenberg, & Ivanoff, 1983)	52	15	0	15
Sex clinic (urology) (Nickel, Morales, Condra, Fenemore, & Surridge, 1984)	256	13	6	18
Sex clinic (urology) (Maatman & Montague, 1985)	300	6	3	9

Risk Factors for Hormonal Abnormalities in
Sexually Dysfunctional Men

A clinician should be alert to information from the medical history or
examination that might indicate a hormonal abnormality. Table 5-2 lists
some of these warning signs. Readers who desire more detailed knowledge
in this area can consult Horwith & Imperato-McGinley (1983); Lipschultz,
Cunningham, & Howards (1983); or Pogach & Vaitukaitis (1983).

Hormones and Female Sexual Dysfunction

We know far less about the impact of hormone abnormalities on women's
sexual function that we do about such problems in men. A woman's life
involves constant variations in hormone levels. Women experience not only
the daily changes of the menstrual cycle, but also pregnancy, menopause,
and treatment with oral contraceptives or replacement estrogens without
any characteristic changes in their sexual desire, subjective arousal, or
ability to reach orgasm. Each hormonal change seems to increase the
variability in women's sexuality, some reporting enhanced function and
others deterioration. No hormonal abnormality has the clear-cut effects on
women that low testosterone has on men. With that caveat, let us look at the
effect of endocrine abnormalities on female sexual dysfunction.

Androgen Abnormalities in Women

When women have androgen levels outside the normal range, few effects on
sexuality can be identified. Such a tiny fraction of women's circulating
androgens is free (unbound to SHBG), that a severe hormonal deficit may
be necessary before sexual function is impaired. Kolodny, Masters, &
Johnson (1979) reviewed clinical observations of small groups of women
who have Addison's disease (adrenal cortex insufficiency) or hypopituita-
rism with reduced ovarian and adrenal function. They concluded that these
women have reduced sexual desire and difficulty reaching orgasm but they
did not in fact gather systematic research data.

In Germany, a group of 61 women with symptoms of hyperandrogenism (acne, hirsutism, menstrual irregularities) were treated with an antiandrogen (cyproterone acetate) (Appelt & Strauss, 1984). Before hormone
therapy, their sexual function was similar to that of women in the general
population. Afterward, however, a much larger percentage (44%) complained of sexual problems, especially loss of desire and difficulty becoming
aroused. More sophisticated, prospective studies are needed to demonstrate
the effect of androgen deficits on women's sexuality.

The effects of hyperandrogenism on female sexuality are controversial.
Kolodny *et al.* (1979) reported that women with polycystic ovaries (Stein-

Table 5-2. Signs that Alert a Clinician to Possible
Hormonal Abnormalities in Men

Medical History
  Genetic abnormalities that affect reproduction
  Disease or injury affecting pituitary or hypothalamus
  Disease or injury of the testicles
  Adrenal or thyroid abnormalities
  Diabetes
  Renal disease
  Sickle cell anemia
  Cirrhosis of the liver
  Alcoholism
  Abuse of opiate drugs
  Obesity or anorexia
  Pelvic irradiation
  Cancer chemotherapy

Physical Examination
  Testicular atrophy
  Gynecomastia (breast tenderness or development)
  Galactorrhea (ability to express fluid from the nipples)
  Visual field abnormalities (signs of a pituitary tumor)
  Sparse body hair
  Decreased beard growth
  Skin hyperpigmentation suggesting adrenal disease
  Signs of thyroid abnormalities
  Low energy level and lack of "well-being"

Medications
  Methyldopa
  Reserpine
  Phenothiazines
  Butyrophenones
  Spironolactone
  Digoxin
  Tricyclic antidepressants
  Benzodiazepines
  Cimetidine
  Opiate medications or synthetic opiates
  Progesterones
  Estrogens

Leventhal syndrome) who secrete excessive amounts of androgens experience increased sexual desire and aggressiveness. A recent comparison of 50 such women with age-matched controls found no differences, however, in sexual history, function, arousability, or activity level (Raboch, Kobilkova, Raboch, & Starka, 1985)

Estrogen Deficiency and Female Sexual Function

Any medical illness that interferes with ovarian function can decrease vaginal blood flow, with a concomitant decline in vaginal lubrication and expansion during sexual arousal. Atrophy of the vagina may occur, too, leaving the mucosa thin and fragile and narrowing the vaginal entrance.

Surgery that removes both ovaries causes an abrupt and severe drop in estrogen, as do pelvic irradiation and many types of combination chemotherapy used to treat cancer. Symptoms of menopause, such as hot flashes and vaginal dryness, are often more severe than during the natural climacteric. Nevertheless, sexual function remains normal or improves in a majority of women who have hysterectomy plus bilateral oophorectomy for benign disease (Dennerstein & Burrows, 1982). Estrogen replacement therapy, if not contraindicated, can also reverse the vaginal changes of menopause (Semmens & Wagner, 1982). If sexual desire and arousability are decreased in estrogen-deficient states, the dysfunction is probably secondary to psychological factors, the underlying disease that led to medical treatment, or the physical discomfort of hot flashes, vaginal dryness, or dyspareunia.

Progesterone and Female Sexual Function

In the last several years, researchers and clinicians have attempted to define a premenstrual syndrome (PMS) characterized by tension, depression, irritability, and breast tenderness in the late luteal (premenstrual) phase of the cycle. Rubinow and Roy-Byrne (1984) have reviewed the evidence for a hormonal etiology for PMS. They conclude that no such evidence exists. Despite the theory that PMS results from a deficiency of progesterone, studies purporting to show such an abnormality are unconvincing. Levels of estrogen and prolactin also rarely differ between women with PMS and controls.

If PMS exists, do women who experience it suffer from sexual dysfunction? A carefully designed study in England measured hormone levels regularly and had women keep daily logs of mood and sexual interest (Backstrom *et al.*, 1983; Bancroft, Sanders, Davidson, & Warner, 1983; D. Sanders, Warner, Backstrom, & Bancroft, 1983). Subjects included 19 women seeking help at a PMS clinic, 18 community volunteers who reported PMS symptoms, and 18 volunteers without PMS. No hormonal differences were found when groups were studied across the menstrual cycle. The PMS clinic group did have a statistically significant decrease in sexual interest before menstruation. A cyclical shift in general well-being, however, accounted for this minor loss of sexual desire.

Hyperprolactinemia and Female Sexual Function

Hyperprolactinemia has received attention as a common cause of infertility and amenorrhea (absent menstruation) in women, but little knowledge is available on prolactin and female sexual function. The data that exist parallel findings in men. In a group of 21 women on chronic hemodialysis for renal disease, those with sexual dysfunction (including lack of desire, difficulty getting aroused, and trouble reaching orgasm) had significantly higher prolactin levels than did sexually functional women. One woman received bromocriptine and experienced an improvement in sexual function (Weizman *et al.*, 1983). In a larger group of 99 women on hemodialysis, an association between hyperprolactinemia and sexual dysfunction was also observed (Mastrogiacomo *et al.*, 1984). In a group of 109 women with hypothalamic or pituitary disorders, 84% with hyperprolactinemia noticed decreased sexual desire, compared with 33% of those who had normal prolactin levels (Lundberg, Hulter, & Wide, 1985, September). Problems with vaginal lubrication and orgasm were also reported in this pilot study.

VASCULAR FACTORS IN SEXUAL DYSFUNCTION

The role of vascular disease in contributing to erectile dysfunction has only been fully appreciated in recent years (Wagner, 1982). Unlike hormonal abnormalities, vascular insufficiency in the pelvis does not primarily affect the desire or orgasm phases of the sexual response cycle. The problems all occur in the arousal phase, although some elderly men with diffuse arteriosclerosis may also have central nervous system complications affecting sexual desire and pleasure. Like researchers who study hormonal factors, those investigating vascular causes of sexual dysfunction have focused principally on men. We begin by reviewing the role of vascular disease in male sexual problems and then look at the data on women.

Vascular Factors in Male Sexual Dysfunction

In discussing vascular disease and erectile dysfunction, it is helpful to examine separately the effects of disease in the large or central pelvic arteries, the finer arteries that branch off to serve the penis, and the venous drainage system of the penis.

Disease in the Large Arteries

Leriche was the first to describe a syndrome of ischemia (inadequate blood flow) to the legs combined with erectile dysfunction (Leriche & Morel, 1948). Blockages or narrowing of the lower end of the aorta or in the common or internal iliac arteries can cause both cramping pain in the legs with exercise (claudication) and difficulty in achieving and/or maintaining erections (Michal, 1982).

How many men with claudication also have erection problems? Based on clinical experience, Michal (1982) estimated the rate to be 40% to 50%.

Metz (1983) reported erectile dysfunction in 46% of 98 consecutive patients under age 70 with arterial disease reducing circulation to the legs. The sexual problem developed gradually in 78% of cases. Although most men could no longer achieve rigid erections, some could still penetrate for intercourse if foreplay was prolonged or if the partner supported the base of the penis with her hand (Metz, Frimodt-Møller, & Mathiesen, 1983c).

In the past, surgery to correct claudication frequently created erection problems as well as causing retrograde ejaculation. Newer techniques avoid damage to sympathetic nerves, and pelvic blood flow can actually be increased rather than decreased. About a third of men report improved erectile function afterwards (Flanigan, Schuler, Kiefer, Schwartz, & Lim, 1982; Forsberg, Olssen, & Neglen, 1982; Metz *et al.*, 1983c).

When the area where the aorta divides into the iliac arteries is partially blocked, a pelvic steal syndrome may occur (Metz & Mathiesen, 1979; Michal, Kramer, & Pospichal, 1978). When the man moves his legs, blood flow reverses in the internal iliac or hypogastric artery, "stealing" blood away from the penile circulation to supply the legs and buttocks. If the man happens to have an erection at that moment, it will detumesce. Typically, a man can achieve firm erections with sexual stimulation as long as he stays relatively still. During the thrusting motions of intercourse in the "missionary" position, however, his leg and gluteal (buttock) muscles need additional circulation and his erection softens. He may notice a cramping pain in his buttocks at the same time. True pelvic steal syndromes are probably quite rare and difficult to diagnose. Nocturnal erections are often impaired (Goldstein *et al.*, 1982) but are more likely to be normal than are erections during sexual activity.

Disease in the Pudendal and Penile Arteries

Michal (1982) believes that lesions of the fine penile arteries are even more common causes of erectile dysfunction than are blockages of the large penile arteries. From a series of postmortem examinations of 30 men aged 19 to 85 years, Ruzbarsky and Michal (1977) concluded that all men over 38 years old begin to show fibrous changes in the small penile arteries. As men age, severe fibrosis, calcification, and thrombi combine to reduce flood flow to the penis, perhaps accounting for the classic observation that older men take longer to achieve erections. Diabetes accelerates this process.

One current view is that vascular erection problems are an "early warning sign" of arteriosclerosis. The changes in blood flow required for erection are so extreme, and the arterial system of the penis is so delicate, that erectile dysfunction may occur before other symptoms such as claudication or angina. We take a more cautious position, however. Ruzbarsky and Michal (1977) had no data on previous sexual function in the men they studied postmortem, so their observations remain theoretical. When a group of diabetics with erectile dysfunction was compared to a well-matched sample of diabetic men with normal erections, results of penile vascular studies were abnormal just as often in the functional group as in men with sexual problems (Buvat *et al.*, 1985b). We need more studies of men at high risk for pelvic vascular disease to see why erectile dysfunction develops in some while others remain sexually adequate. We also must compare older men at high versus low risk for vascular disease to see if rates of sexual dysfunction truly differ between the two groups.

Venous Abnormalities and Erectile Dysfunction

The venous drainage system of the penis is complex and poorly understood. Good evidence exists that venous drainage decreases during erection, helping to maintain the high pressure in the cavernous bodies (Wagner & Green, 1981). It is unclear, however, whether the veins are mechanically compressed during erection or valves inside the veins are constricted by the autonomic nervous system (Delcour, Wespes, Schulman, & Stryven, 1984).

Several research groups believe that excess venous drainage can cause erectile dysfunction. Delcour *et al.* (1984) found that excess venous drainage was present in two thirds of a group of men with abnormal NPT but no other obvious, nonvenous causes of erection problems. These researchers blame incompetence of large veins such as the deep dorsal vein for most such problems. Virag, Zwang, Dermange, and Legman (1981) concur, but Danish researchers have emphasized the presence in some men of abnormal fistulae (leaks) between the cavernous bodies and the spongy body of the penis, allowing excess venous drainage to occur (Ebbehøj & Wagner, 1979).

Peyronie's Disease

Peyronie's disease is an abnormal curvature of the penis only visible during erection. It is caused by a fibrous plaque, or scar, that forms between the two layers of tough tissue (tunica albuginea and Buck's fascia) surrounding the cavernous bodies of the penis. The true cause of the scarring is unknown, but Peyronie's disease is included here because some clinicians attribute it to a poor local supply of blood (Metz, Ebbehøj, Uhrenholdt, & Waner, 1983b: Michal, 1982) and because the plaques, once formed, can further disturb the circulation of the penis.

Many men are so embarrassed by the symptoms of Peyronie's disease that they do not seek help from their physician. Statistics on the incidence of Peyronie's disease are therefore probably underestimates. Michal (1982) has suggested that 1% of men have Peyronie's plaques. We diagnosed Peyronie's disease in 3% of a series of 308 male cancer patients referred for sexual counseling (Schover *et al.*, 1987) and 6% of men seen in a sexual dysfunction clinic (Jensen, Colstrup, Wagner, Nystrup, & Hertoft, 1983). We do know that it is more common in middle-aged men (O'Donnell, Leach, & Raz, 1982) and perhaps in men genetically predisposed (Willscher, 1983). Penile plaques (and similar scarring on the palms, Dupuytren's contractures) may occur when these vulnerable men are exposed to penile trauma, beta-blocking medication, or phenytoin. Repeated small traumas to the penis during medical procedures performed in the urethra (Kelami, 1985) or even from vigorous sexual stimulation may eventually cause scarring. As more men use repeated papaverine injections to treat erectile dysfunction, penile scarring or fibrosis are being observed in that group as well (Larsen, Gasser, & Bruskewitz, 1987).

When the penile curvature begins, some men experience pain with erection. The penis sometimes bends at such an angle that intercourse becomes uncomfortable or even impossible. With time, the scarring may stabilize, but sometimes progresses, preventing the penis from becoming rigid with erection (Willscher, 1983). Recently Metz *et al.* (1983b) observed abnormal drainage from the cavernous bodies during artificial erection in 13 of 15 men with Peyronie's disease and erectile dysfunction. In a few, the leaks could be localized to the area of the plaque. These researchers believe that the scarring itself may provide a route for abnormal drainage or perhaps that the fibrosis damages nerves that regulate venous drainage in the penis.

Risk Factors for Vascular Erectile Dysfunction

Factors that put a man at risk for vascular erectile dysfunction are listed in Table 5-3. Most men develop some pelvic arteriosclerosis with aging, but men at higher-than-normal risk for arterial disease appear to have increased rates of vascular erectile dysfunction (de Tejada, Goldstein, Heeren, & Krane, 1985; Goldstein *et al.*, 1982a; Michal, 1982; Virag, Bouilly, & Frydman, 1985). The importance of smoking history in men evaluated in an impotence clinic was emphasized in a recent series of 178 men. Not only was there an excess of heavy smokers compared to the general population, but smokers were more likely to have abnormal Doppler studies (Condra, Morales, Owen, Surridge, & Fenemore, 1986a).

Some younger men also have vascular erectile dysfunction. For example, pelvic fracture injuries may disrupt penile blood flow, especially in the pudendal arteries (Michal, 1982; Sharlip, 1981). Men who have never been able to achieve rigid erections usually have severe anxieties about intimacy and sexuality and are best treated with sex therapy. When a young man cannot achieve firm erections in any situation, however, the clinician should be alert for the rare case in which a congenital vascular factor is present.

Men who receive high doses of pelvic irradiation, usually as a treatment for prostate cancer, may also be at risk for vascular erectile dysfunction. Goldstein, Feldman, Deckers, Babayan, and Krane (1984) found that 15 of

Table 5-3. Signs that Alert a Clinician to Vascular Factors in Erectile Dysfunction

Medical History
  Over age 50
  Hypertension
  Diabetes
  Cardiac disease
  Claudication
  Pelvic irradiation
  Smoker
  Pelvic fracture
  Osteoarthritis
  Repeated urethral manipulation for medical procedures (Peyronie's disease only)
Physical Examination
  Weak pulses in legs or ankles
  Hair loss on lower legs
  Unusually cool temperature, penis or lower legs
  High lipid levels
  High cholesterol levels
  Dupuytren's contractures (Peyronie's disease only)
  Fibrosis of outer ear cartilage (Peyronie's disease only)
Medications
  Phenytoin (Peyronie's disease only)
  Beta-blockers (Peyronie's disease only)
  Medications used to treat hypertension, cardiac disease, and diabetes are commonly taken
    by men with vascular erectile dysfunction and may have sexual side effects, but they do
    not contribute to the underlying vascular pathology (e.g., antihypertensives disturb the
    neurological regulation of blood flow)

23 such men had vascular erection problems after treatment. They believe that radiation may accelerate arteriosclerosis, especially in men who smoke or are hypertensive. Radiation may also do direct damage, scarring and narrowing arteries. A weakness in their data, however, is the lack of assessment of penile blood flow before radiation. Men with prostate cancer are an elderly group, already likely to have vascular disease. Another research team found no vascular changes in a small sample of men examined before and after pelvic radiotherapy (Mittal, 1985).

Vascular Factors in Female Sexual Dysfunction

Although it seems logical that the same risk factors promoting vascular erection problems in men would interfere with vaginal lubrication and expansion in women, little evidence to that effect is available. Vaginal blood flow and lubrication do decrease after menopause (Semmens & Wagner, 1982). Perhaps premenopausal women are protected from pelvic arteriosclerosis by estrogen. After menopause, however, pelvic vascular disease may account for the more severe vaginal atrophy and dryness some women experience. We need physiological studies comparing groups of women at high risk for pelvic arteriosclerosis (smokers, hypertensives, diabetics, women with high lipid levels) with age-matched controls. Since women can usually make intercourse comfortable by using extra lubrication, their arousal phase dysfunctions receive less medical attention than parallel problems affecting men's erections.

NEUROLOGICAL DISEASE AND SEXUAL FUNCTION

Since the nervous system plays such an important role in regulating sexual function, neurological disease can affect desire, arousal, or orgasm. Little is known about the effects of pathological states on areas of the brain or neurotransmitters involved in sexual desire. Table 5-4 lists some suspected neurological risk factors for low desire, but this chapter focuses on periph-eral neurological causes of erectile dysfunction, female arousal phase dysfunctions, and male and female orgasm phase problems.

Neurological Causes of Erectile Dysfunction

Table 5-5 outlines risk factors for neurological erectile dysfunction. Of all groups of chronically ill patients, men with spinal cord injuries have been most thoroughly studied in terms of sexual function. The degree of erectile function a man retains depends on the area of the cord that has been injured

---

Table 5-4. Possible Factors Affecting The Neurological Regulation of Sexual Desire

Medical History, Low Desire
  Frontal lobe pathology
  Temporal lobe pathology
  Diffuse cortical atrophy (dementing processes)
  Parkinson's disease

Medications, Low Desire
  Opiate medications or synthetic opiates
  Alcohol
  Beta-blockers
  Reserpine
  Methyldopa
  Phenothiazines
  Butyrophenones
  Tricyclic antidepressants
  Benzodiazepines
  Lithium

Possible Central Aphrodisiacs
  Yohimbine
  L-Dopa
  Bromocriptine

Table 5-5. Signs that Alert a Clinician to Neurological Factors in Erectile Dysfunction

---

Medical History
 Diabetes
 Alcoholism
 Chronic obstructive lung disease
 Spinal cord injury
 Lumbar laminectomy
 Radical pelvic cancer surgery (prostatectomy, cystectomy, abdominoperineal resection)
 Internal urethrotomy, external sphincterotomy, or history of urethral rupture
 Neuromuscular disease
 Neurogenic bladder or bowel dysfunction
Physical Examination
 Weak or absent genital reflexes
  Bulbocavernosus
  Cremasteric
  Scrotal
  Internal anal
  Superficial anal
 Neurological abnormalities in the S2 to S4 nerve root distribution
 Reduced penile sensory thresholds to light touch, electrical stimulation, or vibration
Medications That May Interfere with Erection at the Peripheral Nervous System Level
 Antihypertensives (particularly guanethidine)
 Calcium-channel blockers
 Beta-blockers
 Neuroleptics (particularly thioridazine and fluphenazine)
 Tricyclic antidepressants
 Monoamine oxidase inhibitors
 Lithium
 Alcohol
 Neurotoxic cancer chemotherapies (particularly vincristine)

(i.e., level within the cervical, thoracic, lumbar, or sacral portions of the spinal cord) and how completely the spinal cord has been damaged. The cord is rarely cut through. Injuries to the anterior (front) segments of the cord are most likely to affect sexual function, especially if both left and right sides of the cord are involved (Torrens, 1983).

Researchers have noted that two spinal areas are important to erectile function. The sacral segments S2 to S4 are the exit points for parasympathetic nerves, whereas the thoracic and lumbar segments T12 to L3 contain the roots of sympathetic ganglia. Nerves originating from these spinal levels eventually combine to form the prostatic plexus. When the cervical or thoracic spine above T12 is injured, the erection reflex arc within the spinal cord remains intact. About 80% of men can obtain an erection from tactile stimulation to the penis, but the tumescence is often fleeting because psychic arousal from the brain cannot provide continuing stimulation. Such injuries usually abolish all sensation on the genital skin as well. Men with injuries high in the cord may experience autonomic dysreflexia if they become sexually aroused. The body can no longer regulate the autonomic activation that normally occurs with any emotional arousal (Amelar & Dubin, 1982), and the result is flushing, sweating, a pounding headache, and a rapid rise in blood pressure.

Injuries to the sacral area of the cord or the cauda equina (literally "horse's tail," the lowest area of the spinal cord where nerve fibers fan out below the sacral vertebrae) result in a much higher rate of erectile dysfunction. Only 30% of men with complete lesions can achieve full erections. Any erection that occurs depends on psychological arousal rather than on tactile stimulation. Presumably the reflex occurs because of input from the T12 to L3 area. Although injuries in these lower areas often prevent erections, the men are more likely to recover some sensation in the genital area.

Men with injuries below the T10 level but above the S2 level often have the fullest and most sustained erections, since both spinal erection centers remain intact (Torrens, 1983). Men with incomplete lesions at any level also have a better sexual prognosis. Less than a third of all men with spinal cord injuries, however, can achieve and maintain erections sufficient for intercourse (Yalla, 1982).

The erection reflex can also be damaged by radical cancer surgery that involves cutting through the prostatic nerve plexus (Walsh & Mostwin, 1984). These operations include radical prostatectomy (removal of the prostate), radical cystectomy (removal of the bladder and prostate), and abdominoperineal resection (removal of the lower colon and rectum). Nerve-sparing procedures during surgery have boosted the percentage of men who recover full erections from about 15 (Schover & Fife, 1985) to over 80 (Walsh & Mostwin, 1984) in the first two types of surgery. Recovery of erectile function still requires up to 6 months, however. Many surgeons have not achieved the success rates reported by Walsh and colleagues. Controversy also continues about whether the surgeon can spare the prostatic plexus yet still perform adequate cancer surgery. Urological procedures such as internal urethrotomy, external sphincterotomy, or repair of a ruptured urethra may occasionally also damage erection-producing nerves where they exit from the prostatic plexus and follow along the urethra (Lue, Zeineh, Schmidt, & Tanagho, 1984).

Neurological diseases including multiple sclerosis (Goldstein, Siroky, Sax, & Krane, 1982b; Lilius, Valtonen, & Wikström, 1976; Minderhoud, Leemhuis, Kremer, Laban, & Smits, 1984; Szasz, Paty, Lawton-Speert, & Eisen, 1984; Valleroy & Kraft, 1984), neuromuscular diseases (Anderson & Bardach, 1983), or Shy-Drager syndrome (Frank & Boller, 1982) may cause neurogenic erectile dysfunction. Clinicians often look for neurological impairment of bowel or bladder function along with erectile dysfunction since the relevant reflex arcs overlap to some extent.

Diseases that cause peripheral neuropathy may also create erection problems. The classic culprit has been diabetes. A careful longitudinal study of young type I diabetics, however, suggests that the erectile dysfunction associated with diabetic neuropathy can improve over time if relationship factors are favorable (Jensen, 1986). In older type II diabetics, vascular disease is more common than neuropathy in patients with erection problems (Jevtich, Edson, Jarman, & Herrera, 1982; Lehman & Jacobs, 1983; McCulloch, Young, Prescott, Campbell, & Clarke, 1984). Studies are needed that use specialized tests of genital nerves, with samples representative of type I and type II diabetics, with and without erectile dysfunction.

Peripheral neuropathy has also been cited as a cause of erectile dysfunction in alcoholics but, in fact, it seems to be quite rare (Jensen, 1984b). Neuropathy may cause erection problems in some men with chronic obstructive pulmonary disease (Fletcher & Martin, 1982) or end-stage renal disease (Procci, 1983).

Medications that Interfere with
Neurological Regulation of Erection

A number of medications are believed to impair erection by disrupting peripheral neurotransmitters. Since our knowledge of the erectile mechanism is still sketchy, the reasons for such side effects are often unclear. We know that alpha-adrenergic blockers, when injected directly into the cavernous bodies, provide erections (Brindley, 1983). The data are confusing, however. When given in oral doses, some alpha-blocking drugs occasionally cause priapism (Mitchell & Popkin, 1983), while others have no effect on erection (Brooks, Berezin, & Braf, 1982; Shilon, Paz, & Homonnai, 1984), and some researchers believe that the alpha-blocking effects of neuroleptic drugs impair erections (Jones, 1984).

Many neuroleptics have been implicated in causing erectile dysfunction. Anticholinergic or calcium-channel-blocking properties of neuroleptics may be at fault in interfering with sexual function (King *et al.*, 1983). Thioridazine (Mellaril) is cited particularly often as causing problems with erection and orgasm (Gould, Murphy, Reynolds, & Snyder, 1984; Segraves, 1982a). Thioridazine may have received more attention because it is so commonly prescribed, however. Unfortunately, studies of sexual function in psychotic patients are often flawed. Psychotic episodes complicate assessment of current sexual practices or premorbid sexual capacity, and it is almost impossible to control for differing doses and combinations of neuroleptics prescribed.

Tricyclic antidepressants and monamine oxidase inhibitors (MAOIs) have been reported to cause erectile dysfunction in some men (Abel, 1985; Harrison *et al.*, 1985; Segraves, Madsen, Carter, & Davis, 1985), again perhaps by their anticholinergic action. Bethanecol, a drug that stimulates cholinergic nerves, may alleviate erectile dysfunction caused by antidepressants (Gross, 1982), but double-blind studies of its effectiveness are not available. The depression itself complicates research in this area. Before taking medication, men often lack desire for sex. After the depression lifts, a chronic erection problem may seem more troublesome than it did previously.

Moss and Procci (1982) critically reviewed the evidence that antihypertensive medications cause erectile dysfunction. Surprisingly little is known about the true incidence of sexual side effects of such medications. Hypertensives are already at high risk for erectile dysfunction because of their vascular disease. Separating the underlying pathology from medication effects is difficult. Guanethidine does seem to cause erection problems in some men, probably by interfering with the peripheral release of norepinephrine. Beta-blockers, in high doses, are associated with erectile dysfunction (Segraves *et al.*, 1985). Vasodilators and diuretics have no clear effect on sexuality, however.

Neurogenic Factors in Female Arousal Phase Dysfunctions

Considering the abundance of literature on spinal cord injuries and erections, the complete lack of knowledge about vaginal expansion and lubrication in quadriplegic or paraplegic women is remarkable (Comarr & Vigue, 1978; Higgins, 1978; Larsen & Hejgaard, 1984; Thornton, 1981). Apparently, all that can be said is that many women still have adequate vaginal lubrication for comfortable intercourse. The degree of genital sensation a woman retains depends, of course, on the level of her spinal cord lesion.

We do have more knowledge about female arousal in diabetics and women with multiple sclerosis. Diabetic women, compared with healthy controls, report decreased vaginal lubrication (Jensen, 1986; Schreiner-Engel, Schiavi, Vietorisz, Eichel, & Smith, 1985; Tyrer *et al.*, 1983), but we do not know whether the cause is psychological, neurological, vascular, or a combination of these factors. Relationships between standard measures of neuropathy and sexual arousal in female diabetics have been weak or absent (Jensen, 1986; Tyrer *et al.*, 1983).

Women with neuromuscular diseases seem to have normal vaginal lubrication with arousal (Anderson & Bardach, 1983). In samples of premenopausal women with multiple sclerosis, however, 12% to 21% report reduced lubrication (Lundberg, 1981; Minderhoud *et al.*, 1984) and many experience unusual vaginal sensations (Lyndberg, 1981) or loss of genital sensation (Valleroy & Kraft, 1984).

Neurological Factors in Male Orgasmic Dysfunction

Our understanding of the effects of neurological disease on men's orgasms has been impeded by many researchers' poor grasp of the components of orgasm and their neurological control mechanisms (Newman *et al.*, 1982).

It is often impossible to tell from published reports whether men had delayed orgasms, dry orgasms, or no orgasmic sensation at all. We examine separately the effects of illness on the sensation of orgasm (mediated by the pudendal nerve and central nervous system), the striated muscle contractions of ejaculation (also controlled by the pudendal nerve), and the smooth muscle contractions of emission (dependent on the short adrenergic neurons of the sympathetic nervous system).

Table 5-6 lists factors that can affect sensory nerve control of orgasmic sensation and ejaculatory contractions. The relationship between the central nervous system and male orgasm is largely unexplored. Two studies of stroke survivors suggest that orgasm is sometimes impaired (Bray, De-Frank, & Wolfe, 1981; Sjögren, 1983). Since most of the men also had erection problems, however, direct neurological effects on orgasm could not be isolated. A more recent case series only reported impaired orgasms in 3 of 50 men post-CVA (cerebrovascular accident) (Hawton, 1984).

Whether a spinal cord lesion affects orgasmic sensation and muscle contractions depends on the level and completeness of the damage. Orgasmic sensation and the striated muscle contractions that propel semen through the urethra are controlled by the pudendal nerve, which in turn depends on outflow from spinal segments S2 to S4 (Kedia, 1983a). The sensation of orgasm occurs in less than 14% of men with spinal cord injuries (Yalla, 1982). Complete lesions above the thoracic level abolish genital sensation, so that even the few men who have ejaculatory contractions from

Table 5-6 Neurological Factors That May Interfere with Male Orgasmic Sensation

---

Medical History
   Damage to cerebral hemispheres[a]
   Spinal cord injury[a]
   Neuromuscular disease[a]
   Peripheral somatic neuropathy (often diabetic)[b]
   Medical illness or treatment that interferes with emission (see Table 5-7)[b]

Physical Examination
   Decreased penile sensory threshold to light touch, electrical stimulation, or vibration
   Absent bulbocavernosus reflex

Medications
   Tricyclic antidepressants[b]
   Monoamine oxidase inhibitors[a, b]
   Neuroleptics (particularly thioridazine),[a, b]
   Phenoxybenzamine[b]
   Trazadone[a]
   Guanethidine[a, b]
   Calcium-channel blockers[b]
   Alcohol[a]

---

   [a]May prevent orgasm completely
   [b]May reduce intensity of orgasmic pleasure

prolonged tactile or vibratory stimulation of the penis do not really experience an orgasm (Amelar & Dubin, 1982). However, men with high, incomplete lesions may have orgasmic sensation.

In men with lumbar or sacral lesions, semen often drips out with a weak or absent sensation of orgasm. Emission takes place because a higher cord center at T12 to L3 is intact, but the striated muscles around the base of the penis are paralyzed. Only 18% of men with complete lower motor neuron lesions have any type of orgasm in which semen appears (Yalla, 1982). Some men with spinal cord lesions who have no genital sensation report "phantom" orgasms (Newman *et al.*, 1982) with pleasure felt in areas other than the genitals.

Diseases that cause peripheral neuropathy rarely seem to prevent orgasm altogether. In fact, many men with organic erectile dysfunction can reach orgasm with a flaccid penis. Diabetic men do not differ from healthy controls in their rate of delayed orgasm or inability to reach orgasm (Jensen, 1986).

It is often difficult to distinguish between subtle neurological deficits and psychological factors that can affect a man's ability to reach orgasm or the intensity of the sensation (Newman *et al.*, 1982). Williams (1985) noted some psychological commonalities but no organic abnormalities in seven healthy men who experienced normal ejaculation but weak or absent orgasmic sensation. Men with erectile dysfunction, no matter what the cause, often complain that orgasms with a flaccid penis are weakened and involve dripping of semen rather than propulsive ejaculation. If the erectile dysfunction improves with sex therapy, orgasms may also return to normal.

Medications Preventing Male Orgasm

Few drugs can delay orgasm or prevent it entirely. Case reports suggest that some men have difficulty reaching orgasm when taking guanethidine (Moss & Procci, 1982), tricyclics (DeLeo & Magni, 1983; Jones, 1984), MAOIs (Segraves, 1982a), or thioridazine (Mitchell & Popkin, 1982). The alpha-adrenergic blocking effects of such medications, usually blamed for preventing orgasm, should theoretically only impair emission. Some of these cases may really represent men who had dry orgasm but were not carefully assessed. Men with dry orgasm often report having no orgasm at all unless terms are carefully defined by the interviewer.

Some psychoactive drugs can cause painful sensations at orgasm, often accompanied by decreases in semen volume or in the force with which semen is expelled. DeLeo and Magni (1983) suggest that incomplete blocking of the alpha-adrenergic nerve transmission leads to a lack of co-ordination between closure of the internal and external urethral sphincter and to painful spasms of the smooth muscle of the prostate and seminal vesicles.

Neurological Problems that Interfere with Male Emission

A number of neurological diseases, injuries, or medications can interfere with the emission phase of the male orgasm (Table 5-7). Emission is a smooth-muscle event, regulated by sympathetic nerves (short adrenergic neurons) and by a spinal center at the T12 to L3 level. When emission is interrupted, a dry orgasm results. The contractions of ejaculation and the sensation of orgasm still take place, but no semen is expelled through the urethra. We use the generic term "dry orgasm" because two different types of events may really be occurring: If the short adrenergic neurons are severely impaired, the smooth muscle of the prostate and seminal vesicles is paralyzed and there is no emission; but if the adrenergic transmission is only somewhat decreased, emission occurs but the opening of the bladder neck into the urethra (internal urethral sphincter) does not close completely. The semen deposited in the upper urethra is propelled backward into the bladder during ejaculatory contractions instead of being pushed outward through the urethra. This is called retrograde ejaculation.

The major reason to distinguish between lack of emission and retrograde ejaculation is in evaluating a man's fertility. Laboratory analyses demonstrating sperm cells and fructose in a man's urine voided just after dry orgasm are evidence of retrograde ejaculation. A wider range of treatment options exists when infertility is due to retrograde ejaculation rather than complete failure of emission (Garcea, Caruso, Campo, & Siccardi, 1982; Lipschultz *et al.*, 1981).

Dry orgasm of either type results from a variety of illnesses and medical treatments. Diabetics (Jensen, 1986) and alcoholics (Jensen, 1979a, 1979b, 1984b)

Table 5-7. Neurological Factors that May Interfere with Male Emission

Medical History
  Diabetes
  Alcoholism
  Surgery to repair aortoiliac area
  Retroperitoneal lymphadenectomy
  Abdominoperineal resection
  Sacral sympathectomy
Medications that Can Prevent Emission or Cause Retrograde Ejaculation
  Tricyclic antidepressants
  Monoamine oxidase inhibitors
  Neuroleptics (particularly thioridazine)
  Phenoxybenzamine
  Guanethidine
  Calcium-channel blockers
  Neurotoxic cancer chemotherapies (particularly vincristine)
Medications that Stimulate Emission or Antegrade Ejaculation
  Ephedrine (alpha-adrenergic stimulators)
  Imipramine

with peripheral neuropathy may have totally dry orgasms or complain of reduced semen volume, indicating partial failure of the internal urethral sphincter. Surgical interventions are even more common causes of neurological damage to emission. Operations to repair the aortoiliac arteries in men with vascular disease or to remove the retroperitoneal lymph nodes in men with testicular cancer damage the sympathetic ganglia that control the short adrenergic neurons in the genital area. During abdominoperineal resections for cancer or sacral sympathectomies, the sympathetic ganglia are damaged lower down, in the area just in front of the sacral spinal cord (Lipschultz *et al.*, 1981).

Medications that Affect Emission

Some medications can cause dry orgasm by alpha-blocking effects (Table 5-7). Alpha-stimulating drugs can sometimes restore normal emission. Imipramine (Tofranil) has been successfully used to treat dry ejaculation (Goldwasser, Madgar, Jonas, Lunenfeld, & Many, 1983). The other class of drugs effective in treating dry orgasm is the ephedrines (Jonas, Linzbach, & Weber, 1979; Lipschultz *et al.*, 1981).

Emission and Orgasmic Sensation

What effect does dry orgasm have on a man's orgasmic pleasure? Newman *et al.* (1982) believe that dry orgasms are always less intense than normal ones. In studies of young testicular cancer patients who have dry orgasms, however (Schover & von Eschenbach, 1985b; Schover, Gonzales, & von Eschenbach, 1986), only about a quarter of men complain of reduced orgasmic pleasure. Reductions in the men's self-reported semen volume account for only 14% of the variance in their orgasm intensity. In healthy men, too, semen volume does not influence the number of ejaculatory contractions or the subjective intensity of orgasm (Levin, 1984).

For men with impaired emission, treatment with alpha-stimulating drugs can increase orgasmic intensity, so perhaps sympathetic nervous system activity plays some minor role in men's perception of orgasm (Jonas *et al.*, 1979; Riley & Riley, 1982).

Neurological Factors and Female Orgasmic Dysfunction

Since women's orgasms correspond to the ejaculation phase of the male orgasm, one would expect that neurological damage to the brain, sacral spinal cord, or the pudendal nerve would be necessary to prevent orgasm. In fact, little is known about orgasm in women with spinal cord disease or injuries (Comarr & Vigue, 1978; Higgins, 1978; Thornton, 1981; see Table 5-8). If women lose sensation in the genital area, they sometimes can still have orgasmic sensations from caressing of their breasts or other remaining erotic zones. The orgasm is often perceived in the area just above the level where sensation is absent. No study has examined the level of spinal cord lesion and a woman's ability to reach orgasm. Thirteen women with neuromuscular diseases (Anderson & Bardach, 1983) did not seem to have unusual problems reaching orgasm, but about a third to a half of women with multiple sclerosis report problems with orgasm (Lilius *et al.*, 1976; Lundberg, 1981; Minderhoud *et al.*, 1984; Valleroy & Kraft, 1984).

Women at risk for peripheral neuropathy do not seem to have unusual rates of inorgasmia. Diabetic women and normal controls do not differ on this dimension (Jensen, 1986; Schreiner-Engel *et al.*, 1985; Tyrer *et al.*, 1983). Alcoholic women also have no excess of orgasmic dysfunction (Jensen, 1984b). It seems that a rather severe degree of neurological damage is necessary to prevent female orgasm.

Medications and Female Orgasm

The pharmacology of female orgasm is surprising because it suggests an influence of the autonomic nervous system. The same medications that affect male erection and emission apparently prevent orgasm in a minority of women. These include thioridazine, imipramine, clomipramine, amoxapine, and the MAOIs (Lesko, Stotland, & Segraves, 1982; Shen, 1982; Shen & Sata, 1983; Sovner, 1983). We do not know whether the women's psychopathology is the true culprit, if the subtle central nervous system effects of these drugs are at fault, or if the dysfunction results from the drugs' peripheral anticholinergic or alpha-blocking effects. The medications may primarily be reducing sexual desire or arousal, but since female orgasm is a more measurable event, the orgasmic dysfunction becomes the target complaint. The new antidepressant trazodone, which decreases prolactin levels and prevents the uptake of serotonin, has been reported to increase desire and frequency of orgasm in 6 out of 13 women (Gartrell, 1986).

Table 5-8. Neurological Factors that May Interfere with Female Orgasm

Medical History
    Spinal cord injury
    Multiple sclerosis

Medical Examination
    Decreased genital sensory thresholds
    Absent bulbocavernosus reflex
    Neurological signs in the S1–S3 distribution

Medications
    Tricyclic antidepressants (particularly imipramine, amoxapine, clomipramine)
    Monoamine oxidase inhibitors
    Neuroleptics (particularly thioridazine)

Women, unlike men, rarely say that their orgasms occur but with reduced intensity (Schover, Evans, & von Eschenbach, 1987). Whether for physiological reasons or because of societal influences, women report orgasm to be more of an "all or nothing" phenomenon.

DAMAGE TO GENITAL STRUCTURE AND SEXUAL FUNCTION

Occasionally injuries or surgical treatments for disease involve loss of a part of the genitals. Although such cases are rare, the patients' capacity to resume sexual activity can teach us a good deal about the robustness of human sexuality and the potential for sexual rehabilitation.

Male Genital Integrity and Sexual Function

In this section we discuss loss of the testicles, penis, or prostate and seminal vesicles, as well as the more common transurethral prostatectomy (TURP).

Loss of Testicles

One or both testicles may be surgically removed (orchiectomy) to treat cancer. Loss of a testicle through torsion or trauma, or removal of an undescended testicle also occur. If a man still has one healthy testicle, as is usually the case, testosterone levels remain in the normal range. Sexual dysfunction after loss of a testicle can be produced by psychological factors, such as anxiety about masculinity or poor body image. Testicular prostheses made of silicone gel can be surgically implanted to restore the appearance and sensation of having two testicles (Schover & von Eschenbach, 1984).

Men treated for metastatic cancer of the prostate may have both testicles removed as a way of reducing serum testosterone to control tumor growth (Bergman, Damber, Littbrand, Sjögren, & Tomic, 1984; Ellis & Grayhack, 1963; Schover, von Eschenbach, Smith, & Gonzalez, 1984). Since patients become hypogonadal, they are apt to experience low desire, erectile dysfunction, and difficulty reaching orgasm. These men obviously cannot have replacement testosterone therapy. Men who lose function of both testicles for other reasons are usually restored to normal sexual function when given testosterone (Bancroft & Wu, 1983; Salmimies *et al.*, 1982).

Loss of the Penis

Loss of the penis occurs most often as a surgical treatment for cancer of the penis or of the distal (endmost) urethra. Fortunately such cancers are rare. If the tumor is restricted to the glans of the penis, a partial penectomy is performed, leaving enough of a penile shaft so that a man can direct his urinary stream away from his body. After a partial penectomy, men still have erections, and the penis is often long enough to allow vaginal penetration. These patients also still reach orgasm with normal sensation and forceful ejaculation of semen (Schover *et al.*, 1984).

For some men, however, a total penectomy is necessary. The urethra is connected to a new opening (perineal urethrostomy) between the man's scrotum and anus. Witkin & Kaplan (1983) have described a sex therapy case in which a man learned how to reach orgasm again after total penectomy. They believed their patient to be unique, but, in fact, we have interviewed a number of men after total penectomy who report having orgasms either in dreams or through caressing of their remaining genital sensory areas by a partner. Since the prostate and seminal vesicles remain intact, these men ejaculate semen through the perineal urethrostomy. Sexual function has not been studied in men who have lost penile tissue through trauma or severe burns.

Loss of the Prostate and Seminal Vesicles

Radical pelvic cancer operations to remove the prostate or prostate and bladder (cystectomy) also entail removing the seminal vesicles (Schover & Fife, 1985). Although all semen-producing glands are absent, men do have dry orgasms after surgery with normal contractions of the bulbocavernosus muscles (Bergman, Nilsson, & Petersen, 1979). In our experience with 112 such patients, the crucial element in learning to reach orgasm again is practice (Schover, Evans, & von Eschenbach, 1986). Many complain that their orgasmic sensation is weakened, but another large group report normal pleasure and a few claim their orgasms are more intense and prolonged than they were before surgery. Of course, most of the men reach orgasm with only a partial erection, unless they have had a penile prosthesis inserted.

A much more common syndrome is the dry orgasm that results from a transurethral prostatectomy (TURP) performed for benign prostatic hypertrophy. In this operation, most of the prostatic tissue is removed through the urethra, leaving the prostatic capsule intact. Since the prostatic nerve plexus is undamaged, prospective studies have found that erectile function, measured by NPT monitoring, remains intact (So, Ho, Bodenstab, & Parsons, 1982). Lue *et al.* (1984) recently suggested that very complete resections may penetrate the capsule, damaging nerves. Another research group, however, found no evidence that the extent of the TURP predicted sexual function after surgery (Møller-Nielsen *et al.*, 1985). About 80% of men do have retrograde ejaculation after a TURP because part of the internal sphincter muscle is removed. If men are not warned to expect dry orgasms, they may experience considerable anxiety and consequently develop other sexual dysfunctions.

Female Genital Integrity and Sexual Function

In women, too, cancer surgery is the most common reason for loss of the vulva or vagina. Since there is no evidence that vaginal or abdominal hysterectomies for benign disease medically impair sexual function, we will not include them in this discussion. Effects of oophorectomy were described earlier in this chapter.

Loss of the Vulva

Radical vulvectomy for cancer of the vulva usually includes removal of the clitoris, inner and outer labia, and the tissue that pads the pubic bone to form the *mons pubis*. Although the vagina remains intact, scar tissue may narrow the vaginal entrance. The urethral opening also becomes exposed, leading to local tenderness and frequent urinary tract infections, especially after sexual activity. Many women cannot control the direction of their urinary streams. Chronic leg edema is also a problem after radical vulvectomy because the lymph drainage system is removed from both groins.

Recent studies of women after vulvectomy agree that many stop having sexual activity (Anderson & Hacker, 1983; Moth, Andreasson, Jensen, & Bock, 1983; Stellman, Goodwin, Robinson, Dansak, & Hilgers, 1984). Psychological distress, impaired body damage, low sexual desire, and difficulty becoming aroused are also common. For the women who do resume sexual activity, it is difficult to predict who will be able to reach orgasm. It seems to depend more on psychological factors than on whether the clitoris is preserved.

Loss of the Vagina

Several surgical procedures in cancer treatment also involve loss of the vagina. Radical cystectomy for bladder cancer includes removing the urethra and anterior vaginal wall. Women who can overcome the discomfort of reduced vaginal size continue to reach orgasm as easily as they did before surgery, despite the loss of the "G spot" (Schover & von Eschenbach, 1985b). Radical hysterectomy for cervical cancer necessitates removing the upper third to half of the vagina. In a prospective study of women undergoing radical hysterectomy (Schover, Fife, & Gershenson, 1985) women and their partners received sexual counseling at the time of surgery to minimize the psychological impact of the changes. At 6-month follow-up, sexual frequency, variety, function, and satisfaction were unchanged. The loss of vaginal depth rarely caused any discomfort during intercourse.

The entire vagina may be removed to treat invasive vaginal cancers or as part of total pelvic exenteration, a radical surgery for local recurrence of cervical cancer that also entails removal of the bladder, urethra, rectum, and reproductive organs. The vagina is reconstructed using flaps of skin and underlying muscle from the inner thighs (Edwards, Loeffler, & Rutledge, 1981). Women can learn to reach orgasm after total pelvic exenteration. The clitoris is usually preserved, so that sensation from the vulva contributes to erotic pleasure. Sexual counseling after vaginal reconstruction is discussed in Chapter 8.

MEDICATIONS WITH SEXUAL SIDE EFFECTS

In this chapter, we discuss medications in terms of their specific effects on the hormonal or neurological aspects of sexual function. Many texts present large tables of medications and their impact on desire, arousal, and orgasm, but we believe it is easier to recall medication effects by understanding where each drug fits into the etiological spectrum. Thus the reader can scan Tables 5-2 through 5-8 to check on the various actions of a particular drug.

Methodology for studying the sexual side effects of medications has been inadequate (Abel, 1985). Many sexual side effects are not reported by patients or assessed systematically by researchers. Physicians may regard sexual problems as too insignificant to record. Some medications have been labeled as causing sexual dysfunction on the basis of a few, poorly substantiated case reports. Others that may have side effects have probably not yet been identified. Drug researchers rarely understand how to define and assess sexual function. Most published data are anecdotal, and double-blind studies are rare. Sophisticated designs, such as studies varying drug dosage, are almost unknown in this area. Even data on patients' age, gender, and premedication sexual function are rarely included, nor are patients compared with unmedicated control groups with the same underlying medical condition. If knowledge about medication effects on sexuality is to increase, sex researchers and drug researchers will need to collaborate more closely.

PAIN AND SEXUAL FUNCTION

Any painful medical condition can interfere with sexual function. Whether the pain is in the genital area or elsewhere, it can distract from erotic thoughts or sensations and limit range of motion. The impact of chronic pain on sexuality is discussed in Chapter 14. For now, we just wish to remind the clinician not to overlook pain as a medical factor influencing sexual pleasure. Opiate pain medication can compound sexual problems because of its central nervous system effects, such as drowsiness and distractability, as well as its impact on the hormonal axis. Prostaglandin synthetase inhibitors, however, do not seem to have sexual side effects.

6

Assessing Sexual Problems in Medical Patients

Now that we have provided an overview of factors interfering with sexual function in men and women with chronic illnesses, we can use the integrative model to develop a schema for comprehensive assessment. This chapter traces the steps in the pathway from identifying a patient's sexual complaint or noting a symptom that may indicate a hidden sexual problem through contracting with patient and spouse to begin a comprehensive sexual assessment. We describe the assessment interview itself and several questionnaires that we find helpful. Our other goal is to provide readers with enough knowledge about physiological assessment of sexual function to coordinate the evaluation, make appropriate referrals, communicate with specialists in the field, and understand the information amassed.

THE FIRST CONTACT

When dealing with sexual material, the clinician's first responsibility is to make sure that the patient has been invited to discuss the topic. As emphasized in Chapter 1, men and women with chronic illnesses rarely ask for help with a sexual problem. When researchers survey groups of chronically ill patients, high rates of sexual dysfunction are observed (Fletcher & Martin, 1982; Jensen, 1981a, 1984b; Kornfeld, Heller, Frank, Wilson, & Malm, 1982; Papadopoulos, Beaumont, Shelley, & Larrimore, 1983; Procci & Martin, 1985; Schover, Evans, & von Eschenbach, 1987; Sjögren, 1983). Nevertheless, few sexual problems are identified in daily clinical practice. How can we reach the 90% of patients with problems who currently receive no help? The key is the primary care team's ability to bring up the topic of sex and to make patients feel comfortable in discussing a problem.

Occasionally a patient does initiate a discussion of sexuality with the primary health care team. In that case, the clinicians can handle the counseling themselves or refer the patient to a sexuality specialist. Far more problems will be identified, however, if the primary care physician routinely asks about sexual health as well as assessing other aspects of the quality of life. No matter how the topic of sexuality is introduced, clinicians need basic training in discussing sexual issues in a supportive, nonjudgmental fashion. Providing sexual counseling in a medical setting, where sexuality is not a focus of health care, calls for special sensitivity and tact.

THE CLINICIAN'S ROLE IN REFRAMING THE PROBLEM

One factor that prevents patients from seeking help for a sexual problem is that they lack a model of sexual health. The clinician knows that illness can impair sexual function for a variety of reasons, but that with insight and flexibility, a patient usually can continue to enjoy lovemaking. The patient, however, often has a model of illness and its impact on sexuality that engenders helplessness and hopelessness.

Examples of common maladaptive beliefs about illness include the following:

- Disease is a punishment for my sins.
- If I ignore my illness, it may disappear.
- Illness is just a stroke of fate, and my job is to accept it.
- Suffering on earth brings happiness in heaven.

Such attitudes often lead to a sense of resignation about staying sexually active:

- Oh well, we had years of good sex. I guess it's over now.
- There is only one normal way to have sex, and if we can't have inter course, let's not even try.
- If I can't have an orgasm, I don't want to get excited.
- Nobody wants to make love with an invalid.

Unfortunately, the patient does not expect the health care team to provide a new model of the world, but rather seeks relief from medical symptoms. Thus, the first step in the evaluation process is to identify the existence of a sexual problem and to convince the patient that an assessment would be worthwhile. Along the way, the care-giver may have to persuade a patient hoping for a physiological cure that the best treatment is psychological or a combination of physiological and psychological approaches.

From Presenting Complaint to
Acknowledgment of a Sexual Problem

Sexual issues are discussed in medical settings when a patient takes the risk of initiating the topic, when the clinician creates a forum for discussing sexuality, or when the patient presents a nonspecific complaint that in fact masks a sexual symptom, and the clinician realizes the true nature of the problem. Let us examine each of these situations in turn, focusing on how the clinician can help the patient acknowledge that further assessment and treatment planning would be of help.

The Direct Sexual Complaint

Often a patient reveals a sexual problem to the health care team, believing that it is related to a medical illness. For example, a man may complain that he has had erectile dysfunction since his prostate surgery or a woman may state that her oral contraceptives have decreased her sexual desire. The clinician must not fall into the trap of prescribing a medical treatment prematurely, but instead should make sure that any physiological risk factors are truly operating in isolation. How was the patient's sexual function before the illness or medical treatment? Are there any current life stresses? How does the patient usually handle stressful situations such as an illness? If the patient persists in taking a narrow view of the causes of the sexual problem, the clinician can say, "I agree that your illness may be a factor in your sex life, but I also think it is important for me to get to know you as a whole person. When people are ill, their personalities and family lives often interact with their physical symptoms, especially in an emotional area like sexuality." Once the clinician understands the nature of the sexual problem, practitioner and patient can discuss what the next step would be in assessing the situation and planning treatment.

Sometimes what sounds like a simple sexual dysfunction actually is quite a more complex problem:

Jim, a 23-year-old engineering student, was referred by his general practitioner to a sexuality clinic because of erectile dysfunction. The physician commented in a fatherly tone that Jim had problems making contact with women.

When Jim met with the psychotherapist, he took a very intellectualized position toward his sexual dysfunction, discussing it as if it were an engineering problem, listing books about sexuality that he had consulted and mentioning several prominent therapists he had previously seen.

Jim told the therapist that when he went to a party, he decided upon entering the room which woman he would like to approach. He always made his choice from a distance and then sent his thoughts "transcendentally" across the room, attempting to seduce her. If the woman reacted to him at all, whether positively or negatively, he felt that she began to control his thoughts and soon believed he was so much under her power that the blood would run backward in his penile arteries. Thus he could not attain an erection.

At this point the interviewer decided to switch the focus from the sexual dysfunction to Jim's general psychological status. Angry that he would not be considered a candidate for vascular surgery, Jim cut the interview short and refused to return for further sessions. At 5-year follow-up, Jim was an inpatient in a psychiatric unit and diagnosed as schizophrenic.

Asking the Patient about Sexuality

When we train health care professionals to assess sexuality, we find most are surprised by patients' openness and gratitude for the opportunity to talk. Many physicians, nurses, and even mental health clinicians fear that patients will resent a question about sexual health or will refuse to disclose such personal information. Although a minority of patients in medical settings do not wish to reveal sexual information, most are glad to receive some basic education about illness and sexuality and perceive a question about their sex lives as an expression of warmth and concern from the clinician.

How can a health professional comfortably bring up the topic of sex? We believe that a question or two about sexuality should be a routine part of history taking and also of follow-up visits when a patient is receiving continuing care. The first question about sexuality can be prefaced by a normalizing statement, to put it into context:

Clinician: I always ask whether patients are having any sexual problems. Your sexual health is one important part of your life. Sometimes an illness or medication can affect sexuality, too. How has your sexual relationship been going lately?

In eliciting sexual material, open-ended questions are more successful than ones that just elicit a brief "yes" or "no":

• What kinds of sexual problems have you had?
• What happens when you and your partner try to make love?
• What influence do you see your health having on your sex life?
• How would you like your sex life to be different?
• What can we do to help you with sexuality?

The Masked Sexual Problem

Because sexuality is such an emotionally charged topic, patients will sometimes mention a nonsexual symptom, hoping either consciously or unconsciously that a sensitive professional will get to the core of the issue. Clinicians should be alert for cues that a sexual problem exists when the patient presents a psychosomatic complaint (i.e., a physical symptom with no clear organic cause), a somatopsychological symptom (i.e., an emotional symptom related to a medical illness that might suggest poor coping), or a purely psychological complaint. Examples illustrate how each of these three types of symptoms can conceal a troubling sexual concern.

A common psychosomatic complaint in women is pelvic pain. Although many subtle and not-so-subtle physical causes exist for pelvic pain, physical findings are sometimes negative. The gynecologist must decide whether to prescribe medical treatment such as hormone therapy or exploratory laparoscopy or to refer the patient for psychotherapy. In our clinical experience, many of these women have traumatic sexual histories. The pelvic pain provides a perfect excuse for avoiding sexual activity and often elicits sympathy from the spouse or other family members. With such powerful reasons to have the pain, what can we offer a woman to help her reach a higher level of integration? And how can the gynecologist enlist the woman's cooperation in entering psychotherapy rather than alienating her so that she seeks further medical evaluation from a different physician?

The gynecologist can begin by agreeing with the patient that the pain is real, no matter what the cause (Jensen & Hejl, 1987). How does the pain affect her daily life activities? How do family members react when she is hurting? What effect has the pain had on her sex life? Has she ever had a frightening or traumatic sexual experience, whether as a child or an adult? If psychological factors appear to contribute to the pain, the rationale for a further assessment can be presented in a supportive way:

Clinician: Pelvic pain is a confusing kind of problem. Sometimes we cannot find a physical problem to fix. If we try anyway, for example, by doing exploratory surgery, we often just make things worse. Your pain is certainly very real. But have you noticed that if you are distracted, for example by a visit from a good friend, or during a funny television show, that your pain is less noticeable? Because pain is sensed in the brain, both your body and your mind influence how severe your pain feels. I would like you to see a mental health professional because we have had good success in the past few years in helping men and women control their pain through psychological skills, like relaxation, imagining pleasant scenes, and trying to live a more active life. You may want to discuss your history, your feelings about sex, and the way you handle stress with the doctor you will see, because all of these areas of your life can have an impact on treating your pain.

An example of a somatopsychological symptom is a young man who recently had an ileostomy for inflammatory bowel disease. He complains that he does not feel like a real man. Although his feelings about his ostomy, his ability to care for it properly, and the disruption of his work life by the recent surgery are all important, he is also giving a message that he is worried about sexuality. It is not enough for the clinician simply to reassure him that he should have good erectile function after his operation. Areas that should be explored include his fantasies about how his girlfriend will react to the sight of his ostomy appliance, whether he has resumed masturbation since his surgery, and his actual skills at keeping his ostomy appliance leakproof and odor-free. If the clinicians do not recognize the clue being so clearly given, this young man may not bring up future emotional concerns with his health care team.

One of the most common psychological complaints in medical patients is depression. When a chronically ill patient complains of being depressed, some physicians offer an antidepressant as an easy and effective solution. Although antidepressant medication can be a helpful adjunct to counseling, medical patients, on detailed questioning, are often more sad or dysphoric than truly depressed. Perhaps a man feels rejected by his wife, who has recently been avoiding sexual contact. He worries that her withdrawal is a reaction to his intermittent erectile dysfunction. The fear of losing her love is compounded by his current dependence on her to help him care for himself and take over many of his usual roles in the family. If the clinician does not explore the psychosocial factors contributing to the patient's depressed mood, he or she may in fact prescribe a medication that will further impair sexual function and thus exacerbate the problem.

From Problem Identification to Agreement on Need for Assessment

Even when patient and clinician agree that a sexual problem exists, they may not be in accord about the next course of action. The clinician would like to begin a comprehensive assessment, including psychological, social, and biological components. Despite skillful reframing of the sexual problem, however, the clinician may not be able to get the patient to understand the integrative model.

One frustration is that patients select their health-care practitioners to fulfill their own expectations. A man with an erection problem who consults a psychiatrist is apt to be quite different in his world view from the one who makes an appointment with a urologist. Since we like to make patients happy, it is tempting to formulate unidimensional treatment plans rather than to take a stand for integrated assessment. We have noticed how discouraged young physicians often feel when they try the holistic model and a patient reacts by seeking help from another clinician. They fear that losing patients will damage their professional reputation, if not their livelihood. It takes years of practice to realize that even the best clinicians alienate a few patients and that one must not sacrifice good care to be congenial.

Some patients are just not interested in remedying a sexual problem. They prefer to forget about that whole area of life.

Joe, a 72-year-old with prostate cancer, acknowledged that he no longer had full erections. He had a long history of hypertension and coronary artery disease as well as the cancer diagnosis. Joe's medications included a beta-blocker and a diuretic. He said that he still thought about sex occasionally, but that his wife, Betty, had never enjoyed it much and seemed relieved when Joe stopped initiating sex 5 or 6 years before. Joe rarely masturbated. He and Betty kissed goodnight but slept in twin beds. He was not frustrated by their lack of sexual contact or even the lack of touching. He said that he was too old to worry about sex.

As Martin (1981) has pointed out, elderly men like Joe were often on the low end of the spectrum of sexual interest even in adolescence and early marriage. When aging and ill health bring sexual dysfunction, they slip easily into celibacy. A sensitive clinician offers help, but must be prepared to back off when a patient does not wish to remain sexually active.

Disinterest is not the only reason why a patient rejects referral for further assessment. Some perceive the clinician's message to take action in coping with illness as an accusation: "You could have prevented your disease if you had acted more responsibly." Since many illnesses are, in fact, related to lifestyle choices such as smoking or diet, the health professional has the delicate task of encouraging patients to change their habits without making them feel guilty about past failures:

Clinician: Yes, I understand that you felt helpless to slow down at work, even though you knew you had changes in your cardiogram. But now that you've been through your heart attack, let's talk about what you *can* do, *now*, to get back into better shape. Part of your rehabilitation is to restore your ability to work, to enjoy your hobbies, to take an active role in your family, and to enjoy sexual intimacy.

Patients also hesitate to take action to solve a sexual problem when a cure would upset the homeostasis of a relationship. The couple who met and married after the husband's spinal cord injury may not be as eager as the clinician imagines to try a penile prosthesis. Perhaps the wife has a history of sexual dysfunction and chose her husband because of his sexual incapacity. The situation is painful as it exists, but the couple needs gentle, supportive counseling, not a sudden surgical intervention, to reach a new equilibrium.

Sometimes acknowledging the sexual problem is all that the patient needs. The clinician should not feel like a failure if the patient refuses further evaluation. For example, the woman who has learned to see her pelvic pain as a reaction to family stress and sexual anxiety may wish to take time to integrate her new knowledge into her self-concept. Perhaps she will choose to become more active in life despite her pain. Perhaps she will accept things as they are. And maybe, next year, she will return to the gynecologist and say, "Remember when you offered to send me to a clinic for my pain? I thought about it, and now I think I'm ready to try." Whatever the outcome, the health care team has given the patient permission to bring up a sexual problem and has delivered the message that sexual health is a legitimate concern.

Primary Care Clinician versus Specialist in Making the First Contact

With the increasing numbers of mental health professionals working in medical settings, it is tempting to let all sexual counseling be the province of the specialist. While working as sexual rehabilitation experts in a cancer center, we found that the great majority of patients sent for consultation only needed 1 to 3 hours of sexual counseling. Although the patient's physicians, nurses, social workers, or other clinicians could have provided such services, any patient with a question about sex was referred to the specialist. Patients, however, prefer a more integrated approach. In a study of diabetics followed in a specialty clinic (Jensen, 1986), the majority wanted sexual education or counseling to be provided by their primary care team, just as they received information about insulin, dietary control, or physical exercise and diabetes. They resisted the idea of needing services from a special sexuality clinic.

Why does the primary health care team fail to provide sexual education and counseling for medical patients? In a survey of general practitioners (Jensen, 1982) recurring themes included the following:

- I know the problems exist, but I don't know how to treat them, so I ignore them.
- I just don't have the time to listen. I see five patients an hour.
- I don't think we have much help to offer these patients, so why bother talking about sex?
- It is still too early to talk about sex. These patients have just . . . (had a heart attack, learned of their cancer, etc.)

We hope that our readers will reconsider these beliefs and that even those who are specialists will teach referring sources to provide basic education and limit consultations to the more complex cases.

Couple versus Individual Patient at the First Contact

We suggest that physicians who follow a group of chronically ill patients schedule at least one yearly couple appointment to discuss the impact of the disease on family life, including sexuality. If this model is followed, most identification of sexual problems will take place when both partners are present. A yearly couple visit has other advantages as well. The physician gains an appreciation of couples' strengths in handling crises instead of seeing the spouse only when a patient is coping poorly and the relationship presumably lacks resources. When a new patient is assessed, the primary team can include the spouse in one of the first appointments to evaluate how the couple is handling the trauma of diagnosis and treatment and to anticipate how they will cope with future health crises (Doherty & Baird, 1983). This approach is preventive, identifying couples with poor coping strategies so that extra support can be given.

Even when physicians schedule periodic couple visits, some patients choose to bring up a sexual issue when they are alone with a trusted health care professional. Feeling too vulnerable to ask for help in front of a partner, a man or woman will often claim that the spouse does not know a dysfunction exists (e.g. "I don't think she realizes I can't get it up," "I haven't told him that intercourse hurts—I just fake it"). The patient may assert that the spouse is too embarrrassed to talk about sex (e.g. "She clams up if someone even tells a dirty joke," "He would just kill me if he knew I was talking about our sex life").

If the spouse is not present when a sexual issue is first discussed, the next step is to get the partner's perspective, unless the patient is not in a committed relationship. If the patient is unmarried but has a committed partner, we like to involve the significant other. New relationships, or those with more fragile bonding, are particularly vulnerable to the stress of illness, especially when sexual function is affected. If the patient does not want to include the spouse in future contacts with the clinician, some diplomacy must be exercised.

Sometimes the patient fears the spouse will be angry that such private material was discussed outside of the marriage. A strong sense of family secrecy is a characteristic of psychosomatic families as described by Minuchin, Rossman, and Baker (1978). If the patient claims to have invited the spouse to come along for a visit, but says that the spouse refused, the clinician must remain skeptical. Using one's professional prestige and calling the spouse, with the patient's permission, is a more powerful technique for setting up a couple interview than relying on the patient's conveying the message. The clinician should explain the purpose of the session (i.e., to discuss the impact of the illness on the couple's daily life and emotions), with a view toward helping the family function more effectively. Sexuality can be mentioned as one area to be addressed during the visit, but not as the main focus.

What if the partner persists in refusing to come in? The professional must consider whether beginning an individual assessment will be an effective next step, or whether scheduling an appointment for the patient alone would simply play into marital gamesmanship. One way to involve a recalcitrant spouse is to proceed, but to instruct the patient to recount what happens in the evaluation in great detail to the partner. The spouse may either become intrigued by the possibility that things could change for the better, or at least become angry at having his or her viewpoint excluded, so that a visit is in order to "tell that guy how things really are around here."

The First Conjoint Contact

When the spouse has not participated in the initial contact, the clinician is faced with the task of forming a therapeutic alliance with the couple as a unit. Several trains of events may lead up to this session:

- The primary care clinician may have met with the patient, but now must include a spouse who is a stranger.
- The couple has been referred to a specialist for therapy, but the referring clinician has not consulted the spouse in the decision process. No couple contract has been made that an integrative assessment is needed.
- Although the spouse did not meet the referring clinician, the couple wished to be seen conjointly by the specialist and, in fact, already considers the problem to be "ours" rather than "mine versus yours."

The third situation is ideal, merely requiring the clinician to outline the plan of assessment and to obtain the couple's agreement. The first two scenarios are more problematic, however. The clinician must reframe the sexual issue as a couple problem before proceeding with the assessment interview. The issues are somewhat different depending on whether the clinician is a primary care professional or a sexuality specialist.

Conjoint Interviewing for the Primary Health Care Team

When a physician is following a patient on a long-term basis and asks to see the spouse, couples may be confused or suspicious as to the purpose of the visit, especially if the spouse knows that sexual issues are to be discussed. We suggest that, besides using the techniques outlined above to get the spouse involved, a physician new to couple counseling involve a nurse or social worker in the session. In Europe this model has been used to help members of the health care team function as cotherapists. In the United States, where economic concerns often limit the amount of time a physician can spend with a patient, nonphysicians whose time is less costly often take over the counseling role. Sharing the first conjoint interview can help members of the health care team develop mutual respect. An initial investment of time by the physician also pays off by strengthening the relationship with the patient and increasing the impact of later, briefer contacts.

In training primary health care professionals, we find that clinicians make some common mistakes when they first conduct a couple interview. We present some guidelines for the inexperienced clinician, trusting that our more seasoned readers will be able to use this advice in supervision and teaching.

Begin by welcoming the spouse, stating overtly that it can be awkward to come in "after the show has started," but emphasizing that the session is an opportunity for both partners to be heard. Let the couple know that you see your role as a neutral consultant.

Take responsibility for setting up the couple session:

Clinician: After hearing John's story, I felt I had to meet you as well, because sexual problems influence both partners in a couple. How do you feel about being here today?

A question about the emotional experience of having a conjoint visit gives the spouse permission to express anxiety or doubts. If the clinician listens empathetically, the spouse usually feels understood, and a sense of trust develops.

Make the agenda overt from the beginning. Begin by restating the problem as you understand it, checking with each partner that your perspective is accurate. If you give the impression of having a secret alliance with the patient, the spouse will be turned off:

Gynecologist: Well Judy, you finally dragged him in. What did you have to do to get him here?

Or consider the internist whose cardiac patient, David, has complained that his wife has lost all desire for sex:

Internist: (*to wife*) Have you guessed why I asked to see you today?
Wife: David! What did you tell him about me?
David: Oh nothing, Dear.

The clinician can emphasize his or her role as advocate for each partner in helping the couple improve their relationship. Since both spouses contribute to a sexual problem, neither partner will be blamed or labeled as the guilty party.

The reward of a couple visit occurs when a covert conflict is recognized and defused.

Mary had had a mastectomy 6 months previously. Her husband, Carl, had found the lump in her breast and urged her to see their family doctor, but Mary insisted on trying herbal extracts touted by the palm-reader she habitually consulted. By the time she did seek medical attention, she not only needed a mastectomy, but also had to have postoperative radiotherapy and chemotherapy. She had recently finished her last course of treatment, and her hair was beginning to grow back. She told her oncologist, however, that Carl had refused to have any sexual activity since her surgery. Although Carl was invited several times to accompany Mary on her follow-up visits, he only showed up after a call from the oncologist.

Carl's nonverbal behavior was markedly belligerent. He sat with folded arms and would not make eye contact with the oncologist and the social worker who were conducting the interview. Mary tried to enlist the clinicians' support by making "I told you so" faces whenever Carl was not watching.

Oncologist: Mary has explained that the two of you had a good sex life until her mastectomy, but that you have not been able to resume sexual activity since that time. I know she has been angry and upset, and she says that the two of you have had a few fights about sex over the past month or two.

Carl: Only two or three a day.

Social Worker: We know that cancer affects the partner as well as the patient. Since you have shared Mary's fears and pain, we wanted to hear your side of the story, too.

Carl: Yeah, pain is right.

Oncologist: Right now you seem angry, but sometimes that is just a way of expressing hurt.

Carl: Well how can you be angry at your wife because she has cancer?

Mary: Are you angry at me?

Carl: If you had listened to me and seen the doctor when we found the lump, you might not have had to go through all this—but you had to try those stupid tea leaves, or whatever they were.

Oncologist: Do you think your anger affects your desire for Mary as a sexual partner?

Carl: Well I've never liked to have sex when I was mad.

Of course Carl and Mary's problem is not "cured" by this interaction, but the cards are on the table and the couple is ready to work on resolving their feelings.

The novice clinician can also benefit from a few more tricks of the trade:

- Take care not to disclose confidential information that the patient has told you, but may not have shared with the spouse. You can ask whether a topic, such as thoughts about resuming sex after an illness, has been discussed at home. You can also ask, "Is there anything either one of you would like to bring up today? I am here to help you talk openly about the illness and your family life."
- Emphasize the couple's strengths and praise their successes in coping with the illness.
- Remember that the initial task is to understand the couple's relationship and to evaluate their readiness to change. Their conflicts have often persisted for years and will not be resolved in one visit. If they agree to try something new, help them negotiate one or two small, positive changes in their daily life routine. Set up a contract that you will follow up with a phone call in a week or two to see how successful they have been in carrying out the plan.

Conjoint Interviewing by the Sexuality Specialist

The sexuality specialist is expert in marital dynamics and is used to reframing a problem from an individual to a couple issue. Still, the specialist must cope with the false expectations a patient has when a referral has not been carefully set up. To avoid the uncooperative patient who wants a physiological treatment and resents being sent to a "shrink" or the patient who wants to be seen individually and is confused or annoyed by the request for a joint visit, the specialist must educate clinicians who are potential sources of referrals.

• Give the primary health care team some pointers on explaining the need for a referral in a way that gives the patient accurate expectations about what will happen.
• Give in-service training in brief sexual assessment and counseling to the primary health care team members.
• Give feedback to referral sources about the appropriateness of the patient for specialty assessment and about the treatment plan formulated. Be careful, however, about violating patients' confidentiality. It is best to ask the patient how much information can be shared with the referring team.

Clinicians who work in sexuality clinics, or even in sexual counseling units that are part of a medical clinic, often lose sight of the select nature of their clientele. This overview of the first contact, although it may seem detailed, was designed to remind clinicians of the gap between the large percentage of men and women with a chronic illness who experience sexual problems and the 5% or 10% who actually get help.

Once the couple agrees that a sexual problem exists and that they want to overcome it, the comprehensive assessment process can begin in earnest.

THE ASSESSMENT INTERVIEW

The most crucial part of the comprehensive assessment of a sexual problem is the semistructured interview. Whenever the patient is in a committed relationship, we prefer to have both partners present at the beginning of the interview. As in the first joint contact, including the partner in the assessment interview conveys several important messages:

• Sexual problems are couple issues.
• Even though one spouse is medically ill, the couple and family have important roles in coping with disease.
• Each person's point of view is important and will be heard.
• Treatment decisions will be made as a team, with input from patient, partner, and clinician.

In medical settings, the assessment interview may need to take place in a hospital room. Privacy, however, is important. If possible, avoid sessions behind flimsy bed curtains, with a roommate listening avidly on the other side.

Setting the Tone of the Interview

For most patients, the interview is their first detailed discussion of a sexual problem with a health care professional. For many, it is a new experience to discuss a sexual problem at all. Should the interviewer focus on sex from the first? We think it depends on the patient's comfort. Men or women who seek help assertively often wish to begin by defining the sexual problem. If the sexual problem was identified by the primary care physician, however, beginning with a more general assessment can build a therapeutic relationship that allows a more open discussion of sexual issues.

Patients have often felt apprehensive about the interview, especially when a referral to a specialist was involved. We find that an introductory statement can set the patient at ease and circumvent thoughts such as, "Why did my doctor send me to a headshrinker? Did he think I'm crazy? I'm a normal person; I don't need counseling." The sexuality specialist can help to normalize the situation:

Clinician: I'm part of your health care team, but I specialize in helping couples deal with the effects of an illness on their relationships. I'd like to find out your reactions to the illness, how you communicate with each other, and how you relate in your sex life. Even the happiest couples usually feel stressed going through an illness together.

The clinician can also demystify the interview process and help the patient feel confident that privacy will be respected:

Clinician: Today I would like to take some time to get to know you as a couple and find out how you are feeling about your illness. We can talk about how your medical treatment has affected your relationship and your sex life. Maybe I can offer you some suggestions on how to make things better. I know I ask you some pretty personal questions, so I'd like to say that I'm careful about what I write in your medical chart. I try to limit my notes to a diagnosis and a treatment plan. As you'll notice, though, I take more detailed notes for my own use. They are kept in a confidential file and are not released without your permission."

The need for such explanations varies with the patient's readiness to be open. Most medical patients have never sought psychotherapy and regard it as stigmatizing, or at least as a very anxiety-provoking experience. With such individuals or couples, beginning the interview with mundane material helps to build an atmosphere of trust. We often begin by reviewing the demographic facts gleaned from the medical chart: where the couple lives, each partner's occupation, ages of children and grandchildren, previous health history, and how the current illness was discovered and treated. Discussing the medical illness allows the clinician to begin to assess emotional styles of coping and the degree of intimacy and communication in the couple's relationship.

Interviewer: From your chart, Renee, it looks like you found the lump in your breast yourself, and you went to see your gynecologist soon after.

Renee: The next day!

Interviewer: How did you handle your fears those first few days?

Renee: I just tried to keep busy. I worked my usual schedule in the store until the day of the biopsy, and I just tried to put the whole thing out of my mind.

Interviewer: (*to the husband Todd*) Did she talk to you about how she was feeling?

Todd: Oh . . . well, she was quieter than usual, I guess. And she was absentminded.

Renee: (*laughs*) I forgot his birthday! We usually have a steak dinner, and I didn't even get him a present.

Interviewer: Did you forgive her?

Todd: Oh yeah (*squeezes his wife's hand*).

This small exchange illustrates patterns of couple interaction. Renee copes by trying to conceal her feelings and carry out her work and family responsibilities. Todd feels powerless to help, given his wife's apparent efficiency, even though he knows she needs support. He collaborates in the denial by telling her everything will turn out fine. These are common coping strategies. The couple's stable relationship is evident in the partners' ability to laugh about the crisis, and the husband's nonverbal expression of affection.

Contrast Renee and Todd with another couple, Dora and Jack:

Interviewer: Jack, how did you first find out you needed a cardiac bypass?

Dora: (*cutting in before her husband can reply*) He knew! He knew he was sick but he kept saying it was indigestion.

Jack: Well I thought it was! Damn doctors, always charging an arm and a leg. Best thing for your health is to stay out of their offices.

Interviewer: It sounds like you'd been having chest pain for a while.

Jack: I thought I was just going a little too heavy on the beer.

Dora: If you didn't drink all that beer, you might not be such a sick man today.

Interviewer: Do the two of you disagree about Jack's drinking?

Jack: Ah, she's always nagging. I only drink a little beer, doc. None of the hard stuff.

Dora: The doctor told him to cut down to one beer a day, and I swear he still drinks a six-pack. (*Turning to her husband*) Isn't one operation enough for you?

Jack: It's my heart, goddamnit, not yours!

Clearly Jack and Dora have no helpful way to provide each other with support. Dora's intrusive concern about Jack's health angers her husband. He lashes back, making his wife feel more distant, persecuted, and self-righteous. Unfortunately Jack does not manage well without his wife's care, as is evident in his heavy drinking and delays in seeking medical attention.

Other useful questions about the illness include the following:

- How have you felt about your medical care?
- How has communication been with your doctors?
- What has helped you get through this crisis?
- What has the family done to support you during this crisis?
- What do you think the outcome of your medical treatment will be?
- How has the illness changed your marriage relationship?

Notice that these questions are open-ended to elicit the maximum amount of information. The clinician should also look for symptoms of individual psychopathology, particularly affective disorders, organic brain syndromes, or maladaptive levels of anxiety or denial.

Assessing the Relationship

Since the discussion of health focuses on the partners' communication, it is easy to change the topic to the relationship itself. Like many marital therapists, we find it useful to ask a couple how they first met and what attracted them to each other (Jacobson & Margolin, 1979, pp. 59–60). Couples who can recall a humorous or romantic anecdote about courtship days and can list each spouse's best attributes are usually functioning well. When marital conflict is severe, partners have difficulty expressing positive sentiments about each other.

> *Interviewer*: How did you and Dora meet?
> *Jack*: I don't remember anymore.
> *Dora*: Yes you do! His cousin introduced us.
> *Jack*: Oh yeah, I guess so.
> *Interviewer*: What made you choose each other to marry? (Silence. Jack rolls his eyes.)
> *Dora*: (*looks at the floor and finally says*) Well, we both liked to dance. He was a good dancer.
> *Interviewer*: Do you still go dancing?
> *Jack*: No, I'm too tired.
> *Dora*: We haven't gone in years.
> *Interviewer*: Well, what's kept you together as a couple?
> *Dora*: Family.
> *Jack*: We can't afford a divorce.

The relationship assessment should cover the couple's leisure activities, how much time the partners spend together, whether they have enough adult time for couple intimacy, how they feel about having separate friends and hobbies, whether they can share emotions, how each expresses caring and affection, how each expresses anger, and areas of conflict and disagreement.

The Sexual Assessment

When seen as part of a relationship assessment, an evaluation of the couple's sexual interaction seems natural. As in the first contact, open-ended questions are helpful, especially with a couple that is not accustomed to discussing sexuality. A general question can be an icebreaker, for example, "Tell me a little about your sex life. How important has sex been as a part of your relationship?"

Other good questions include the following:

- Who usually gets things started when you make love?
- How can you tell when your partner is in the mood for sex?
- What kinds of disagreements do you have about when to have sex or trying new kinds of touching?
- If you want a certain kind of caress, how do you let your partner know?
- How has your illness affected your fertility and your feelings about having children?

During the sexuality assessment, the clinician can use the multiaxial diagnostic system presented in Chapter 3 as a guiding principle. The sexual questionnaires discussed later in this chapter also outline important areas to assess. By the end of the interview, the clinician should be able to describe each partner's function across all phases of the sexual response cycle.

Questions about sensitive sexual issues are less threatening when prefaced by a normalizing statement.

Clinician: Couples vary tremendously in the kinds of touching they include in foreplay. Some partners enjoy kissing each other's genitals, but others feel uncomfortable with the idea. What has been your experience with oral sex?

Sometimes, too, the clinician can explain why it is necessary to ask a very personal question:

Clinician: I always ask spouses whether they have helped each other reach orgasm through hand caresses or oral sex, rather than during intercourse. I want to know because some illnesses make intercourse difficult, but couples can still enjoy other kinds of lovemaking. How do each of you reach orgasm?

When clinicians learn techniques of sexual assessment, they often wonder what kind of language to use. Will patients be most comfortable with street slang, or should the interviewer be dignified and use medical terms? We think the answer is "neither of the above." As in the examples we provide, we try to use common, everyday words for sexual organs and activities. If we use a latinate word such as *ejaculation* or *clitoris*, we check to make sure the patient understands our meaning. We only use street slang if a patient has very limited education and comes from a subculture where the everyday language of sex is unique.

One way to help each partner feel acknowledged in the assessment process is to ask the man and woman to state their two or three most important goals for the sexual counseling. Is their concern to keep sexual function intact during medical treatment, to get information on what sexual side effects to expect, or to correct sexual problems that already exist? When the assessment is complete, feedback to the couple should address their goals.

Individual Interviews

Some couple therapists avoid seeing partners individually because they fear that hearing a marital secret will interfere with their nonallied position (Jacobson & Margolin, 1979, pp. 129–131). We think that it is usually helpful to have some time alone with each partner, however. Some sexual topics, such as masturbation or the content of sexual fantasies, are so taboo in our society that a majority of couples have never discussed them. We prefer to assess those areas of sexuality individually, at least in the beginning of the therapy relationship. We also prefer to know if one partner is bisexual or is having an extramarital affair, since such information is vital to the therapy process. If we cannot work with the couple because of one partner's secret sexual preferences or lack of commitment to the relationship, at least we can recommend appropriate treatment alternatives without wasting time. If one therapist is seeing the couple, the "split" interview can be introduced as follows:

Clinician: Now I'd like to spend a few minutes with each of you alone. Some areas of sexuality can be easier to discuss without your partner. I will hold what you say in confidence, although I might ask your permission during the interview to bring something up when we all get back together.

When a male–female cotherapy team is performing an assessment, the male therapist can interview the husband and the female the wife. Some patients may find it easier to share very sensitive material with a same-sex clinician, although a skilled therapist can do a good job in the great majority of cases regardless of gender.

The split interview is especially useful for assessing sexual attraction to the partner, the existence of concurrent sexual relationships, masturbation practices (for example, does a sexual dysfunction persist in masturbation as well as in partner sex?), content of sexual fantasies, and any subjects a partner seemed reluctant to discuss during the couple interview. Even when a couple appears to have a conventional relationship, the clinician should always ask about each partner's history of sexual trauma, such as molestation, incest, rape, and about family violence in past and current relationships. We always include one general question in the split interview: "Is there anything I have not covered that you think I ought to know?"

Although we prefer to conduct most of the assessment in a joint interview, we have learned to be flexible. In medical settings, the partner is not always available for the first appointment. Some patients also prefer to be seen alone, either because they feel so vulnerable sexually or because they are involved in more than one sexual relationship. If couple issues are important, the therapeutic alliance formed in an individual assessment interview may provide support for a patient to ask the partner to participate in treatment.

For unmarried patients who are not in a committed relationship, the individual assessment interview can follow the basic outline of the couple assessment. It is especially important to find out single patients' resources for emotional support during the illness, their history of close relationships, and their beliefs about the impact of the illness on future dating, marriage, and parenting.

QUESTIONNAIRE ASSESSMENT

Questionnaires are a valuable part of a sexuality assessment when precise research data are being gathered, or when a clinician wants a quantitative measure of pretreatment to posttreatment changes. In everyday clinical work, using questionnaires can also reduce expensive clinician time spent in conducting a structured interview and/or provide unique information that can be compared with standardized norms and used to plan therapy. We regard questionnaires as a supplement to the assessment interview and rely most heavily on our clinical judgment of the face-to-face contact with a patient or couple.

In medical settings, patients are often less willing to complete reams of questionnaires than they are in sex therapy clinics. Not only may some medical patients regard sexual issues as less salient, but those who are acutely ill may be fatigued and irritable. Therefore, we choose our instruments both for utility and brevity.

Standardized Psychological Inventories

We do not routinely administer commonly used psychological tests such as the MMPI or a neuropsychological battery. We do advocate referral for neuropsychological assessment whenever the interview reveals signs of cognitive impairment. An MMPI may add clarifying information if a question of psychosis exists or if a reconstructive operation is planned and the clinician fears the patient might react by having a psychotic break or committing suicide.

We never advocate using cutoff scores on any one inventory, or even a formula involving several tests, as the exclusive basis for a treatment decision, such as whether to prescribe antidepressant medication or to proceed with elective surgery. Psychological testing has failed dismally, for example, to discriminate between men with psychogenic and organic erection problems (Schover & von Eschenbach, 1985a). Psychological testing is most helpful when used to answer a specific question or to clear up a confusion in diagnosis after the interview.

In a medical setting, large groups of patients may need to be screened for psychological distress. Sometimes a clinician cannot offer a full assessment to everyone and wishes to identify a target group of especially needy patients. For screening purposes, we have used the BSI (Derogatis & Melisaratos, 1983) a 53-item self-report questionnaire that can be completed in 10 or 15 minutes and asks about symptoms over the past week. The scales include somatization, obsessive–compulsive symptoms, interpersonal sensitivity, depression, anxiety, hostility, phobic anxiety, paranoia, and psychoticism. We use the norms for men and women from a community, nonpatient sample, because they are more appropriate for medical patients than norms from a psychiatric clinic population. Norms for men and women over age 60 are also available (Hale, Cochran, & Hedgepeth, 1984).

Questionnaires Designed for Medical Patients

With the recent meteoric rise in the popularity of health psychology, several inventories have been designed for use in medical settings. They assess patients' ability to cope with illness and their need for psychological intervention. The two most comprehensive are the Millon Behavioral Health Inventory (MBHI) (Green, 1982) and the Psychosocial Adjustment to Illness Scale (PAIS) (Derogatis, 1983b). Since our main focus is the sexuality and relationship assessment, we prefer the PAIS because it is brief, rests on common sense, and does not make high-level inferences about personality. The scores delineate a profile of the level of distress within each of the following domains: Attitudes about health care, vocational environment, home environment, sexual relationships, relations with the extended family, social environment, and psychological adjustment. A global summary score is also calculated. Norms are available for several different populations of medical patients.

Marital Questionnaires

A number of inventories have also been developed to assess the marital relationship. For our purposes, the interview is usually sufficient. We find quantitative scores more helpful in research than in daily clinical practice. If a clinician is screening a large number of couples, however, and can only perform a complete assessment on those in distress, we recommend the Dyadic Adjustment Inventory (DAI) (Spanier, 1976). In addition to identifying unhappy partners, the DAI, because of its detailed questions, can guide the clinician during the interview in assessing areas of conflict. It is designed to be relevant for dating partners or homosexual dyads, not just for heterosexual married couples. The DAI is a good measure of change in relationship happiness when given before and after couple therapy.

An Inventory Assessing Couple Issues and Illness

In the course of longitudinal research on sexuality and diabetes, one of us (SBJ) has developed a questionnaire designed to measure the impact of illness on a couple's relationship: the Disease Acceptance Scale (Jensen, 1985a, 1985b, 1986). Although validation studies using different groups of patients are still in progress, we present the questionnaire in Figure 6-1 as an evolving research instrument that can also provide useful clinical information.

Patient and partner separately indicate how much they agree or disagree with 16 items about emotional reactions to illness. Each spouse then specifies how well the items apply to the other. The partners' combined answers create a profile of the impact of illness on the relationship and whether patient and partner agree in their perceptions.

Questionnaire Assessment of Sexuality

When using questionnaires to assess sexual function, we must be especially sensitive to the clinical setting. In a sexual dysfunction clinic, patients expect detailed questions about their sex lives and are usually willing to complete explicit questionnaires even before meeting their therapist. In a hospital or medical clinic, however, we do not advocate beginning an assessment by handing out a sexual questionnaire. If the clinician wants to see questionnaire results before the assessment interview, a member of the team can meet the patient, explain the usefulness of the sexual items and make sure the patient understands that the answers will be confidential. Otherwise, the questionnaires can be held until after the interview.

One extremely detailed and complete interview outline, designed for sex researchers, is the Sexual Behavior Assessment Schedule (Meyer-Bahlburg & Ehrhardt, 1983). A less comprehensive questionnaire that can be used as a self-report measure or as an interview guide is the Sex History Form (SHF), developed at the Sex Therapy Center at Stony Brook (Schover *et al.*, 1982). Table 6-1 lists the SHF questions and normative data gathered in 1980 from 92 couples living in the New York City area. Subjects responded to a newspaper advertisement for couples in stable relationships

Figure 6-1. Disease acceptance scale.

Below are a series of statements about emotional reactions to illness. For each item, indicate how much you agree or disagree that it applies to your experience.

Patient Version	Totally agree	Partly agree	Partly disagree	Totally disagree
1. I worry too much about my illness.				
2. I often feel sad or in low spirits because of my illness.				
3. My moods shift frequently.				
4. Daily life is made difficult by limitations and routines imposed by my illness.				
5. I feel bitter and angry at fate because I became ill.				
6. My partner sometimes uses the illness against me.				
7. I have become more health conscious and take better care of myself.				
8. I am worried and anxious about the future.				
9. I worry whether our relationship can withstand the long-term stress of having an ill mate.				
10. I feel that my illness is visible.				
11. I have difficulty talking about my illness and the problems it brings.				
12. I am always tired.				
13. I lack full information about the influence my illness has on relationships.				
14. I think the most important thing is to adapt to an illness.				
15. Problems should be discussed with an outside authority (such as a physician, psychologist, etc.)				
16. I believe that my children will inherit my illness.				
17. My partner worries too much about my illness.				
18. My partner often feels sad or in low spirits because of my illness.				
19. My partner's moods shift frequently.				
20. My partner finds daily life difficult because of limitations and routines imposed by my illness.				
21. My partner feels bitter and angry at fate because I become ill.				
22. I sometimes use my illness as an excuse.				
23. My partner has become more health conscious and takes better care of him/her self.				

Figure 6-1. Continued

	Totally agree	Partly agree	Partly disagree	Totally disagree
Patient Version				
24. My partner is worried and anxious about the future.	___	___	___	___
25. My partner worries whether our relationship can withstand the long-term stress of having an ill mate.	___	___	___	___
26. My partner feels that my illness is visible.	___	___	___	___
27. My partner has difficulty talking about my illness and the problems it brings.	___	___	___	___
28. My partner is always tired.	___	___	___	___
29. My partner lacks full information about the influence my illness has on relationships.	___	___	___	___
30. My partner thinks the most important thing is to adapt to an illness.	___	___	___	___
31. My partner thinks problems should be discussed with an outside authority (such as a physician, psychologist, etc.).	___	___	___	___
32. My partner believes that my/our children will inherit my illness.	___	___	___	___
Partner Version				
1. I worry too much about my partner's illness.	___	___	___	___
2. I often feel sad or in low spirits because of my partner's illness.	___	___	___	___
3. My moods shift frequently.	___	___	___	___
4. Daily life is made difficult by limitations and routines imposed by my partner's illness.	___	___	___	___
5. I feel bitter and angry at fate because my partner became ill.	___	___	___	___
6. My partner sometimes uses the illness against me.	___	___	___	___
7. I have become more health conscious and take better care of myself.	___	___	___	___
8. I am worried and anxious about the future.	___	___	___	___
9. I worry whether our relationship can withstand the long-term stress of having an ill mate.	___	___	___	___
10. I think my partner's illness is visible.	___	___	___	___

Figure 6-1. Continued

Patient Version	Totally agree	Partly agree	Partly disagree	Totally disagree
11. I have difficulty talking about my partner's illness and problems it brings.	___	___	___	___
12. I am always tired.	___	___	___	___
13. I lack full information about the influence my partner's illness has on relationships.	___	___	___	___
14. I think the most important thing is to adapt to an illness.	___	___	___	___
15. Problems should be discussed with an outside authority (such as a physician, psychologist, etc.)	___	___	___	___
16. I believe that our children will inherit my partner's illness.	___	___	___	___
17. My partner worries too much about illness.	___	___	___	___
18. My partner often feels sad or in low spirits because of his/her illness.	___	___	___	___
19. My partner's moods shift frequently			___	___
20. My partner finds daily life difficult because of limitations and routines imposed by his/her illness.	___	___	___	___
21. My partner feels bitter and angry at fate because he/she became ill.	___	___	___	___
22. I sometimes use my partner's illness as an excuse.	___	___	___	___
23. My partner has become more health conscious and takes better care of him/herself.	___	___	___	___
24. My partner is worried and anxious about the future.	___	___	___	___
25. My partner worries whether our relationship can withstand the long-term stress of having an ill mate.	___	___	___	___
26. My partner feels that his/her illness is visible.	___	___	___	___
27. My partner has difficulty talking about his/her illness and the problems it brings.	___	___	___	___
28. My partner is always tired.	___	___	___	___
29. My partner lacks full information about the influence his/her illness has on relationships.	___	___	___	___

Figure 6-1. Continued

Patient Version	Totally agree	Partly agree	Partly disagree	Totally disagree
30. My partner thinks the most important thing is to adapt to an illness.	___	___	___	___
31. My partner thinks the problems should be discussed with an outside authority (such as a physician, psychologist, etc.).	___	___	___	___
32. My partner believes that his/her children will inherit his/her illness.	___	___	___	___

to participate in sex research. The couples had an average age in the early 30s and were lower-middle to upper-middle class. Jewish and Catholic couples were overrepresented in our sample. Of course older pople, or those with chronic illnesses, would differ in their level of sexual activity and function from this reference group. The norms here simply offer a comparison with a young, healthy, urban sample.

Information from the SHF can be used to identify patients with sexual dysfunction and to focus an interview assessment, increasing the accuracy of the multiaxial diagnosis. When both partners in a couple fill out the questionnaire individually, discrepancies between their answers clarify their disagreements about sexuality and the accuracy of their perceptions of each other.

Even more detailed information can be gathered on couple dimensions by using the Sexual Interaction Inventory (SII) (LoPiccolo & Steger, 1978). The SII asks how often each of 17 sexual activities is part of a couple's sexual routine and also how often an activity should ideally be included. Patients rate their own and their partner's actual and ideal pleasure in engaging in each type of sexual caress. The SII can only be scored if both partners fill out a questionnaire.

Although the SII is quite helpful in planning sex therapy and measuring changes from before to after treatment, it takes 30 to 40 minutes for the patient to complete. Another drawback for older or more conservative couples is that the booklet depicts the sexual activities in explicit line drawings. Although the illustrations ensure that the patient knows which sexual behavior to rate, many couples in medical settings would find the SII offensive. The SII scoring procedures are rather cumbersome unless the clinician has a computer available, but the profile includes scales measuring the accuracy of each partner's view of the other's preferences, each partner's general level of pleasure, acceptance of one's own sexual enjoyment, acceptance of the mate's degree of pleasure, satisfaction with sexual variety, and

Table 6-1. Sexual History Form and Norms

	% of Men	% of Women
1. How frequently to you and your mate have sexual intercourse or activity?		
1) more than once a day	2	1
2) once a day	2	3
3) 3 or 4 times a week	36	40
4) twice a week	30*	24*
5) once a week	16	21
6) once every two weeks	9	9
7) once a month	2	2
8) less than once a month	3	0
9) not at all	0	0
2. How frequently would you like to have sexual intercourse or activity?		
1) more than once a day	12	3
2) once a day	29	20
3) 3 or 4 times a week	42*	51*
4) twice a week	12	16
5) once a week	4	10
6) once every two weeks	0	0
7) once a month	0	0
8) less than once a month	0	0
9) not at all	0	0
3. Who initiates having sexual intercourse or activity?		
1) I always do	11	2
2) I usually do	38	8
3) my mate and I each initiate about equally often	40*	39
4) my mate usually does	10	48*
5) my mate always does	1	3
4. Who would you like to have initiate sexual intercourse or activity?		
1) myself, always	0	0
2) myself, usually	10	0
3) my mate and I equally often	78*	63*
4) my mate, usually	11	33
5) my mate, always	1	4
5. How often do you masturbate?		
1) more than once a day	1	0
2) once a day	4	2
3) 3 or 4 times a week	12	7
4) twice a week	12	14
5) once a week	13	9
6) once every two weeks	10*	12
7) once a month	10	9*
8) less than once a month	13	18
9) not at all	23	30
6. How frequently do you feel sexual desire? This feeling may include wanting to have sex, planning to have sex, feeling frustrated due to a lack of sex, etc.		
1) more than once a day	40	13
2) once a day	37*	29
3) 3 or 4 times a week	14	32*
4) twice a week	9	11
5) once a week	0	4

Table 6-1. Continued

	% of Men	% of Women
6) once every two weeks	0	4
7) once a month	0	4
8) less than once a month	0	1
9) not at all	0	1
7. For how many years have you and your mate been having sexual intercourse?		
1) less than 6 months	1	1
2) less than 1 year	3	3
3) 1 to 3 years	11	14
4) 4 to 6 years	20	18
5) 7 to 10 years	34*	33*
6) more than 10 years	30	31
8. For how long do you and your mate usually engage in sexual foreplay (kissing, petting, etc.) before having intercourse?		
1) less than one minute	1	2
2) 1 to 3 minutes	7	10
3) 4 to 6 minutes	13	12
4) 7 to 10 minutes	27	24
5) 11 to 15 minutes	30*	32*
6) 16 to 30 minutes	19	15
7) 30 minutes to 1 hour	3	4
9. How long does intercourse usually last, from entry of the penis until the male reaches orgasm (climax)?		
1) less than one minute	1	0
2) 1 to 2 minutes	6	12
3) 2 to 4 minutes	16	21
4) 4 to 7 minutes	28	34
5) 7 to 10 minutes	22*	11*
6) 11 to 15 minutes	10	10
7) 15 to 20 minutes	9	3
8) 20 to 30 minutes	6	4
9) more than 30 minutes	3	4
10. Does the male ever reach orgasm while he is trying to enter the woman's vagina with his penis?		
1) never	63*	75*
2) rarely, less than 10% of the time	31	21
3) seldom, less than 25% of the time	3	4
4) sometimes, 50% of the time	2	0
5) usually, 75% of the time	0	0
6) nearly always, over 90% of the time	0	0
11. Overall, how satisfactory to you is your sexual relationship with your mate?		
1) extremely unsatisfactory	4	2
2) moderately unsatisfactory	3	3
3) slightly unsatisfactory	6	2
4) slightly satisfactory	6	4
5) moderately satisfactory	43*	44*
6) extremely satisfactory	39	44
12. Overall, how satisfactory do you think your sexual relationship is to your mate?		
1) extremely unsatisfactory	7	2

Table 6-1. Continued

	% of Men	% of Women
2) moderately unsatisfactory	4	2
3) slightly unsatisfactory	6	10
4) slightly satisfactory	7	8
5) moderately satisfactory	47*	42*
6) extremely satisfactory	30	36

13. When your mate makes sexual advances, how do you usually respond?

1) usually accept with pleasure	92*	77*
2) accept reluctantly	4	13
3) often refuse	3	10
4) usually refuse	0	0

14. When you have sex with your mate do you feel sexually aroused (i.e., feeling "turned on," pleasure, excitement)?

1) nearly always, over 90% of the time	83*	63*
2) usually, about 75% of the time	8	23
3) sometimes, about 50% of the time	8	11
4) seldom, about 25% of the time	1	3
5) never	0	0

15. When you have sex with your mate, do you have negative emotional reactions, such as fear, disgust, shame or guilt?

1) never	74*	65*
2) rarely, less than 10% of the time	19	26
3) seldom, less than 25% of the time	6	6
4) sometimes, 50% of the time	1	2
5) usually, 75% of the time	0	0
6) nearly always, over 90% of the time	0	0

16. If you try, is it possible for you to reach orgasm (sensation of climax) through masturbating?

1) nearly always, over 90% of the time	80*	56*
2) usually, about 75% of the time	2	4
3) sometimes, about 50% of the time	4	6
4) seldom, about 25% of the time	3	11
5) never	2	3
6) have never tried to	8	20

17. If you try, is it possible for you to reach orgasm (sensation of climax) through having your genitals caressed by your mate?

1) nearly always, over 90% of the time	42	46
2) usually, about 75% of the time	26*	21*
3) sometimes, about 50% of the time	13	11
4) seldom, about 25% of the time	9	12
5) never	4	9
6) have never tried to	6	1

18. If you try, is it possible for you to reach orgasm (sensation of climax) through sexual intercourse?

1) nearly always, over 90% of the time	97*	42
2) usually, about 75% of the time	2	20*
3) sometimes, about 50% of the time	0	12
4) seldom, about 25% of the time	1	18
5) never	0	9
6) have never tried to	0	0

Table 6-1. Continued

	% of Men	% of Women
19. What is your usual reaction to erotic or pornographic materials (pictures, movies, books)?		
1) greatly aroused	33	31
2) somewhat aroused	62*	58*
3) not aroused	3	3
4) negative—disgusted, repulsed, etc.	1	8
20. Does the male have any trouble in getting a full erection during sexual activity?		
1) never	48	64*
2) rarely, less than 10% of the time	44*	30
3) seldom, less than 25% of the time	7	4
4) sometimes, 50% of the time	0	0
5) usually, 75% of the time	0	1
6) nearly always, over 90% of the time	1	1
21. Does the male lose part or all of his erection before completing sexual activity?		
1) never	56*	63*
2) rarely, less than 10% of the time	30	32
3) seldom, less than 25% of the time	11	2
4) sometimes, 50% of the time	0	1
5) usually, 75% of the time	1	1
6) nearly always, over 90% of the time	2	1
22. Does the male ejaculate (climax) without having a full, hard erection?		
1) never	48	71*
2) rarely, less than 10% of the time	40*	18
3) seldom, less than 25% of the time	7	8
4) sometimes, 50% of the time	3	2
5) usually, 75% of the time	1	1
6) nearly always, over 90% of the time	1	0
23. Is the female's vagina so "dry" or "tight" that intercourse cannot occur?		
1) never	48	53*
2) rarely, less than 10% of the time	29*	30
3) seldom, less than 25% of the time	16	13
4) sometimes, 50% of the time	6	4
5) usually, 75% of the time	2	0
6) nearly always, over 90% of the time	0	0
24. Do you feel pain in your genitals during sexual intercourse?		
1) never	76*	40
2) rarely, less than 10% of the time	22	35*
3) seldom, less than 25% of the time	0	18
4) sometimes, 50% of the time	2	7
5) usually, 75% of the time	0	1
6) nearly always, over 90% of the time	0	0
(WOMEN ONLY — QUESTIONS 25, 26, & 27)		
25. Can you reach orgasm (sensation of climax) through stimulation of your genitals by an electric vibrator or any other means such as running water, rubbing with some object, etc.?		
1) nearly always, over 90% of the time	—	44

Table 6-1. Continued

	% of Men	% of Women
2) usually, about 75% of the time	—	4
3) sometimes, about 50% of the time	—	4*
4) seldom, about 25% of the time	—	8
5) never	—	4
6) have never tried to	—	35
26. Can you reach orgasm (sensation of climax) during sexual intercourse if at the same time your genitals are being caressed (by yourself or your mate or with a vibrator, etc.)?		
1) nearly always, over 90% of the time	—	52*
2) usually, about 75% of the time	—	15
3) sometimes, about 50% of the time	—	9
4) seldom, about 25% of the time	—	0
5) never	—	1
6) have never tried to	—	23
27. When you have sex with your mate, including foreplay and intercourse, do you notice some of these things happening: your breathing and pulse speeding up, wetness in your vagina, pleasurable sensations in your breasts and genitals?		
1) nearly always, over 90% of the time	—	88*
2) usually, about 75% of the time	—	8
3) sometimes, about 50% of the time	—	4
4) seldom, about 25% of the time	—	0
5) never	—	0
(MEN ONLY)		
28. Do you ever ejaculate semen without a pleasurable sensation of orgasm (climax)?		
1) never	64*	—
2) rarely, less than 10% of the time	28	—
3) seldom, less than 25% of the time	3	—
4) sometimes, 50% of the time	2	—
5) usually, 75% of the time	0	—
6) nearly always, over 90% of the time	2	—

*Median response.

the couple's overall level of agreement about their sexual interaction. The norms for the SII are based on a young, middle-class reference group. Older or more sexually conservative patients may appear to have elevated (i.e., maladjusted) scores, especially on the Pleasure Mean scales, yet be satisfied with their sexual relationship.

Most other sexual inventories have been designed for research purposes. Although they are useful in measuring differences between groups of patients, they add little to an interview assessment for planning couple therapy. For example, in research using the Derogatis Sexual Functioning Inventory (DSFI) (Derogatis, 1983a), a group of diabetic women was found to use significantly fewer types of sexual stimulation and to have less sexual "drive" than healthy, age-matched controls (Schreiner-Engel *et al.*, 1985). The DSFI, however, is a very long questionnaire, with complicated instructions. We do not believe that the costs in patient fatigue and noncompliance are justified by the clinical information it contributes.

MEDICAL ASSESSMENT

The medical portion of a comprehensive assessment should be guided by the same cost–benefit considerations as the psychological testing. A thorough medical history and a general physical examination are the equivalent of the assessment interview. Then the nature of the sexual dysfunction and the risk that it is due to organic factors will determine which specialized tests to pursue. Invasive and expensive technology should only be used when the results contribute to important decisions about treatment.

The Importance of the Medical History

The first step in a medical assessment is finding out the patient's history of major illnesses and surgical procedures and listing current medications. It is also crucial to assess the use of alcohol and recreational drugs. A physician should take the medical history, but nonphysicians should remain alert, too, for unexplored etiologic factors, since many physicians are still not aware of the range of causes for sexual dysfunctions.

For men over age 50, low sexual desire and erectile dysfunction are clearly related to general health (Slag *et al.*, 1983). In a study of 112 men with bladder cancer, a disease that should not affect sexual function in itself, the number of noncancer medical risk factors for erectile dysfunction was correlated at the .001 level with a man's erectile capacity before radical surgery was performed. Cardiovascular disease and antihypertensive medication were each significant predictors by themselves of sexual dysfunction. Men who had better erections and were more sexually active before cancer surgery were more likely to be alive and free of tumor at follow-up, further underlining the importance of sexual health as an indicator of general vitality (Schover *et al.*, 1986a).

The Physical Examination

Any medical evaluation of a sexual problem should include a thorough physical examination. Although the examination is general, the physician who conducts it should be aware of the sexual problem and make a special effort to spot relevant physiological problems. Sometimes in the couple interview a sexual dysfunction with a possible organic cause in the partner of the chronically ill patient is identified. Ideally, in that case, both partners should have a medical examination. For both men and women, the general medical evaluation should include routine blood chemistry testing and a review of physical systems. A brief neurological examination (Zorgniotti, 1984) and screening for signs of endocrine abnormalities are especially important.

For men, the examination should include palpation of the ankle, dorsalis, popliteal, and femoral pulses to assess the peripheral vascular system. The examiner should elicit the major genital reflexes (Wagner & Green, 1981, pp. 94–96), palpate the penis for plaques or scarring, and examine the scrotum for masses.

Assessment of a woman with sexual dysfunction should of course include a pelvic examination. Since we know so little about neurological and vascular factors in problems of female sexual arousal and orgasm, the pelvic examination usually focuses on assessing vaginal atrophy or physical sources of dyspareunia.

Dyspareunia is one of the most common sexual problems in women with chronic illnesses (Fordney, 1978). The clinician should obtain a careful description of the nature of the pain, that is, whether it occurs on penetration or with deep thrusting, what types of sexual stimulation evoke the pain, if the pain is localized or generalized, sharp or diffuse, and whether soreness persists after intercourse. The gynecologist looks for vaginitis (Fordney, 1978) or scarring in the genital area and tries to reproduce the pain by pressure or movement in the vagina during the examination. Other findings may include evidence of endometriosis or pathology of the uterine ligaments, the occurrence of vaginal muscle spasms during the examination, or occlusion of a Bartholin gland duct (Sarrel, Steege, Maltzer, & Bolinsky, 1983).

Vaginal atrophy resulting from hormonal insufficiency is one of the most common causes of dyspareunia. Leiblum, Bachmann, Kemmann, Colburn, and Swartzman (1983) have developed an index of vaginal atrophy for research purposes that can also be a useful guide for clinicians. The gynecologist rates genital skin elasticity as poor, fair, or excellent and pubic hair as sparse or normal. The labia are judged to be full or atrophic and dry. The vaginal entrance is described as less than one finger wide, or one or two fingers wide. The vaginal mucosa varies from thin and friable, to smooth, to normally rugated. Vaginal depth is rated as shortened or normal.

The pelvic examination performed to assess female sexual dysfunction is thus much more detailed than the usual annual gynecological evaluation. Clinicians who treat sexual dysfunction should collaborate with a gynecologist interested and skilled in assessing sexual problems.

All of the examinations described in this section are noninvasive and can be obtained as part of routine medical care. In the last few years, however, a number of specific medical tests have been developed to find the causes of sexual problems. Many of these require equipment or skills that are only available from a few specialists.

Specialized Examinations for Male Sexual Dysfunction

The availability of lucrative medical treatments for erectile dysfunction, including hormonal therapy, the penile prosthesis, and penile revascularization, has fostered the development of new technologies to assess the erection reflex. The goal of specialized examinations has been to select patients with organic erectile dysfunction to undergo medical therapy. Men who have low sexual desire or difficulty reaching orgasm are also occasionally candidates for these complex evalautions. A big business flavor pervades the treatment of "impotence." Before referring a man for expensive, time-consuming, and sometimes invasive tests, clinicians should ask the following questions:

- Will the results of this test make a real difference in planning treatment?
- What are the risks and side effects of this test?
- How much will this test cost the patient? Is it covered by insurance?

We will not attempt to give instructions on performing each examination. We do review the various tests available, however, and comment on their usefulness. Clinicians interested in more detailed "how-to's" can consult the sources we cite.

Nocturnal Penile Tumescence Monitoring

The measurement of men's erections during sleep has been touted as an "unequivocal direct test" that discriminates between organic and psychogenic erectile dysfunction (Karacan & Moore, 1982). Unfortunately, both the results of NPT monitoring and the proper procedures for carrying it out are far more controversial than they first appear. The earliest mention of using sleep erections to diagnose the cause of erectile dysfunction was in 18th-century French and German divorce cases (Benedek & Kubinec, 1982). The testimony of a male friend or a surgeon that the husband had had a nocturnal erection was used to contest a wife's suit for divorce on the grounds of impotence. Impotence was one of the only grounds for divorce for a woman, and winning the case allowed her to recover her dowry. Now NPT is sometimes used in workmen's compensation cases, to prove that an on-the-job injury damaged erections.

The modern sleep laboratory evaluation of NPT usually consists of 2 or 3 nights' observations. The patient's sleep stages (indicated by brain waves), eye movements, leg movements, and respiration are monitored continually by electrodes connected to a polygraph. This complex evaluation can reveal whether a man is spending a normal amount of time in REM sleep and if NPT recordings are influenced by sleep apnea (abnormal respiration) or nocturnal myoclonus (repeated leg jerks). The erections themselves are assessed by two mercury-filled strain gauges that record circumference changes at the base and tip of the penis.

The normality of NPT depends on the number of erections per night, the duration of each episode, whether the erections occurred during REM sleep, and the degree of penile circumference change. Circumference is only an indirect measure of whether an erection would be sufficient for penetration, however. Many men can achieve partial erections that would not be rigid enough for intercourse. Since blood pressure inside the cavernous bodies of the penis continues to increase even beyond the point of maximum circumference change, a measure of rigidity is needed (Dhabuwala, Ghayad, Smith, & Pierce, 1983). Researchers have now developed devices that continuously monitor penile rigidity and not just circumference changes (Bradley, Timm, Gallagher, & Johnson, 1985; Virag, Virag, & Lajujie, 1985). Studies on the reliability and validity of these new instruments are still in progress.

Measuring rigidity is not the only major problem with NPT monitoring. As Condra *et al.* (1986b) pointed out, the reasoning used to validate NPT testing has been circular. Researchers assume that a man with abnormal NPT has organic erectile dysfunction. NPT results are used to validate other examinations, such as penile blood flow studies. Then correlations between penile blood flow and NPT results are cited as evidence for the usefulness of NPT as a diagnostic tool. Meanwhile, nobody has proved the first premise. Men who are depressed have transient decreases in NPT that resolve when their mood lifts (Roose, Glassman, Walsh, & Cullen, 1982). Schiavi, Fisher, Quadland, and Glover (1985) also found that young diabetic men with normal erections had abnormally small increases in penile circumference during NPT episodes. In the same study, two nondiabetic subjects who complained of erectile dysfunction and had clearly abnormal NPT for 3 nights responded to sex therapy by achieving normal erectile capacity. Condra *et al.* (1986) also demonstrated discrepancies between clinical improvements in erectile function and results of repeated NPT testing. Thus NPT monitoring results in some false positives and negatives.

If measuring NPT in a full-scale sleep laboratory often yields equivocal results, imagine what happens when clinicians try to use shortcuts. Take-home NPT monitors measure penile circumference without assessing sleep parameters. Home monitors can overestimate erections because leg movements interfere with the recordings (Marshall, McGrath, & Schillinger, 1983). Another potential danger would be underestimating a man's erectile capacity if he had little REM sleep, for example, because of sleep apnea.

Perhaps it makes more sense to screen nocturnal erections by using a truly simple and inexpensive method. The "stamp test" (Barry, Blank, & Boileau, 1980) consists of a strip of postage stamps glued at the ends to fit snugly around the midshaft of a man's flaccid penis. The patient wears undershorts during sleep to minimize the chance of breaking the stamps accidentally. A full erection should tear open the stamp ring. Of course the stamp test tells nothing about the number of erections that occurred during the night or their duration. We also do not know how often a partial erection is sufficient to break the stamps.

The Dacomed snap-gauge™ is a somewhat more standardized and costly version of the stamp test. Simultaneous recordings of NPT with strain-gauges in the sleep laboratory suggest that an erection that breaks all three snaps on the gauge is probably full and of reasonable duration (Ek, Bradley, & Krane, 1983). Our clinical experience with older men who report good sexual function is that many do not break all three snaps. The results of snap-gauge testing are probably most helpful when a man breaks all the snaps on 2 nights. If no snaps break, he may have an organic problem or perhaps is not sleeping efficiently.

The snap-gauge test is helpful as one component of a screening battery of physical examinations for erectile dysfunction. A full sleep laboratory evaluation should be reserved for men whose problems remain obscure even after testing with some of the more convenient and inexpensive assessments that we describe below. In any case, NPT monitoring should no longer be regarded as the "gold standard" of evaluation of erectile dysfunction

Measuring Erections during Sexual Stimulation

A number of researchers have tried to measure men's erections during various types of sexual stimulation. If a man can achieve a full, lasting erection in the waking state, the problem is presumably psychogenic and expensive NPT testing is unnecessary. When strain-gauges are used, the patient can undergo sexual stimulation in privacy. Of course a man's failure to respond to erotic materials may just reflect the same psychological processes that interfere with his erections in other sexual situations. Two comparisons between NPT monitoring and daytime assessment suggest that measuring erections during sexual stimulation can be a helpful addition to a comprehensive assessment (Melman, Kaplan, & Redfield, 1984; Zuckerman *et al.*, 1985).

Vibration has also been used as a sexual stimulus (Godec, 1985; Wagner, 1985). As with visual erotic stimulation, not every man responds with erection, and failure may be caused by psychological inhibitions. It may also be worthwhile to use new techniques of measuring penile rigidity during visual or vibratory stimulation, since many men with organic damage to the erection reflex can attain nearly full erections in sexual situations but would still have difficulty with intercourse.

Noninvasive Vascular Assessment of Erectile Dysfunction

The advent of NPT testing led to a sharp increase in the percentage of cases of erectile dysfunction that were labeled organic. The use of noninvasive vascular examinations has had a similar impact. The question for both techniques remains: Is there an epidemic of organic erection problems or an epidemic of organic diagnoses based on unreliable criteria? We believe that many men over 50 do have organic pathology that contributes to their sexual dysfunction, but we also advise against using any one type of assessment to make treatment decisions. Noninvasive vascular testing has had the same uncritical aceptance as NPT monitoring enjoys.

The actual research data, however, are not overwhelming. Again, circular reasoning is rife. The typical publication has been a report on a large series of men referred to a setting such as a vascular laboratory that attracts a sample at high risk for vascular diseases (Metz, 1983; Virag *et al.*, 1985; Wabrek, Shelley, Horowitz, Bastarache, & Giuca, 1983). Only men with erectile dysfunction are assessed and—lo and behold—an association is observed between erection problems and poor penile circulation.

Although we know that penile blood pressure decreases with age, control groups of older men with good erectile function have been small, even when included in studies (Abelson, 1975; Kempczinski, 1979; Kerstein, Gould, French-Sherry, & Pirman, 1982; Metz, Christensen, Mathiesen, & Ostri, 1983). How many men who would be labeled abnormal by noninvasive vascular testing actually are functioning well sexually? Better normative data are needed.

Another problem is the reliability of the tests themselves. Finding the fine penile arteries is difficult. Currently, the most popular technique is to use a Doppler ultrasound probe to measure systolic blood pressure and to record the wave pattern of blood flow in each of the four penile arteries (left and right dorsal and cavernosal) (Jevtich, 1983). Several formulae have been used to assess whether penile blood pressures are within normal limits. A conservative method is to average the pressures in all four arteries and divide that value by the brachial (arm) systolic blood pressure. If this penile/ brachial index is below 0.60, vascular pathology is likely to be present. Values above 0.80 are considered normal by most clinicians. Values between 0.60 and 0.80 are more equivocal. The Doppler probe can also be connected to a chart recorder to produce a pulse waveform on a strip of paper. The waveform can be rated as abnormal or normal using objective scoring systems that depend on its shape and amplitude (Jevtich, 1983; Metz *et al.*, 1983a; Stauffer & DePalma, 1983; Velcek, 1980).

Noninvasive testing can also be used to assess blood flow to the penis under more dynamic conditions. Like a local "stress test," these examinations measure how well the pelvic vascular system can adjust to minute-to-minute changes in blood flow during sexual arousal or movement. One such method is the hyperemic stress test (Bell, Lewis, & Kerstein, 1983). When blood flow to a distant part of the body is temporarily restricted, for example by a tourniquet, a healthy vascular system reacts with a sharp increase in blood flow as soon as the interference is removed. A blood pressure cuff is inflated around the base of the penis for 5 minutes and then released (Jevtich, 1983; Kedia, 1983b). The penile pulse waveform is recorded until the amplitude (height) of the pulse wave returns to its original level. In healthy men, the amplitude doubles after the stressor. In men with vascular disease, the pulse may not increase at all, and, if it does, it may take much longer than the normal 2 minutes to return to baseline levels.

Another kind of stress test has been used to screen for the "pelvic steal syndrome" (see Chapter 5; Goldstein *et al.*, 1982a). The examiner obtains baseline Doppler penile and brachial systolic blood pressures and then asks the patient to exercise his leg and buttock muscles. As soon as the period of exercise is over, a second set of Doppler measurements is taken. The postexercise penile/brachial index should not decrease more than 0.15 from the original ratio.

Currently, a thorough vascular evaluation might include obtaining a penile-brachial systolic index, a postexercise Doppler reading, and a post-ischemic hyperemia test. For a skilled examiner, such testing should only take perhaps 15 minutes, and can add a useful estimate of vascular capacity to the comprehensive evaluation.

Invasive Vascular Assessment of Erectile Function

The noninvasive vascular tests we have just described have the advantage of being safe and inexpensive, but their disadvantage is their question-able accuracy. Invasive examinations give far more exact information on the state of the pelvic vascular system. They are costly, however, and can have dangerous side effects. Invasive vascular testing has increased our basic knowledge about the physiology of erection. For clinical purposes, however, invasive examinations should be reserved for the small group of men who are candidates for angioplasty or reconstructive vascular surgery.

In order to visualize the arteries that bring blood to the penis, a tiny tube (catheter) must be threaded into the internal iliac artery. Usually a man is given general anesthesia and the catheters are inserted in the groin area. When older men with abnormal Doppler findings are tested, the great majority have narrowed areas or blockages in the system of arteries that brings blood to the penis (Jevtich & Maxwell, 1983).

As usual, however, we lack data on older men with good erectile function. We doubt that a one-to-one relationship exists between findings from an arteriogram and a man's sexual function. Some elderly men may maintain adequate erections in spite of having pelvic vascular disease that looks just as severe on an arteriogram as that in men selected for revascular-ization or penile prosthesis surgery (Hawatmeh, Houttuin, Gregory, & Purcell, 1983).

Since vascular disease often affects the smallest arteries just above and within the penis while the larger arteries remain free from blockage, recent efforts have concentrated on visualizing the arteries and veins within the penis itself. The blood vessels are so tiny that they are easier to see on a radiograph when they are dilated, that is, during an erection.

Jevtich and Maxwell (1983) have advocated injecting saline solution directly into one cavernous body. They recorded how much fluid was needed to produce a full erection. The resulting "artificial" erection could be measured for circumference changes and observed for signs of abnormal curvature of the penis, as in Peyronie's disease. Even if the only surgery under consideration is implantation of a prosthesis, the surgeon can benefit from knowing in advance that scarring exists. A dye can then be injected through the needle and a series of four radiographs (cavernosograms) obtained to determine the shape of cavernous bodies and to check for abnormally fast drainage through the venous system of the penis (Delcour, Wespes, Schulman, & Struyven, 1984).

Artificial erections can also be created by using an electronic pump to infuse a saline or radiographic contrast medium into the penis (Newman & Reiss, 1984). The rates of flow needed to achieve full erection and to maintain it are considered measures of the vascular system's integrity. Buvat, Lemaire, Dehaene, Buvat-Herbaut, and Guieu (1986b) have found that artificial erection is predictive of sexual dysfunction only if flow rates to maintain erection are very elevated, or if a venous abnormality is combined with an arterial or neurological deficit.

Papaverine Testing

The latest technical fad is to inject papaverine into the cavernous bodies to assess vascular erectile dysfunction. Men who have severe vascular disease should not show a normal response, that is, a full, rigid erection. Buvat, Buvat-Herbaut, Dehaene, and Lemaire (1986a) found only fair correlations with NPT testing or with invasive vascular examination results, however. A special duplex ultrasound instrument can measure how much the penile arteries dilate during a papaverine-induced erection and how fast blood flows into the penis. This test could make the penile arteriogram obsolete, since no anesthesia is needed (Lue, Hricak, Marich, & Tanagho, 1985a). Another variation is to follow the papaverine injection with an injection of radiographic contrast medium to perform a cavernosogram and monitor penile venous drainage (Lue, Hricak, Schmidt, & Tanagho, 1986). As usual, the investigators report no normative data on older men with good erectile function. Although the actual injection is not very painful, papaverine can produce local bleeding, infection, flushing and dizziness, or priapism, an erection that will not detumesce without emergency medical intervention.

Neurological Evaluation of Male Sexual Dysfunction

The complex interaction between the various parts of the nervous system in producing the normal sexual response has limited the development of useful neurological assessment devices. Most available tests measure the function of the pelvic sensory nerves. We currently have no direct way to monitor autonomic or peptidergic nerves involved in erection or ejaculation and orgasm.

Even tests of the sensory nervous system are often indirect. Sensory thresholds of the penis can be measured quite accurately by using an electrical square-wave generator attached to a hand-held stimulating electrode. The electrical signal is turned upward until the patient can feel a very mild tingling. The threshold to vibration can also be measured by using a small device that vibrates at varying frequencies. Men who have peripheral neuropathy may actually have reduced ability to sense penile touch. It is unclear how well such tests correlate with erectile function, especially since normal aging can also reduce sensory threshodls (Wagner & Green, 1981, p. 96).

Problems with the neurological control of urination and with erection often appear simultaneously in men with diabetic neuropathy or multiple sclerosis. Some researchers have used cysmetrograms, a measure of the neurologic control of bladder function, to assess erectile dysfunction, but results have been of doubtful value (Buvat et al., 1985b; Jensen et al., 1983). Although the innervations of the bladder and penis overlap, they are not identical. The test is uncomfortable and involves putting a catheter into the bladder, with the usual risks of infection and soreness afterward.

Other indirect measures of autonomic nervous system function include beat-to-beat variation of heartbeat in response to deep breathing and measures of blood pressure changes with exercise or changes in posture (Hilsted & Jensen, 1979; Jensen, 1986; Lindenberg, Hjardem, Kelbaek, Munkgaard, & Jensen, 1981; Slag et al., 1983). Tests for autonomic neuropathy were only marginally correlated with erectile function in male diabetics, however (Jensen, 1986).

Perhaps in the future we will be able to stimulate the autonomic nerves around the prostate directly with an electrical signal to produce an erection, but such techniques are still in the realm of science fiction except for experiments performed during surgery (Hager, 1983; Lue, Schmidt, & Tanagho, 1985b). The neurological tests available that monitor nerves directly involved in erection all focus on the sensory pudendal nerve or on its final branch, the dorsal nerve of the penis. None of the techniques is as simple, painless, and clearly related to erectile function as noninvasive vascular testing. The first test to be widely used was the sacral electromyogram (EMG) (Ertekin & Reel, 1976). A needle electrode is inserted into the bulbocavernosus muscle, behind the scrotum. A mild electrical shock is delivered to the glans of the penis and the speed of the reflex muscle contraction is recorded. A reflex speed that is abnormally long or an absence of reflex activity is diagnostic of pathology in the pudendal nerve reflex arc. Sacral EMG latency does not correlate one-to-one with clinical symptoms (Siroky, Sax, & Krane, 1979). Wabrek (1985) found only a 9% rate of abnormal sacral EMG tests in 100 men consecutively referred for evaluation of erectile dysfunction. Melman and Frye (1983) found that the sacral EMG results were not in agreement with other findings from a comprehensive evaluation of erectile function, including NPT monitoring and visual sexual stimulation in 46 men.

Undaunted by the limited usefulness of the sacral EMG, its proponents have gone on to complicate the procedure by adding recording electrodes over the lumbar spinal cord and on the scalp (Goldstein, 1983). Then the reflex latency can be averaged over many stimulations of the glans penis and divided into two segments: penis to sacral spinal cord and sacral cord to cortex. Normative data are available, but the subjects were all under age 40, not an ideal control group for men with erectile dysfunction (Haldeman, Bradley, Bhatia, & Johnson, 1982). The results of the evoked potential tests appear to correlate with clinical syndromes such as spinal cord injuries or neuropathies (Ertekin, Akyurekli, Gurses, & Turgut, 1985). This uncomfortable and expensive form of assessment will probably prove more useful, however, for basic research or testing of special cases than as a routine part of treatment planning.

Hormonal Evaluation of Male Sexual Dysfunction

Hormonal abnormalities are frequent enough in men with sexual problems to justify ordering screening assays as a routine part of their comprehensive medical evaluation. Nickel *et al.*, (1984) recommend a single test of serum testosterone as the most economical adjunct to a careful history and medical examination. We agree, but also suggest adding a serum prolactin assay when symptoms include a global loss of sexual desire or a loss of ability to reach orgasm. Buvat *et al.* (1985a) advocate prolactin testing in all men with erectile dysfunction, since a man with a prolactin-secreting tumor occasionally has a normal testosterone value. Some centers routinely screen levels of FSH and LH. Since such tests do add up in expense, we prefer to reserve them for cases in which the testosterone value is abnormal and a more definitive workup is needed.

The Utility of the Comprehensive Medical Workup for Male Sexual Dysfunction

The array of technology available to evaluate male sexual dysfunction is so impressive that it is easy to lose sight of the goal. How useful are all these tests in determining the best treatment? The literature is full of anecdotes and even some studies (Blaivas, Nagler, White, & Barbalias, 1982; Schiavi *et al.*, 1985) suggesting that sex therapy often effectively remedies sexual problems even when organic causes have been identified. Yet in the United States, men are so accustomed now to medical solutions for erection problems that psychotherapy is seldom offered or accepted as a treatment if a suspicion of physiological pathology exists. Even when men are referred for psychotherapy, insurance companies pay limited mental health benefits compared with their good coverage of costly elective operations.

Some examinations are performed because they are intrinsically interesting to the physician or researcher performing the workup. What use is it, however, to put a 63-year-old man through the pain and expense of an arteriogram when his only medical treatment option with a good chance of success is a penile prosthesis? What does a penile cerebral evoked potential test add to our rehabilitation plans for a man with multiple sclerosis or a spinal cord injury other than several hundred dollars in medical bills and 2 hours of discomfort?

We hope that our review of available tests will help clinicians choose those that are practical and relevant considering a patient's medical history. Many centers have published their suggested medical evaluation for erectile dysfunction. Table 6-2 summarizes our current beliefs about the elements of a comprehensive medical screening.

Specialized Examinations for Female Sexual Dysfunction

In comparing the lack of progress in medical evaluation of women's sexual problems with the sophisticated technology developed for men, we do not know whether to be indignant or relieved. Without the impetus of a medical treatment like the penile prosthesis, less attention has been given to solving the problems of measuring female sexual arousal and orgasmic potential.

Table 6-2. Suggested Screening Evaluation for Erectile Dysfunction

---

Medical history
Thorough physical examination
Routine blood chemistry
Serum testosterone
Elicitation of genital reflexes
Measurement of genital sensory threshold
Doppler penile/brachial index
Postexercise Doppler index
Penile postischemic hyperemia
Dacomed snap-gauge or Rigiscan testing for 2 nights
Visual or vibratory sexual stimulation in the laboratory

Women are also socialized to look for emotional solutions to relationship issues rather than technical answers.

With demographic and attitudinal shifts, however, more sexually active women are postmenopausal and more may be vulnerable to chronic illnesses such as cardiovascular disease. Without "medicalizing" women's sexual problems to an unhealthy degree, we could still devote more attention to identifying the role of hormonal, vascular, and neurologic factors in causing dysfunction. New medical treatments may be an outgrowth of better knowledge.

Hormonal Assessment and Female Sexual Function

The decision to prescribe estrogen replacement for a postmenopausal woman is usually based on her medical history, risk for osteoporosis or cardiovascular disease, and clinical symptoms such as hot flashes or vaginal atrophy and dryness. Sometimes estrogen or LH and FSH levels are measured in a perimenopausal woman to see whether ovarian failure has begun. At our current state of knowledge, knowing precise levels of serum estrogen, androgens, and progesterone does not help a clinician understand the cause of a woman's sexual problem.

Vascular Assessment of Female Sexual Function

Why do some postmenopausal women and diabetic women (Schreiner-Engel *et al.*, 1985) experience more vaginal atrophy and loss of lubrication capacity than others? Is it a hormonal difference, perhaps based on percentage of body fat, or is it a difference in the health of the pelvic vasculature or the neurologic control of vaginal blood flow? We do not have a way to measure vaginal blood flow in the resting state, analogous to the Doppler penile pressure and flow measures. Changes in vaginal blood flow can be monitored, but only during sleep or sexual arousal, and the clinical significance of individual differences in women is still a mystery.

Many women with sexual problems are not willing to have their vaginal blood flow measured during a period of erotic stimulation in the laboratory. Those who do volunteer to undergo testing while masturbating, watching an erotic film, or having a sexual fantasy may not be able to achieve high levels of arousal, particularly if sexual anxieties or a lack of desire for sex are their presenting complaints. If vaginal blood flow does not increase with erotic stimulation, the cause might just as well be psychological as physiological.

Even in women who can get aroused in the laboratory, measuring vaginal blood flow changes is problematic. The most common instrument used is a vaginal photoplethysmograph. The patient can insert this tampon-shaped probe in privacy into her own vagina. The photoplethysmograph measures light reflected from the vaginal walls, which darken in color with increased blood flow (Semmlow & Lubowsky, 1983). Unfortunately, the photoplethys-mograph is quite sensitive to movement and, because of interference from pelvic muscle contractions, may not be able to measure blood flow changes at high levels of excitement (Amberson & Hoon, 1985). The reliability of the probe itself has also been questioned (Beck, Sakheim, & Barlow, 1983).

A device less sensitive to movement is the heated oxygen electrode, which measures changes in vaginal temperature and surface oxygen during sexual arousal (Amberson & Hoon, 1985; Levin & Wagner, 1985). These indirect indicators of vaginal blood flow can be measured accurately throughout the sexual response cycle, including orgasm. However, the electrode cannot be used for more than an hour or two because the suction device holding it to the vaginal wall may cause irritation. The electrode thus is not suitable for sleep studies.

Other researchers have tried to measure temperature within the vagina (Fugl-Meyer, Sjögren, & Johansson, 1984) or in the labia (Henson, Rubin, & Henson, 1982) as a reflection of blood flow. No ideal measure has yet been found (Hoon, 1984).

If vaginal blood flow changes analogous to NPT episodes occur during REM sleep, a more acceptable test for physical abnormalities might be developed. In fact, increases in vaginal blood flow have been recorded during REM sleep using measures of vaginal temperature (Fisher *et al.*, 1983) and pulse amplitude (Rogers, Van de Castle, Evans, & Critelli, 1985). Studies are needed comparing women with good sexual function to women at high risk for pelvic vascular problems, such as diabetics or women with postmenopausal vaginal atrophy (Semmens *et al.*, 1985).

Neurological Assessment of Female Sexual Function

The technology used to diagnose neurological causes of sexual dysfunction in men has rarely been applied to women. Sensory thresholds of various parts of the female genitals have not been carefully measured. The bulboca-vernosus reflex can be elicited in a woman by pinching the glans of the clitoris. Brindley and Gillan (1982) claimed that absence of the reflex was highly predictive of failure to become orgasmic during behavioral sex ther-apy for lifelong inorgasmia. However, other researchers, using more precise measurement techniques, have not found the female bulbocavernosus reflex diagnostically helpful. Blaivas, Zayed, and Labib (1981) found that results of both manual and EMG tests of the bulbocavernosus reflex were normal unless a lesion existed in the sacral spinal cord, but that the tests were less reliable in women than in men. Haldeman *et al.* (1982) found that women's cortical evoked responses to stimulation of the clitoris were not as marked as men's cerebral responses to a penile stimulus. They believe the difference resulted from technical difficulties in stimulating the pudendal nerve accu-rately in a woman.

One other approach to measuring sensory nerve function is to monitor contractions of the pelvic muscles during sexual arousal and orgasm using a pressure-sensitive probe placed in the anus or vagina (Bohlen *et al.*, 1982). Although this technology is promising, these measures, too, must take place during sexual stimulation, limiting applicability in medical settings.

Indirect measures of peripheral sensory or autonomic neuropathy in diabetic women have not been useful in predicting sexual function (Jensen, 1986; Tyrer *et al.*, 1983). Perhaps when the role of neurological mechanisms in promoting vaginal expansion and lubrication and female orgasm is better understood, clinically useful examinations will be developed.

7

Counseling for Sexual Problems in Medical Patients

Once an assessment is complete, the clinician must decide what kind of treatment to offer. If the answer is psychotherapy, should counseling be conducted by one therapist or a cotherapy team? Are couple sessions optimal, or would individual or group therapy be more helpful? Will a few sessions be enough, or is a formal, longer-term treatment program needed? Could the therapist be a member of the primary care team, or are the issues so complex that the case should be referred to a mental health specialist with training in sexual counseling? This chapter addresses the selection of treatment format when psychotherapy is the chosen modality and then describes techniques of sexual counseling both for the typical brief therapy case and for the patient who needs intensive therapy.

LEVELS OF THERAPEUTIC INTENSITY

As Jack Annon (Annon & Robinson, 1978) has pointed out, clinicians treating a sexual problem can intervene on several levels of therapeutic intensity. Annon's PLISSIT model of sexual counseling identifies four levels of intervention. *Permission* is the process of encouraging a patient to discuss a sexual problem. We have already discussed the permission level of counseling in the previous chapter. Annon's next level is giving *limited information* to the patient, such as educating a couple about the sexual response cycle or telling them about the sexual side effects of a medical treatment. Therapy intensifies when the clinician also provides *specific suggestions*, such as instructing the couple in sensate focus techniques or helping a patient find comfortable positions for intercourse after a back injury. Annon's final level of intervention is *intensive therapy*, corresponding to formal treatment programs for sexual dysfunction such as those used by sex therapists.

Annon's model provides a good description of treatment options for sexual problems in medical patients. We find, however, that the limited information and specific suggestion levels can be combined into a treatment category we call *brief sexual counseling*. Such therapy is primarily educational in nature and is the appropriate treatment for the large majority of patients seen in medical settings, that is, men and women who have good relationships but are undergoing sexual or marital stress related to an illness. Their anxieties and sexual problems can usually be ameliorated in fewer than five counseling sessions. Members of the primary care team can learn to provide brief sexual counseling, although basic skills in interviewing patients and in handling sexual issues are necessary.

Intensive therapy is the province of the mental health clinician who has training in sex and marital therapy. Patients should be referred to a specialist if they have had chronic sexual dysfunctions or marital conflicts; if they have a history of a major psychiatric disorder, chronic substance abuse, or appear to be psychologically fragile; if they have undergone an illness with a severely debilitating impact on sexuality, (e.g., becoming quadriplegic or having radical pelvic cancer surgery); or if brief counseling fails to remedy a sexual problem.

After deciding on the intensity of therapy, the clinician must consider the format of the sessions. How many therapists and how many patients should be present?

SINGLE THERAPIST VERSUS COTHERAPY TEAM

Masters and Johnson (1970) created sex therapy using the cotherapy model. They believed that each partner in a heterosexual patient couple needed a same-sex therapist as an advocate. We do not regard the need for cotherapy in such absolute terms. Cotherapy teams in fact have both advantages and drawbacks, whether the treatment modality is sex therapy, marital work, or family therapy.

Cotherapy is a luxury for two therapists who work well together. They can combine impressions of a case and help each other through difficult moments in the session. While one focuses on the couple's verbal interaction, the other clinician can tune in to nonverbal cues, entering into the process when a different perspective is needed. Cotherapy is also an excellent vehicle for training. Two inexperienced therapists can join forces in practicing new techniques. Their separate views of the session provide rich material for supervision.

Cotherapy is not a panacea, however. Perhaps its most salient disadvantage is its expense. In the United States, cotherapy has become a luxury, affordable only for training clinics or for private practitioners with a very wealthy clientele. When cotherapists' styles diverge, cotherapy can also become a liability. If one therapist is much more active and directive, the second may feel angry and excluded. A novice may also be intimidated to the point of paralysis by seeing cases with an experienced and self-confident clinician. When both therapists are used to taking an active stance, combining forces may result in a power struggle to direct the session. To an observer, the patient becomes an audience for the cotherapists rather than being the focus of the treatment.

We do agree with Masters and Johnson's idea that a cotherapy team for a sex therapy case should include a male and a female clinician. Imagine a heterosexual couple seeking treatment for the man's erection problem. The husband would probably feel outnumbered by his wife plus two female therapists. Gender issues are even more obvious in the case of a woman with an orgasmic dysfunction being seen in couple therapy by two male therapists. Perhaps an exception might be a homosexual couple, who could feel comfortable with two same-sex therapists.

A few studies have examined the effectiveness of a single therapist versus a cotherapy team in remediating sexual dysfunctions. J. LoPiccolo, Heiman, Hogan, and Roberts (1985) and Arentewicz and Schmidt (1983) found that outcomes were equivalent with a single therapist or cotherapists. J. LoPiccolo *et al.* (1985) also carefully controlled for the gender of the single therapist, balancing it against the gender of the partner in the couple who had an identified sexual problem. Therapist gender did not predict treatment outcome. Although these studies suggest that cotherapy has no measurable advantage, all therapists were working in training settings where extensive team supervision was the rule. We must be cautious in extrapolating the findings to the more common setting, where each therapist depends exclusively on his or her own clinical judgment.

CHOOSING AMONG INDIVIDUAL, COUPLE, AND GROUP MODALITIES

Although sex therapy was built around a couple-treatment format, clinicians soon discovered that patients do not always appear with a convenient significant other. Masters and Johnson, believing strongly that couple therapy was the only effective way to treat sexual dysfunction, tried providing sexual surrogate partners for patients who could not supply a spouse or lover. They, and other clinicians, became disenchanted by the legal and ethical complications inherent in finding a sexual partner for a patient, although a few centers still use surrogates (Apfelbaum, 1984). In a medical setting the use of surrogate sexual partners would be even rarer than in an unaffiliated sexuality clinic or in a private practice. Even when the surrogate is a trained body therapist, the question remains whether experience with an expert sexual partner who is paid to be supportive will alleviate anxiety in the more usual situations of meeting a potential mate and initiating a sexual relationship.

Individual and group therapy have been used successfully as alternatives to the couple format in treating sexual dysfunctions (Mills & Kilmann,

1982; Zilbergeld, 1980). An individual approach is not only a way to offer help to a man or woman who is not in a committed relationship; for some patients, individual therapy is the treatment of choice for a sexual dysfunction. Patients with poor social skills or a low tolerance for intimacy may need help just to prepare for having a sexual relationship. Individual therapy can also give a patient the time and freedom to work through a past sexual trauma before focusing on current relationship issues.

Terry, a 35-year-old homemaker with three children, was referred to a psychologist after cryosurgery for dysplasia. Terry complained that dyspareunia was ruining her sex life with her husband, Will. Terry and Will had separated after he got drunk and beat her so severely that she had to be hospitalized for a concussion. Now, 2 years later, Will was back living with his family, but had not made a commitment to stay. The physical violence had not recurred, but Will continued binge drinking and became angry and verbally abusive to Terry when he was intoxicated.

On questioning, Terry said that the dyspareunia had been noticeable for 3 years, beginning during her last pregnancy. Pain occurred not only during sexual intercourse, but also episodically several times weekly, limiting Terry's ability to keep up with household chores and to care for her children.

Terry mentioned spontaneously in the assessment interview that her father had died when she was an infant. She told the therapist, with a grimace, that her mother's second marriage was to a man who was an alcoholic. Picking up on Terry's nonverbal cues, the therapist asked if the stepfather had molested her sexually. It turned out that Terry had been coerced into an incestuous relationship from age 11 to 15, when she left her mother's house to live with an aunt. Will knew about the incest, but did not believe it explained Terry's pain, since she had enjoyed sex when the couple first married.

The therapist believed, however, that the history of incest was significant. In fact, Terry's pain began when her oldest daughter showed signs of puberty. Terry feared that Will might molest their daughter, and kept constant vigilance over the situation, although she never discussed it with her husband.

Individual therapy sessions with Terry focused on her tendency to put herself in a victim role and to use physical pain to ask for nurturance instead of being assertive about her needs. Experimental techniques, such as speaking to the empty chair or writing a letter from her adult self to her child self, helped Terry resolve her feelings about the incest. Although her pain improved, she and Will continued to argue about sexual frequency. At that point in treatment, the therapist invited Will to come in and began to use sex therapy techniques with Terry and Will as a couple.

Individual sex therapy includes the use of behavioral homework exercises, just as in joint sex therapy. Without an available partner, however, the body work often centers on self-stimulation.

Greg, a 19-year-old student, lost a leg at age 15 in a motorcycle accident. Although he was well-liked on campus and sang in his college glee club, Greg rarely dated. He worried that women would spend time with him out of pity rather than because they felt attracted to him.

Greg had attempted to have intercourse on only one occasion and had ejaculated prematurely. Greg needed some basic information on sexuality and a chance to role play meeting women and asking for a date. Once he began to have a more active social life, the therapist provided support and encouragement for Greg's efforts to keep sexual experimentation to a comfortable pace. Greg used techniques to delay ejaculation in a series of masturbation exercises (Zilbergeld, 1978). He was later able to learn to delay ejaculation during sexual activity with a partner.

Group therapy has also produced good results when used to treat sexual dysfunctions (Mills & Kilmann, 1982). Group members may be men or women who have similar sexual problems (Andersen, 1983) or couples who are trying to improve their sexual communication and enrich their sex lives (J. LoPiccolo & Miller, 1978).

In medical settings, group sex therapy not only is economical and effective for patients without partners, but also can promote peer support among men and women who have experienced similar medical problems. The potential of groups in providing sexual education and treating sexual dysfunctions has rarely been tapped for medical patients. Christensen (1983) describes a four-session group for mastectomy patients and their husbands. It would be simple and logical to add sexuality "modules" to patient education and family support groups in cancer centers, cardiac rehabilitation programs, ostomy societies, diabetes clinics, and other similar settings.

When behavioral homework exercises are assigned to group members, their experiences with the assignment are discussed at the next meeting. Comparing notes enhances the opportunities for learning, because some patients find the homework helpful while others cannot carry it out or do so only with difficulty.

Women in a group for mastectomy patients were asked to spend 15 minutes at home viewing themselves nude in the mirror. They were instructed to focus on their whole body, not just on the mastectomy scar, and to find three things that were attractive about their appearance.

Four of the women carried out the exercise with no difficulty. They felt saddened by their loss of a breast but could also see good things about their bodies. One woman did not find time during the week to do the homework, and the group helped her to disclose her fears about really looking at herself. The sixth group member had spent half an hour crying after the exercise— the first time she had allowed herself to cry in the 4 months since her surgery. Her experience led into a discussion of the need to mourn for a lost body part and of the reactions of the women's husbands or lovers to their sadness after mastectomy.

As we go on to decribe techniques of brief sexual counseling and intensive sex therapy for patients with chronic illnesses, we usually focus on couple therapy. Readers should be aware, however, that the same homework exercises or ways of interacting with patients can easily be modified for use in an individual or group format.

BRIEF SEXUAL COUNSELING FOR MEDICAL PATIENTS

Brief sexual counseling is the most common type of psychotherapy we use with patients who have a chronic disease. Brief sexual counseling includes several components that can be combined to fit patients' needs: educating patients about effects of illness and medical treatment on sexual function; helping patients change their maladaptive beliefs about sexuality and illness; encouraging couples to resume noncoital and coital sexual activity by prescribing sensate focus exercises and enhancing sexual communication skills; resolving mild couple conflict related to illness; and teaching patients to minimize distraction from physical handicaps such as dyspareunia, limited strength or range of motion, alterations in sexual function, or ostomy appliances, urinary catheters, limb prostheses, and so on.

Brief sexual counseling can usually be accomplished in one to five therapy sessions. Because this type of intervention is most appropriate for patients who are coping adequately with their illness and have stable relationships or social support, brief counseling can often be successfully provided by a member of the primary care team such as a physician, physician's assistant, nurse, medical social worker, or even a physical or occupational therapist. If a trained sex therapist is available and the primary care team does not want to assume responsibility for brief counseling, then the specialist can provide such limited intervention as well as offer intensive sex therapy.

Sex Education

Perhaps the most crucial task of brief sexual counseling is to help men and women understand their own reproductive physiology and the impact that an illness or medical treatment has had on it. Sex education has a long history in sexology; in fact in many nonindustrialized nations providing knowledge about contraception, abortion, and the sexual rights of minorities is still the primary task.

Even in the United States and Europe, sexual knowledge in the general population lags far behind the level of information easily available in the media. For example, a Danish survey of 40-year-old women revealed that a third could not explain the origin of menstrual blood (Garde & Lunde, 1982). In our clinical experience, men rarely know the prostate's location or sexual function and women often cannot find the clitoris and are surprised to learn that their vaginas expand during sexual arousal. We cannot thus assume that our patients understand basic genital anatomy or function.

Sexual education is best provided to both partners in a couple simultaneously, so that they share all new information. Support groups for patients or couples with a particular illness are ideal settings for presenting educational material on sexuality and illness and then leading a discussion of members' personal experiences and emotional reactions.

Because genital and pelvic anatomy is confusing to patients, we begin education with a brief review of each part and its function during the sexual response cycle. For women we include the vulva, labia, clitoris, urethra, vagina, anus, cervix, uterus, ovaries, and fallopian tubes. For men we discuss the penis, urethra, prostate, seminal vesicles, vasa deferens, Cowper's gland, anus, and the functions of the testicles in producing sperm cells and testosterone. We find it most helpful to use lifelike genital models* to illustrate the various areas. Many patients, especially women, have never viewed their own genitals carefully in a mirror. Looking at the models and touching them has a desensitizing effect. If the clinician has no model available, photographs and diagrams can be used instead from the many sexuality texts in print. We then suggest that the partners try genital self-examination at home and afterward give each other "guided tours" of their genital anatomy.

We use the simplest language we can to explain how hormones do or do not influence sexual desire, what produces an erection, how the vagina and external genitals swell and lubricate during sexual arousal, the process of orgasm and the normalcy of coital and noncoital orgasms, and the resolution phase. We often turn to the patient or couple with questions about their experiences to see if they have understood us:

• Have you noticed a few drops of moisture at the tip of your penis before you ejaculate?
• Has your vagina ever felt tight and dry when you began intercourse?
• Have you ever seen your cervix in a mirror during a pelvic examination?

This discussion is an excellent time to assess patients' attitudes about masturbation or variety in sexual caressing and their ability to talk openly about sex. Changes in genital anatomy or function as a result of illness, surgery, or medication can also be explained as an integral part of the lesson:

---

*A catalogue is available from Jim Jackson & Company, 33 Richdale Avenue, Cambridge, MA, 02140.

Clinician: When you had your fibroid tumors, your uterus was enlarged. They grew inside it, here. Some women find intercourse painful when they have large fibroids. How was it for you? Did any one position hurt less than another? Do you still have pain now that you've had your hysterectomy?

Of course your uterus and cervix were removed, but because you are not due for menopause for another 10 years, we left your ovaries and fallopian tubes in place. Your ovaries will continue to make the hormones estrogen and progesterone. Those hormones circulate in your bloodstream, helping your vagina stay stretchy and produce moisture during sexual excitement. Estrogen also protects you from osteoporosis by keeping your bones strong and prevents hardening of the arteries.

Not only will your sexual desire remain normal now that you've had a hysterectomy, but you also should be able to reach orgasm just as easily as ever, and your pleasure will feel the same. How did you usually reach an orgasm before your hysterectomy? Have your orgasms changed in any way?

Some clinicians prefer to use slide shows or films to educate patients about sexual anatomy and function. We like the tactile dimension of the models and the opportunity to interact with the couple along the way as we present new information. A film or slides can be helpful supplements, however. When patients are undergoing mutilating surgery, such as a vulvectomy or an abdominoperineal resection, seeing photos of how the area looks after healing can benefit them, especially if the partner has not been encouraged to view the surgical scars during hospitalization.

A few sex therapists have advocated giving couples a sexological examination (Hartman & Fithian, 1972). Each partner in turn is put on the examining table and the clinician illustrates how the genitals function, using a mirror so that both patient and partner can see. The clinician actually stimulates the genital area to produce erection or vaginal expansion and lubrication, or asks the partner to do so. We think such examinations are often unnecessarily intrusive. They are most natural and helpful when the clinician is a physician or nurse and uses the examination to show patient and partner changes that have occurred after an illness or treatment. Even then, we think the couple will benefit most if explanations with genital models are used first to prepare the couple for the in-person inspection. After the examination, time should be set aside to discuss emotional reactions.

Timely education can prevent anxiety that interferes with a patient's resuming sex or actually causes a sexual dysfunction.

Morton, a retired salesman, had an uneventful recovery after a transurethral prostatectomy. On his return visit, however, he complained to his surgeon that his sex life was ruined. "I wish I'd never let you talk me into this operation!"

The surgeon asked what the actual problem was. Morton was afraid that he would be unable to have erections and so had only initiated sex once since surgery. Although he was able to have intercourse, he was surprised by his dry orgasm in spite of having signed an informed consent form before surgery that stated he understood the likelihood of having retrograde ejaculation.

The surgeon called in Morton's wife and went through the procedure again for the couple, using a cross-sectional model to explain why retrograde ejaculation occurred and what happened to the semen. He explained that the feeling of orgasm might be different, but should still be satisfying. He reassured the couple that a transurethral prostatectomy does not impair erections. Both partners thanked the doctor and a week later Morton called to say that sex was back to normal.

Education can also be used to alert a patient that a new medication could have sexual side effects. Physicians often hesitate to mention such a possibility, fearing that patients will become anxious and develop a psychogenic sexual problem. We believe that excessive anxiety can be avoided, however, if the patient is told that the sexual problem is uncommon and can be treated by reducing the dosage or changing the type of medication. Then the patient is more likely to ask for help for a sexual dysfunction instead of being bewildered or angry.

Judith had been on a tricyclic antidepressant for 2 months when she requested that her psychiatrist meet with her and her husband, Paul. Judith and Paul agreed that her depression had lifted greatly, but were upset because on their first attempt at sexual activity for several months, Judith had vaginal dryness and pain. She had never experienced such problems before and said that her desire for sex had returned to normal levels. Paul, however, was afraid that he had rushed his wife into resuming sex before she was ready.

The psychiatrist told the couple that Judith's medication could be reducing vaginal lubrication. She gave the couple samples of some lubricants to try and also reduced Judith's antidepressant dose. As Judith's need for medication decreased, the couple reported that her lubrication had returned to normal, but that they kept a lubricant in their bedside drawer, "just in case."

Changing Sexual Attitudes and Beliefs

Educational approaches are also useful when patients hold maladaptive beliefs or attitudes about sexuality and illness. Examples include accepting myths about sexuality and illness, as discussed in Chapter 4, or having a narrow concept of sexual normalcy. In Chapter 2 we pointed out that couples cope well with an illness when they can be playful in their sex lives, regard intercourse as just one aspect of a good sexual interaction, and are willing to experiment with a variety of sexual techniques.

Educational books or films on sexuality can be helpful therapeutic adjuncts when couples maintain a performance-oriented, intercourse-centered model of sex that does not leave room for fatigue or disability. The power of the media rests in reassuring people that sexual attitudes and practices are extremely diverse.

Clinicians can also use cognitive-behavioral techniques to alter patients' beliefs and self-statements. One homework assignment is for a man or woman to monitor and record all automatic, irrational thoughts about sex, such as:

- A man should always have an erection during lovemaking.
- Sex is a failure unless both partners reach orgasm.
- If we can't have intercourse, it's not worthwhile to get aroused.
- No man would want a woman with an ostomy.
- People over 65 shouldn't care about sex anymore.

Once the thoughts have been identified, partners can collaborate to create adaptive self-statements to replace them, for instance:

- Sex feels good whether or not the man has an erection.
- I don't always have to have an orgasm to feel sexually satisfied.
- Sex can be fun even without intercourse.
- My ostomy covers a few square inches of my body. The rest of me looks as good as ever.
- Sex is part of life no matter how old you are.

The partners can practice summoning up these positive beliefs about sexuality as they try out new sexual behaviors. They can remind each other not to fall into negative thinking in sexual situations.

When only one partner in a couple believes a sexual myth, counseling can often be short and effective.

Henry owned a small grocery in a rural town. In his mid-50s, Henry had been a bachelor until 8 years previously when he married Lisa, a widow who was 10 years younger. Henry sought help for an erection problem after reading a newspaper article about penile revascularization. Henry had mild hypertension, well-controlled by diet and a thiazide diuretic.

Henry and Lisa were referred by the local vascular surgeon to a university-based sexual dysfunction clinic. Henry was surprised that his wife was to be included in the assessment, especially since he had not discussed the problem with Lisa at all. She agreed to accompany him, after he explained the chain of events, but told Henry that she thought the idea of surgery was ridiculous.

At the interview, Henry complained that his erections did not occur spontaneously anymore and hung at an angle instead of standing out straight. He feared that Lisa would leave him for a man her own age if he was not the "bull" she married. Lisa was able to assure Henry that he was her beloved husband, and she had no thoughts of leaving. She told him he was the best lover she could imagine and that she enjoyed caressing his penis until it became erect. Effects of aging on men's erections were also explained to the couple.

At 1-year follow-up, Henry and Lisa phoned in to cancel their appointment. They were busy in the store, but wanted the therapist to know that they had very pleasurable sex once or twice a week and had almost forgotten their visit to the clinic until they received the appointment card for their return visit.

Changing patients' attitudes becomes a sticky issue when therapist and patient see sexuality from different religious or cultural contexts. Sometimes, however, the clinician can respect the patient's beliefs but still help him or her view a sexual problem from a different perspective:

Achmed was a university student from a wealthy Arab family. He lived in the college dormitory but socialized mainly with other Arab students. A year before his assessment, Achmed had sustained multiple fractures in an auto accident. He was seen by a neurologist after his recovery because he still had frequent headaches, fatigue, and difficulty concentrating. A computerized tomographic (CT) scan of the brain was normal, as was a complete neurological examination. The neurologist discovered, however, that Achmed was very concerned about erectile dysfunction, and so referred the young man to a sex therapy clinic.

Achmed told the sex therapist that he had only had two sexual experiences with a partner. In his homeland he was taken at age 16 by his father and older brothers to a brothel for his sexual initiation. He was unable to get an erection, and while he was lying despondently in the prostitute's bed, a hanging carpet was shoved aside, allowing his family members to laugh at Achmed's shame. A year later he had a similar fiasco when he went to a house of prostitution while traveling with pals in Europe. He had not made any further attempts at sexual intercourse for 5 years.

Achmed reported that he almost always felt sexually frustrated and had daily, full, waking erections, even after his accident. He did not masturbate because he believed that it not only was unmanly, but could also cause spinal curvature and hairy palms.

Achmed was given education about sexual anxiety and arousal. He was also told that physiological tests showed his sexual function to be normal. Although the clinician discussed medical facts about masturbation with Achmed, he made no effort to get the young man to try self-stimulation, though normally that might be a first step in an individual treatment program. In fact, Achmed was so elated by the knowledge that he was physically normal that he decided to try dating for a while rather than beginning sex therapy. He almost danced out of the clinic. Several months later he reported that he had had several successful sexual experiences. His headaches and fatigue had disappeared and he was doing well in his college courses.

Helping Couples Stay Sexually Active

When a patient becomes ill or undergoes a medical treatment such as surgery or cancer chemotherapy, the frequency of sexual activity often decreases sharply. Many couples do not experience an actual sexual dysfunction, but one or both partners fear that sexual activity would be unhealthy. Sometimes the trauma and physical weakness of the illness leave little energy for sexual interaction. Because many illnesses are chronic, the couple needs to adapt and resume normal life activities.

Brief sexual counseling can often help patients resume their sex lives. The sensate focus exercises that are the keystone of most sex therapy programs (H. S. Kaplan, 1974; Masters & Johnson, 1970) provide an ideal framework for returning to sexual activity in a gradual, unpressured way.

Sensate focus exercises require each partner to take turns giving and receiving touch, always focusing on one's own pleasurable sensations. At first the breasts and genitals are off limits for the touching, removing pressure for the partners to become sexually aroused. Orgasms are also banned during initial sensate focus exercises, and the session is not to lead into sexual activity of a more genital sort. As the couple relaxes and becomes comfortable with the intimacy and sensual pleasure of touch, the breasts and genitals are gradually included in the areas to be caressed. First, these zones are just to be explored with brief, light touch. In later sessions partners can help each other reach orgasm through manual or oral stimulation.

Vaginal penetration is the next step, but the man is instructed to lie still while the woman, sitting on top of him, gently places his penis in her vagina. After a few moments in which both partners focus on the sensation of penetration without movement, the couple disengages and continues the session with touching, as before. The next try at penetration, in a subsequent session, can include gentle pelvic thrusting by the woman, but unrestricted intercourse is not included until both partners are ready for it.

Sensate focus exercises are modified slightly in treatment programs for inability to reach orgasm, erectile dysfunction, premature ejaculation, or dyspareunia, but the basic sequence described above is usually maintained. For couples without sexual dysfunction who are just trying to feel comfortable sexually after an illness, some steps can be combined, depending on the partners' responses to the sessions.

Table 7-1 presents written instructions for the first sensate focus exercise, which could be given to a couple to take home. Although a series of sensate focus sessions is often presented in self-help books (e.g., Schover, 1984, pp. 187–193), we believe couples are most likely to follow instructions accurately when the clinician presents the exercise in the session, allowing time to make sure that the couple understands and to elicit their comments and questions. Clinicians who have never given instructions on sensate focus can practice by tape recording themselves 10 times, using slightly different versions of the initial exercise procedure to find the most comfortable format.

When a clinician assigns a sensate focus exercise, the next session should begin with a detailed discussion of where each partner touched the other, caresses that were pleasurable and those that were aversive, emotional reactions, and erotic zones. Any problems in carrying out the exercise should be analyzed so that next week's assignment can be designed to avoid the same obstacles. We often ask patients to keep a diary of when the session occurred, types of touching used, thoughts and feelings during the session, and ratings from 1 to 10 of their own sensual pleasure and their estimates of the partner's degree of pleasure. An alternative is to have each partner draw his or her own body from a front and back view, using colored crayons to represent the degree of pleasure felt from touch in various zones. The partners can also draw each other in the same way, guessing how the mate would color his or her pleasure.

Clinicians and patients can underestimate the difficulty of sensate focus. The exercises sound simple but often evoke intense emotions.

Aaron and Wendy had been married for 36 years when he was diagnosed as having cancer of the rectum and had an abdominoperineal resection. Wendy was present while Aaron learned colostomy care, but he felt self-conscious about his pouch when the two were lying in bed or kissing.

To help the couple feel comfortable again with intimate touch, they were assigned sensate focus exercises. The first two sessions, not including genital caressing, were very positive experiences for both partners. They felt closer than they had in months and Aaron forgot he was wearing an ostomy appliance during moments of the second session.

When genital touch was to be added to the instructions, Aaron and Wendy were cautioned not to focus on those areas, but just to explore them briefly, learning what kinds of sensations each could experience. Wendy began in the "giver" role. When she lightly stroked Aaron's penis, her husband sat up abruptly and said he had had enough. He would not discuss his negative reaction until the therapy session, when he revealed that the touch had evoked intense anxiety about whether his erections would recover after surgery. He felt that "all this touching" was useless unless he could have intercourse again.

The therapist helped Wendy express her anger at Aaron's emotional withdrawal, leading to a problem-solving discussion of how Aaron could enlist his wife's help the next time he became anxious instead of shutting her out.

Another technique that can help couples resume sex is communication training. Many partners never discuss sex verbally and rarely even give each other nonverbal cues about the kinds of sexual touching that would feel best. They have evolved a stereotyped sexual routine that is satisfying enough so that neither is willing to take a risk to change it. As we discussed in Chapter 2, when an illness disrupts that routine, such couples lack the skills to be flexible and try having sex in a new way. Sometimes intercourse is made difficult or impossible by an organic impairment of erection or by dyspareunia, but partners could enjoy noncoital caressing to orgasm.

The key to changing a sexual routine is good communication. Communication training includes role-playing exercises during therapy sessions and homework assignments. We counsel couples to be specific in asking for the type of touch they would prefer. We show them how to guide the partner's hand in where and how to caress. We suggest they find comfortable words to use in referring to genital zones so that they can ask to be touched verbally. Requests should be framed positively, rather than in a "don't do that" mode. Sexual communication should focus on the present rather than bringing up the partner's past failures and shortcomings. Partners should show appreciation to one another for efforts to change.

Sometimes we ask one partner to give the other a hand or foot massage during a counseling session, instructing the partner receiving touch to guide the giver verbally and nonverbally. We can observe the effectiveness of the partners' communication and help them try new techniques when the message fails to get across. As part of sensate focus exercises, we often ask the receiver to describe for the giver the three most enjoyable caresses used and the one touch that was least preferred (Table 7-1). In early sensate focus sessions we limit communication to a period after the touching. Later, however, verbal and nonverbal communication are encouraged during the exercise.

Couples may benefit from role playing in the therapy session how they would like the partner to initiate sex, or how to ask for a new type of sexual stimulation. Not only is the skill of asking emphasized, but also each partner's right to refuse a sexual request.

Resolving Mild Couple Conflict

Because an illness disturbs couples' daily lives, partners who normally get along well find themselves irritated with or withdrawn from each other. To assess the impact of an illness on a couple's allocation of everyday tasks and

Table 7-1. Sensate Focus Instructions

This is an exercise designed to help couples enrich their ways of touching each other and tune in to the pleasurable feelings they can experience all over their bodies. This exercise should be done at least two times before you move on to the next step in the program.

Setting the Scene

This exercise will take about an hour of your time. Often couples find that they need to plan ahead and make a date to do the exercise together. You might want to take turns in planning time to do the exercise. Before you start actually touching each other, it is nice to set this special time apart from the rest of your daily routine. Some couples do that by spending some time relaxing before the hour that they schedule together. You might want to take a shower together, take a bubble bath, put candles in your bedroom, or put soft music on your record player. The partner who schedules the exercise should also be the one responsible for setting the scene. This exercise should be done in a private place where you will not be interrupted. If you feel comfortable together in the nude, you will probably want to do this exercise with all of your clothes off. If nudity does not feel comfortable for you, you might want to keep on some underwear.

Instructions for the Exercise

In this exercise, you are going to take turns being the giver and the receiver. The person who is the receiver starts by lying on his or her stomach. The giver is going to spend at least 15 minutes touching the receiver all over the back of the body. In this exercise, however, we are going to ask you not to touch your partner's breasts or genital area.

Your job as receiver is just to tune in to the feelings you experience in your body. Notice the places that you like to be touched, and the kinds of touch that are most pleasant for you. You do not have to worry about whether your partner is getting bored, or is enjoying your body. If you find yourself being distracted by thoughts about your partner, try to tune back into the sensations that you feel as you are being touched.

As giver, your job is also to tune in to your own feelings. Notice the different textures and temperatures of your partner's skin. Notice the parts of the body that you enjoy touching the most. Try to be as creative as you can in thinking of different ways to touch your partner. You can use a light, teasing kind of touch, circular strokes, or more of a massage type of touching. You can touch your partner with your hair, with your hand, or even kiss occasionally. Try not to worry about whether you are giving your partner the kinds of caresses that he or she likes the best. Your job is to just enjoy being the giver. The first time that you do this exercise, the receiver should not tell the giver how to touch. The only time the receiver does any talking is to ask the giver to stop doing something that hurts or feels very unpleasant.

When you have spent at least 15 minutes as the giver touching the back of your partner's body, you can ask your partner to turn over and lie on his or her back and then continue the touching. Spending 15 minutes on each side of the body does not mean that you have to have a timer by the bed. These are just some guidelines for you. We do ask you to spend a longer time than usual in touching your partner because this should be a special experience that gives you a chance to tune in to your feelings. Again the job of the giver is to enjoy touching the partner's body. As the receiver, you do not have to do anything except notice your own sensations.

When you have spent a total of half an hour being the receiver, and both your back and your front have been touched and stroked, take a 5-minute break. During this break, tell your partner, in as much detail as possible, the three kinds of touching that you liked the best and the one touch that you liked the least. It is important to keep the balance of your feedback positive. That's why we suggest saying three positive things and only one negative thing. Please do not give your partner a very general statement like, "I really liked it when you touched me on my front side." Try to make your feedback as specific as possible. For example: "I really liked it when you touched my left shoulder with that gentle circular motion." Or "It gave me the shivers when you stroked the inside of my thigh very lightly."

For the second half of the exercise, the giver and receiver switch roles. Now the partner who was the receiver takes a turn spending 15 minutes touching the partner's back and then another 15 minutes touching the partner's front. Again after the second partner has been the receiver, take the 5-minute break and have the receiver give the three positive comments and one negative comment.

Table 7-1. Continued

A Note on Sensuality versus Sexual Arousal

The goal of this exercise is not to get sexually excited or turned on. The goal is to enjoy touching, without feeling that you have to perform for your partner or have an orgasm. For that reason, we ask you not to go from this exercise into a more sexual kind of touching. Please do not end your hour by switching over to kissing, sexual touching, or having intercourse. Save that for another time. This exercise is to help you to unlearn some of your old sexual habits. It should also be useful in helping you to tell each other more clearly what kinds of touching feel the best.

---

adult time together, we suggest the clinician use the couple worksheets presented in Chapter 2, Figures 2-1 and 2-2. Another way to evaluate couple conflict is to have each partner separately fill out the Relationship Time Line in Figure 7-1. In the therapy session, the clinician can compare the partners' perceptions of their relationship happiness over time, discussing crucial events in the relationship history and how they affected marital roles, intimacy and time together. When marital conflict is chronic and severe, referral to a specialist is in order. For many couples, however, marital issues related to ilness are fairly trivial and can be dealt with in brief counseling.

The asessment of current marital conflict related to an illness often leads to problem solving (D'Zurilla & Goldfried, 1971). The first task is to agree on a definition of the problem.

Bud and Marie were a couple in their 30s. Marie had been diagnosed as having rheumatoid arthritis 5 years earlier. She recently had had hip replacement surgery and had severe deformities of her fingers. The partners agreed that bickering had increased because Bud resented taking over household chores, especially in the evenings when he was tired from work and wanted some adult time to talk with his wife.

The next step is to brainstorm and generate a variety of solutions to the problem, even ones that appear impractical on the surface.

Bud and Marie, with the therapist's help, thought of five possible solutions.

- The couple could hire a part-time housekeeper.
- Marie could get a job and Bud, in turn, could work fewer hours.
- Bud could learn to keep his resentment inside.
- Marie could plan her day more efficiently.
- The couple could get their two children (aged 10 and 8) to help more around the house.

The therapist guides the couple in imagining potential outcomes for each solution chosen, trying to paint a realistic picture.

The line below represents your relationship happiness from the day you met until the present. The "+" point represents perfect satisfaction and the "−" point represents dissatisfaction to the point of separating. Please draw the ups and downs of how you perceive your relationship happiness, dating the beginning of the line and the most significant points along the way. In the last section, predict how happy you will be in this relationship a year from now.

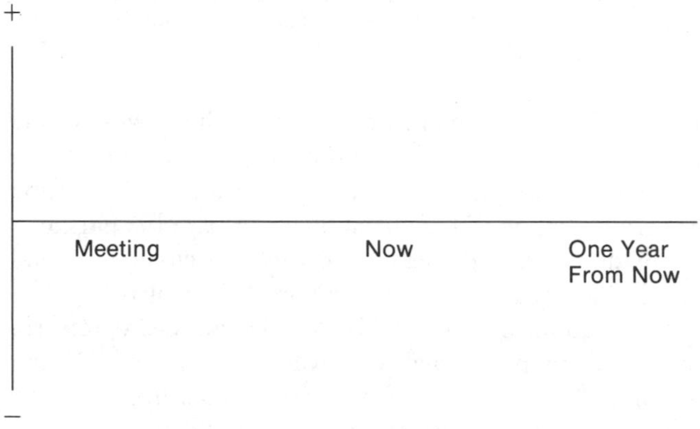

+

Meeting   Now   One Year
                                                  From Now

−

Figure 7-1. A relationship time line.

- If Bud and Marie hire a housekeeper, their budget will not cover other necessities of life.
- Marie's only real job skill is typing, and she can no longer function as a secretary. She has no way of contributing significant earnings to the family income without more education.
- Bud has tried to ignore his anger, but it always comes out either in couple arguments or when he leaves tasks undone and Marie nags him.
- Marie could reduce the 1 or 2 hours she spends each day on the phone with her mother and sisters, or visiting with neighbors. She could also get advice from a physical therapist on making household chores easier.
- The two older children do not even make their own beds or do the dishes. The therapist could help Bud and Marie set up a system for making weekly allowance and recreation time contingent on the children getting chores done.

Finally, therapist and couple choose the best solution or solutions and make a contract to try them out:

Marie agreed to call the physical therapist at her rheumatologist's clinic. Bud said he would make a chart of chores for the children and a simple system of rewards and penalties.

If the options chosen do not work, it is necessary to go back to the drawing board. Usually the therapist's most difficult task is to get the couple to define the problem clearly so that it can be broken up into specific behaviors that can be changed. The problem-solving approach can be combined with marital contracting (Jacobson & Margolin, 1979), in which each partner agrees to change his or her behavior in some ways to please the other.

Minimizing Distraction from Physical Handicaps

When a disease strikes, patients who always functioned well sexually may have to contend with a physical handicap. Brief sexual counseling cannot rid them of the medical problem, but the therapist can often help patient and partner minimize the impact of a physiological impairment on sexual activity.

Some illnesses actually produce a sexual dysfunction such as erection problems or alterations in a woman's vaginal caliber, depth, or lubrication. When intercourse becomes painful or impossible, sensate focus exercises and communication training may help a couple stay sexually active and learn to reach noncoital orgasms. Many couples use the techniques of sexual stimulation that were part of their past sexual routine. Some, however, want to learn new ways of providing erotic stimulation (Schover, 1984, pp. 193–201). Besides teaching partners skills and enhancing their comfort with manual and oral caressing, therapists can suggest the use of sexual aids such as vibrators.

A 72-year-old cardiac patient and his hemiplegic wife wanted to continue noncoital sexual activity. Each, however, had difficulty reaching orgasm without a long, fatiguing period of manual caressing. Their therapist helped them use a sexual aids catalogue to order a quiet, hand-held vibrator that came with several attachments. Both were more easily orgasmic after experimenting with their new erotic toy.

Treatment of female dyspareunia, especially after menopause, is discussed in Chapter 8. Clinicians should remember that mild dysparcunia is often eased by liberal use of a water-based lubricant and a shift to intercourse positions that allow the woman to control depth of penile penetration and angle and speed of thrusting.

Illness may bring chronic fatigue, shortness of breath with exertion, nongenital pain, or limitations in mobility. With some creativity, however, couples can continue to enjoy sexual activity. Rather than having impromptu sex, partners may need to schedule lovemaking at the time of day when fatigue and pain are least severe, or when pain medication is in effect, if the patient does not become too drowsy. Because our society holds an ideal that sexual desire should occur on a whim rather than on schedule, couples need support and encouragement to make such changes. Some intercourse positions minimize shortness of breath by allowing a relaxed, upright posture with use of pillows for support. Couples with traditional beliefs that the man must always initiate lovemaking and direct the stimulation may also respond to attitude change techniques.

Pain and limitations on range of motion can distract from the pleasure of lovemaking. Sometimes the frustration is so severe that a couple discontinues sexual activity completely, although some practical advice on pain control and positioning could go a long way to overcoming the handicaps.

Martha was a 66-year-old farmer's wife. She had always worked hard on the couple's land. Her only contacts with the health care system had been at the births of her five children. She began to have severe arthritic pain in her hips and knees, however, and went to see her general practitioner, a woman physician.

At the first visit, the doctor examined Martha and prescribed a prostaglandin synthetase inhibiting medication (ibuprofen). Martha returned after a month. Although her pain had decreased, Martha felt her ability to walk and do household chores was so limited that she wanted hip replacement surgery. The general practitioner also thought a gynecological examination was in order but discovered that Martha could not assume a position that would allow a complete pelvic inspection. She asked Martha how her arthritis had influenced her sex life.

Martha was silent for a moment and the young physician worried that she was offended. Perhaps this elderly couple had discontinued sexual activity years ago. But Martha had another story to tell:

"You know Ken and I have been married for 45 years, and we've always enjoyed sex, even though our sex life is maybe a little routine. Now that my hips have gotten so bad, we can only do it from behind, and I've just never felt right about that position—I feel like a dog. I was hoping you'd ask, but I was just too embarrassed to bring it up."

Martha had her operation and was given instructions on comfortable positions for intercourse (Chapter 14). She has not returned to her local doctor's office. The two women did run into each other at the supermarket, however. Martha thanked her doctor for all her help, and gave her a discreet wink.

Some patients have to learn to manage changes in their bodies, such as ostomies, urinary catheters, or limb protheses. Health care professionals such as enterostomal therapy nurses or physical therapists who manage such patients' rehabilitation often act as frontline sexual counselors and can offer valuable information to other clinicians working with these groups.

For the patient with an ostomy (Schover, 1986c), practical advice can include emptying a pouch before sexual activity; keeping the appliance from flapping during vigorous movement by taping it down, turning it sideways, or wearing a sexy undergarment that leaves the genital area free; buying a mini-sized urinary pouch for sexual occasions, or for patients who can irrigate a colostomy, wearing a small ostomy cap or safety pouch; planning sexual activity at a time of day when a colostomy or ileostomy is least active; and avoiding foods that cause strong urinary odors or promote flatulence. Couples can minimize the risk of leaks by avoiding intercourse positions that exert friction on the ostomy faceplate.

Men and women with limb prostheses, or even mastectomy patients who use a breast prosthesis, must choose whether to wear them during sexual activity. After mastectomy, some women prefer to wear a nightgown with their breast prosthesis, but others find nudity less cumbersome. For a person with a limb amputation, the choice affects not only appearance and feelings of wholeness but also mobility. For some, the limb prosthesis may afford a greater ability to move actively during lovemaking, but for others the harness attaching the prosthesis may be an esthetic liability or a practical problem if it covers erotic zones. Pillows can be used to prop up a part of the body that lacks normal support.

Brief Sexual Counseling Skills
for the Novice Therapist

When primary care clinicians have not had extensive training in psychotherapy, we find that remembering a few principles of good interviewing can ease first attempts at brief sexual counseling:

- There is no correct way of doing psychotherapy. The clinician has a whole kit of tools and must choose the one that appears best for the job at hand.
- You can be a responsible therapist without taking control of everything that the patient does.
- Ask fewer questions than you usually do, and focus on "hows" rather than "whys." If you do ask a question, make sure it gets answered, even if it gets lost at first.
- Even by being silent, you are being therapeutic if you remain aware of what is going on.
- The patient's surface emotions are not always the important ones. Anger is a good mask for hurt or anxiety, and depression often hides anger.
- Be aware of covert verbal and nonverbal messages expressed between spouses or between the patients and you.
- When you observe a marital "game," consider whether it would be most helpful to bypass it or to point it out directly.
- If you interpret the meaning of the patient's behavior, wait until he or she is ready to listen. Frame the interpretation tentatively so that the patient does not feel scolded but can explore it with you.
- Structure a session so that you can reach some closure by the end of the time allotted. Do not try to resolve intense emotional issues in the last 5 minutes.

- Remember the limitations of your power as a therapist. You need to make the patient your ally in order to produce change.
- When patients' reactions become annoying or frustrating, remember that defense mechanisms are just their best efforts to cope with a stressful world.

INTENSIVE SEX THERAPY FOR
PATIENTS WITH CHRONIC ILLNESSES

Intensive sex therapy for patients with chronic illnesses is based on techniques that have been set forth in several textbooks (Arentewicz & Schmidt, 1983; H. S. Kaplan, 1974, 1979; Leiblum & Pervin, 1980; J. LoPiccolo & LoPiccolo, 1978). We cannot include all the skills of sex therapy here, but rather refer interested readers to the resources just listed.

We do discuss how intensive sex therapy can be applied to patients with a chronic illness, focusing on the skills needed by the sexuality specialist. The primary care clinician should find this section helpful as well in deciding when a patient could benefit from a sex therapy referral.

Sex therapy has been characterized as a behavioral treatment, and, in fact, draws heavily on techniques such as *in vivo* desensitization of anxiety, communication training, and assigning behavioral tasks that gradually increase in difficulty. We are typical of modern sex therapists, however, in using cognitive, psychodynamic, and humanistic psychotherapy styles as we conceptualize a case and carry out the treatment. We might point out a patient's irrational beliefs about sexual performance such as, "A man should always delay his orgasm until his partner has climaxed at least once." A man with low sexual desire might be urged to recount his memories of his relationship with his mother, focusing on what he learned about intimacy with women. The therapist might ask a woman who was sexually molested as a child to put her attacker in the "empty chair" and tell him how she felt.

Clinicians sometimes ask when to recommend marital therapy rather than sex therapy. We rarely make such a distinction. A sexual problem cannot be treated in couple therapy without also working on relationship issues. Often the sexual problem is just one aspect of marital conflict but was perceived by the couple as the most acceptable reason for seeking help (Clulow, 1984). An experienced clinician can use the sexual dysfunction as an entry point into treating wider issues. Sometimes, of course, marital conflict is so severe that the couple needs to decide first whether to remain together before they can commit themselves to changing their sexual interactions.

Nina and Bruce had been married for 13 years when he had a myocardial infarction. The couple had two children, aged 6 and 10, but Bruce did little parenting, spending 12 to 16 hours a day at his office. The couple was referred for sex therapy because Nina had little desire for sex after Bruce came home from the hospital.

Although it was obvious that the couple had many disagreements, the partners seemed receptive to counseling about the safety of sexual activity after a heart attack. They completed 2 weeks of sensate focus exercises, but, during the third therapy session, Nina announced that the focus on her feelings about Bruce had forced her to realize that she wanted a divorce. She made it clear that she had considered divorce before Bruce's illness because she hated his workaholic lifestyle.

Seeing him return to his same old habits despite his heart attack was the final straw. The focus of therapy shifted to deciding on a marital separation.

Sex therapy looks simple when viewed as a collection of homework exercises that can be plugged in to treat various dysfunctions. We believe, however, that sex therapy is one of the more difficult psychotherapies because the clinician needs to be expert in individual psychopathology, couple and group dynamics, and sexual physiology. The brief sexual counseling techniques outlined in the last section are within the grasp of the primary care clinician who has had a minimal amount of psychotherapy training. Intensive sex therapy, however, calls for a mental health professional who has had specialized supervision in couple therapy and sexuality issues.

Structuring Intensive Sex Therapy

Patients with chronic illnesses are accustomed to medical treatments that are structured, action-oriented, and time-limited. Sex therapy shares these features—a fact that can be stressed in presenting the treatment to patients who may have always regarded psychotherapy as stigmatizing.

The Spacing of Sessions

Research and clinical experience (Heiman & LoPiccolo, 1983) suggest that the spacing of sex therapy sessions can be flexible, depending on the patient's circumstances. Most clinicians schedule one session a week, allowing time for patients to complete several homework exercises. When an individual or couple is in crisis or is unusually fragile, a twice-weekly format can be used.

We believe it optimal for patients to be treated in a setting close to home, so that behavioral exercises take place in the usual environment and new learning can be integrated into daily life routines. Some medical patients receive treatment in regional centers, however, or live in areas where a sex therapist is not available. For such cases, scheduling daily sessions of sex therapy for an allotted period at a clinic can also be effective and reduces expensive intermittent trips. Special attention should be paid during the homecoming period, however, to factors in the home environment that interfere with generalization of the gains made during therapy at a specialized clinic.

No matter where sex therapy takes place or the spacing of sessions, a short-term (3 months) and a long-term (1 year) follow-up should be scheduled routinely at the end of treatment.

The Therapy Contract

When patients begin therapy, whether the format is individual, couple, or group, they should reach a clear agreement with the therapist on the number of sessions expected, how termination will be accomplished, the goals of therapy, and homework procedures. Some therapists might find this degree of structure limiting, but we believe it not only makes therapy effective, but also helps medical patients feel more comfortable.

An average duration for sex therapy is 15 to 20 sessions. Some therapists make an initial contract with the patient that sex therapy will last (for example) 15 sessions, with the option at Session 13 of extending treatment if goals have not quite been met. Another option is to contract for 5 or 6 sessions at a time, evaluating at the last agreed-on session whether to continue. The therapist must be aware that setting time limits can induce anxiety that needs to be discussed and allayed, although time boundaries also can make therapy more efficient. Without them, problems often expand to fill as many sessions as are available.

Therapist and patients agree that termination of treatment will always be discussed with both partners (or all group members) present and that a phone call does not obviate having a termination session. Thus patients have the right to withdraw from therapy at any time, but the therapist also has the right to make sure that some sense of closure is attained.

Another way to boost the efficiency of therapy is to set goals. In the first session of therapy, each patient can be asked, either on the spot or as homework, to list the three most important sexual changes wanted for self and partner. This goal setting can be expanded to include the three most imortant changes in marital patterns as well, so that each partner in a couple would specify six personal goals and six partner goals. In addition, the patient rates the importance of each goal on a 5-point scale.

When patients identify goals, the therapist can help them to be specific (i.e., "I would like to have sex twice a week," instead of "I want more sex"); to be positive (i.e., "I would like my partner to ask for the kind of touching he wants," vs. "My partner should stop being so passive"); and to be practical (i.e., "I would like to have an afternoon a week of child care," vs. "I want my husband to do 50% of all child care").

Partners can negotiate a final set of mutual goals that will be used periodically to evaluate the progress of sex therapy. The therapist can use a large sheet of paper to write down the goals and have it available to hang up at future sessions.

Homework assignments can include sensate focus exercises, masturbation exercises, or assignments that build communication and negotiation skills. Homework is assigned at the end of each therapy session. We like to write down the assignment, making a carbon copy for the patient or couple to take home. We keep the original for our file. In a group, each member writes down his or her copy of the assignment as it is presented and discussed. Homework assignments are always based on discussion with the patients. If a therapist suggests an activity that is impractical or distasteful to the patient, the patient has not only the right but the responsibility to protest so that an alternative can be proposed. Therapist and patient agree that once the homework is assigned, the patient will carry it out.

Homework is usually the first item on the agenda at the next session. Some therapists ask patients to tell what occurred in detail, whereas others have patients hand in written diaries of the homework as we suggested in the section on sensate focus. Each partner's records can be read by the therapist before the session while the couple is in the waiting room. Written diaries help to focus attention on the most important issues from the past week.

An example is given in Table 7-2. Marilyn, a 39-year-old woman with multiple sclerosis, is trying to become more reliably orgasmic. Marilyn and her husband, Norman, have engaged in 5 weeks of a sensate focus program, enjoying the exercises. Marilyn has been reaching orgasm more easily in her own masturbation. The first time that each partner is allowed to reach orgasm during the exercise, however, they hit a roadblock. Marilyn and Norman keep separate diaries of their homework exercises, using standard forms provided by the therapist. The therapist can compare Marilyn's homework record to Norman's. Her diary reveals she was angry at Norman for watching a movie when she wanted to do the homework. He does not perceive her anger, but, instead, believed that her genitals were sore or unusually sensitive because of her disease. Information from the homework sheets can be used in session to discuss how each partner expresses anger and the influence of mood on Marilyn's sexual arousal.

Treatment Programs for Specific Sexual Dysfunctions

Sex therapists have developed sequences of homework assignments designed to remedy specific sexual dysfunctions. Such programs are outlined in *Human Sexual Inadequacy* (Masters & Johnson, 1970) and *The New Sex Therapy* (H. S. Kaplan, 1974). Every sex therapist should be familiar with techniques such as the stop–start program for premature ejaculators (Perelman, 1980), directed masturbation training to enhance women's orgasmic capacity (Heiman, LoPiccolo, & LoPiccolo, 1976), or the series of exercises used to treat erectile dysfunction (H. S. Kaplan, 1974; Zillbergeld, 1978).

Table 7-2. A Homework Sheet from the Case of Marilyn and Norman

Date: Thursday, 3/10   Week of Therapy: __6__

Activity	Time	Pleasure rating, self (1 least, 10 most)	Estimated pleasure rating, partner (1 least, 10 most)	Thoughts and Feelings
Sensate focus including orgasms for both partners: I began by caressing Norman's back, and then spent time on his front. I rubbed his penis for 5 minutes until he ejaculated. Then he stroked my back, and afterwards my stomach. He rubbed my clitoris for a while, but I wasn't very excited. After a few minutes I told him to stop.	11: pm	3	9	I was mad because we were supposed to go to bed at 10:00, but Norman insisted on watching a dumb TV movie. By the time he came to bed, I was too tired to enjoy the touching. I think he doesn't really care if I have orgasms. He just wants me to give him pleasure.

When marital conflict is a factor, we tend to use a variety of approaches including elements from Stuart (1976), Jacobson and Margolin (1979), and Segraves (1982b). Cases are almost always more complex than in the textbook, requiring therapeutic creativity rather than rote application of a standard treatment program.

Patients who are chronically ill are particularly likely to present a complex challenge, and their sexual dysfunctions vary widely (Schover *et al.*, 1987). To illustrate the techniques of sex therapy with medical patients, each chapter of Part 2 contains an intensive case relevant to a disease in focus. We hope readers will be able to combine the structured material in this chapter and the clinical examples in Part 2 in formulating treatment plans for their own patients.

Outcome Research on Sex Therapy

Sex therapy has specific goals, making outcome research more feasible than for many other types of psychotherapy. Most studies have used populations from sexual dysfunction clinics, however, rather than medical patients. Although they have criticized Masters and Johnson's (1970) methodology, Zillbergeld and Kilmann (1984) have concluded, on the basis of more recent research, that sex therapy is reasonably effective and is the psychotherapy of choice for sexual dysfunctions. Studies of short-term outcome have been encouraging (Heiman & LoPiccolo, 1983; J. LoPiccolo *et al.*, 1985), although results are better when measured in terms of overall sexual satisfaction or general adjustment on sexual questionnaires than when based on symptom reversal. A 3-year follow-up study of 38 couples was somewhat less optimistic, especially for couples whose presenting complaint was low sexual desire (De Amicis *et al.*, 1985). Sexual satisfaction remained at a sustained level of improvement, however.

Schover *et al.* (1987) were able to obtain therapist ratings of outcome in 118 cancer patients sent for consultation to a specialized sexual rehabilitation clinic. At least from the clinician's perspective, symptoms were rated as at least somewhat better in 63% of cases. Results were more positive when patients had more sessions of therapy. Unfortunately, only eight patients had formal sex therapy, so the data do not really address the effectiveness of intensive treatment in medical settings.

Future researchers should use outcome measures such as structured interviews, sexual questionnaires, and even psychophysiological assessment of sexual arousal in the laboratory to compare sexual function and satisfaction before and after the various levels of therapeutic intervention used with patients who are chronically ill and have sexual problems. Only by illustrating that sexual counseling can prevent and remedy problems in these groups will sex therapists be accepted in medical settings.

8

Combining Sexual Counseling with Medical Treatments

All too often, both physicians and patients search for the "magic pill" that will "cure" a sexual dysfunction. Clincians become inured to having the suggestion of sex therapy greeted with disappointment, or even revulsion, and to the eternal question, "But doctor, isn't there some medicine I could take, or an operation to fix it?" Now that medical treatments do indeed exist for some problems, we have to work doubly hard to counteract the "quick-fix" mentality, with its risk that patients will have more successful intercourse but be left with dysfunctional sexual relationships. The answer may be to say, "no" to an inappropriate medical treatment or to combine brief sex therapy with appropriate medical treatment, in keeping with the integrative model.

In recent years, each new medical discovery—estrogen replacement for women, testosterone therapy for men, the penile prosthesis, yohimbine, or papaverine injections—has been hailed as *the* answer to sexual dysfunction. Often such treatments have the powerful backing of pharmaceutical or medical equipment manufacturers. For example, the maker of several penile prostheses publishes a quarterly newsletter *Colleagues in Urology*. In a recent issue (Staff, 1985), its "Medical Marketing" column carried a story on "impotence support groups." Urologists who wished to increase their numbers of penile prosthesis operations were urged to set up self-help groups for men with erection problems. Rather than helping couples explore various solutions for sexual dysfunction, the meetings sounded like forums for recruiting new operative cases. "The bottom line is revenues," said a clinical nurse specialist who coordinates one of the organizations. A urologist commented, "The patient is worried about the success of implant surgery, and what better way to convince him than to have a man and his sexual partner at the meeting who will talk his ears off about how wonderful it is."

Psychotherapists are not comfortable marketing treatments. In fact, our task is often to deflate the unrealistic expectations of men and women who have seen a television program or read a magazine article about the latest neoorganic craze. Medical treatments are successful for some sexual dysfunctions. A man or woman who has high self-esteem and a strong, intimate relationship but has become dysfunctional because of a medical illness may not need psychotherapy. The majority, however, can use preparation and counseling in choosing a medical therapy as well as help adjusting to their improved sexual function. Even an organically caused problem can distort and stress dyadic interactions.

This chapter outlines the risks and benefits of the more widely used medical treatments for sexual problems and demonstrates how sexual counseling can help patients who undergo them.

HORMONE REPLACEMENT THERAPY FOR MEN

For men with abnormally low levels of testosterone, doses of replacement hormone improve sexual function. Sexual desire, erections, and sexual activity have increased in frequency with hormone therapy but not with placebo in double-blind studies (Davidson *et al.*, 1979; Salmimies *et al.*, 1982). Similarly, when hyperprolactinemia is normalized by pituitary surgery or by medication, sexual symptoms often disappear (Muir *et al.*, 1983; Ruilope *et al.*, 1985; Weizman *et al.*, 1983). There is an art to hormone therapy, since effective doses vary from man to man. Until recently, injectable forms of testosterone were considered more effective than oral forms, which are partially metabolized by the liver before they can affect target tissues (Benkert, Witt, Adam, & Leitz, 1979). An effective oral medication (testosterone undecanoate) is now available in Europe but not in the United States (O'Carroll & Bancroft, 1984).

If hormone therapy were given only when appropriate, it would be uncontroversial. The problem is that androgens have been prescribed indiscriminately for men with normal baseline testosterone levels. In our experience, when a patient complains of any sort of sexual problem—low desire, premature ejaculation, or erectile dysfunction—many internists, family practitioners, or even urologists in the United States will give him hormones without checking his serum testosterone first. Unnecessary hormone therapy is not only ineffective in changing sexual function (Benkert *et al.*, 1979; O'Carroll & Bancroft, 1984), but it can also cause liver damage, atrophy of the Leydig cells, benign hypertrophy of the prostate, and, most dangerously, growth and metastasis of an undiagnosed prostate cancer. Both physicians and patients must be educated about the risks and limitations of hormone therapy (Schover, 1984, pp. 120–123).

Sometimes, even after hormone levels are normalized, a sexual dysfunction does not resolve. Years of sexual disinterest or awkwardness take their toll on a relationship. Couple therapy may be of help even if a hormonal abnormality persists. For example, when the assay for prolactin became available, Schwartz, Bauman, and Masters (1982) analyzed frozen blood samples from a series of patients and found, retrospectively, that eight men treated with sex therapy had been hyperprolactinemic. Nevertheless, sexual symptoms were at least ameliorated in all cases and sometimes reversed by psychological treatment. We are not advocating psychotherapy instead of hormone therapy, but it certainly can be a helpful adjunct to medical treatment.

Wayne was a 52-year-old business executive. Two years previously, he had surgery to remove a prolactin-secreting pituitary adenoma. He was maintained on a regimen of replacement hormones, but still felt little desire for sex and was unable to attain full erections. Wayne and his wife, Jackie, had a warm and loving relationship, but for the past 12 years, as Jackie commented, "We're affectionate all during the day or evening, but touching stops when we get to the bedroom door." Both partners were interested in improving their sex life now that the medical treatment had removed the apparent cause of Wayne's long-term dysfunctions. Neither Wayne nor Jackie, however, knew how to break down the barriers and begin sexual touching again.

The couple participated in sex therapy for 15 sessions. They discussed their difficulty in putting priority on time for intimacy and privacy together, their guilt and struggle to adjust to having a bisexual son, their feelings about aging and their own sexual attractiveness, and how to communicate their sexual wishes more clearly to each other.

Homework assignments followed the usual sequence of sensate focus exercises but started off very slowly with cuddling in the bedroom with pajamas on. Wayne and Jackie enjoyed their renewed freedom to touch, and Wayne began to get erections during the sensate focus sessions. Jackie found some private time to masturbate to orgasm and to get in touch with her sexuality through reading and fantasy.

Therapy reached a plateau, however, when the couple confronted Wayne's lack of "lust." Even as a teenager, he had not been highly interested in sex, and now he could enjoy touching but felt little desire to initiate it. Jackie openly expressed her sadness at her husband's lack of desire, albeit in a loving way. Wayne felt helpless to change. Finally, husband and wife agreed that they would try to maintain the gains they had made in intimacy, but current family and work responsibilities precluded further work on their sexual relationship.

Although the case of Wayne and Jackie was not a complete success, it illustrates that medical factors are often not the only reason a sexual problem persists.

HORMONE REPLACEMENT THERAPY FOR WOMEN

Clinicians who treat many women over age 50 in couples with sexual dysfunction are impressed by the wide individual variation in postmenopausal symptoms. Some women are truly miserable without hormone replacement, having frequent hot flashes that embarrass them during the day and interrupt their sleep. They may experience vaginal dryness, tightness, pain with orgasm, and postcoital bleeding and irritation. Others sail through menopause with hardly any noticeable effects. Women who discontinue sexual activity for several years and then resume intercourse may have more vaginal atrophy and discomfort than women who remain consistently sexually active (Leiblum *et al*, 1983), but the role of sexual inactivity in causing vaginal atrophy will remain unclear until prospective studies are completed. As yet, we have no other clues as to why some postmenopausal women are more prone to atrophy.

The decision to give hormonal therapy to a postmenopausal woman is usually based not only on her symptoms, but also on the risks treatment entails. Side effects can include increased blood pressure in a minority, especially smokers; changes in liver function; gall bladder disease; and, most importantly, an increased risk of uterine cancer in those who take estrogens for over 2 years (American Council on Science & Health, 1983; Cutler, Garcia, & Edwards, 1983). Evidence for increased rates of breast cancer is contradictory, with most studies suggesting no additional risk with the lower doses of estrogen now prescribed, especially if progestogens are added to the therapy. Improvements in hormone regimens have also reduced the risk of uterine cancer (S. M. Levy, 1983, p. 33). On the positive side, replacement estrogens protect older women against osteoporosis and cardiovascular disease. These benefits become crucial to younger women who lose ovarian function as a part of medical treatment, for example after pelvic cancer surgery or radiotherapy or during chemotherapy for a malignancy.

Oral or vaginal doses of replacement estrogens clearly promote improvements in vaginal blood flow, pH, and lubrication, ameliorating sexual function (Semmens & Semmens, 1984). For women at low risk of cancer, the benefits of hormonal therapy are unquestionable. For women at high risk, for example those with a history of breast cancer, perhaps conservative behavioral treatments could alleviate enough postmenopausal symptoms to make medical intervention unnecessary.

A comprehensive behavior treatment program for a symptomatic postmenopausal woman might include several components:

- Progressive muscle relaxation training can decrease hot flashes without medication (Germaine & Freedman, 1984). Hot flashes not only interfere with a woman's general well-being, but may also reduce sexual desire or activity (McCoy *et al.*, 1985). Women with very severe hot flashes may also get some relief from nonhormonal medications like clonidine (Germaine & Freedman, 1984).
- Couple counseling, including sensate focus exercises and communication training, can help the woman and her partner take more time for love-

making, compensating for the slowing of the sexual response with age. Noncoital stimulation to orgasm is an alternative to intercourse when a woman has dyspareunia or a man cannot achieve erections firm enough to penetrate a dry, tight vagina.

• Water-based vaginal lubricants provide enough moisture to make intercourse comfortable again for many women. K-Y jelly and Ortho Personal Lubricant are common in the United States, but some newer lubricants such as Lubrin, a suppository, and Transi-Lube, a foam, have a thinner texture and are less apt to dry out during lovemaking.

• Vaginal dilators, used several times a week, have effectively reduced pain during intercourse for some women. It is unclear whether the dilators really expand the vagina or if they help because women learn to relax the pubococcygeal muscles while inserting the dilator, giving them a sense of mastery over the genital pain (Fordney, 1978). Many older women will not use a dilator because they associate it with masturbation. Sometimes asking the husband, during sensate focus exercises, to insert just one, and eventually two or three lubricated fingers into his wife's vagina can be a helpful alternative.

Young women who lose ovarian function prematurely may refuse to take hormones because they fear that estrogen causes cancer. Since the risk of osteoporosis and cardiovascular disease from premature menopause far outweighs the cancer risk from estrogens, they need counseling and reassurance. Despite recent publicity on osteoporosis, many women, young and old, do not know how important it is to get adequate dietary calcium and to do regular, weight-bearing exercise such as walking, bicycling, or jogging. Women who have ovarian failure in their 20s, 30s, or 40s need advice on preventing bone loss and vaginal atrophy. For this population, sexual counseling and advice on general health are inseparable.

THE PENILE PROSTHESIS

The penile prosthesis ushered in a new era of medical treatment for erectile dysfunction. Powdered rhinoceros horn and rubber tourniquets around the base of the penis have been replaced as nostrums by silicone devices, implanted with the aid of the most advanced surgical technology. The array of options includes hinged, malleable, and inflatable models, with several companies competing for the market. At least 20,000 penile prosthesis operations take place yearly in the United States. Physicians in Europe have been less eager to sanction the wide-scale use of the prosthesis. In some countries, including Denmark, medical ethics committees question the appropriateness of surgery, except for a small group of patients with obvious and severe organic deficits (Jensen, 1984a).

What is a penile prosthesis, and what can it accomplish? A silicone device surgically implanted into the cavernous bodies can make the penis rigid no matter what caused erectile dysfunction. It cannot, however, restore sexual desire, improve sensation on the penile skin, or change a man's ejaculation or capacity to reach orgasm. Since the prosthesis is positioned outside the spongy body which surrounds the urethra, the surgery does not affect urination unless a severe complication occurs.

Three basic types of prosthesis are used (Figure 8-1). The semirigid version gives a man permanent penile rigidity. His penis hangs at about a 45-degree angle and is flexible enough to permit him to bend it upward and conceal it under clothing. Many men wear briefs made for athletics, with heavy elastic in the crotch to minimize the bulge created by the prosthesis. A semirigid prosthesis consists of two silicone rods, sized to fit the individual's penis and inserted into twin spaces created by dilating the spongy tissues of each cavernous body (Small, 1983). Spinal or local anesthesia is sometimes used so that the procedure can be performed with a very brief hospital stay (Kaufman, 1982).

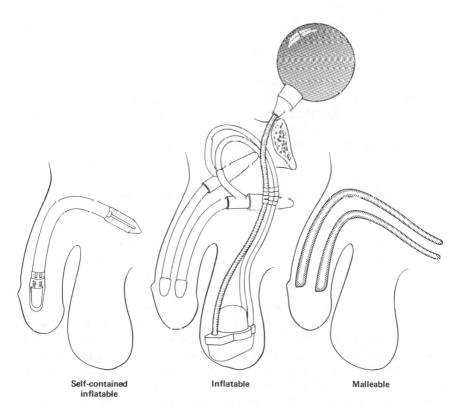

Self-contained
inflatable   Inflatable   Malleable

Figure 8-1. Three types of penile prosthesis.

Prosthesis designers have made concealment of a semirigid prosthesis easier by adding a hinge to the silicone so the penis bends more easily at its base, filling each silicone rod with a core of silver or stainless steel wire so the penis remains fixed in the bent or straight position as desired, or incorporating a mechanism that snaps the rod into stiff or limp positions. Rates of infection or physiological complications are similar for all models, generally ranging from 5% to 10%. Men are sometimes dissatisfied because their erections are shorter and thinner than normal. The penis may feel cool to the touch at the tip, and, unless a man still retains some penile blood flow, the glans does not become swollen or warm with sexual arousal.

Urologists also can choose between two inflatable models (Fishman, Scott, & Light, 1984; Merrill, 1984). Short-term complication rates vary widely in different case series but seem to be 5% to 15% with the latest versions in large centers where surgical teams are experienced in the procedure. Some urologists believe, however, that most men will eventually need a surgical revision of their inflatable prostheses (Merrill, 1984). Two balloon-type cylinders are placed in the cavernous bodies and are connected with tubing to a reservoir, positioned under the muscle of the groin, and a pump, placed in the loose scrotal skin above the testicles. A man operates the pump by locating it under his skin and squeezing it between his fingers, forcing the saline solution from the reservoir into the penile cylinders. The result is a thicker penile shaft than that produced with a semirigid prosthesis, but the penis remains shorter than in a normal state of erection. To deflate his penis, a man pushes a release valve on the base of the pump, returning the fluid to the reservoir.

A new version of the inflatable prosthesis is the self-contained prosthesis, consisting of two cylinders, each with its own pump and release valve. When fluid is in a deep chamber located in the base of the cavernous body, the penis is semiflaccid. The penile shaft becomes rigid when fluid is pumped into a middle chamber. Although the tumescence produced is not as full as that achieved with the more complex inflatables, surgeons find that surgical revisions are fewer and easier to perform.

If the goal is to create a rigid penis, the prosthesis is an overwhelming success. Our goal, however, is to facilitate satisfying sexual relationships. Although the penile prosthesis is just one possible ingredient in sexual satisfaction, it has been treated as if it were the entire recipe.

This attitude has shaped the evaluation process. Urologists attempt to classify erection problems as either psychogenic or organic. Once an organic "cause" has been identified, doctor and patient often assume that sex therapy would be useless, and, indeed, that psychological and relationship factors are superfluous and can be ignored. Yet, even an organic sexual dysfunction affects a man's self-esteem and a couple's interaction. For example, wives commonly blame the problem on their unattractiveness or lack of sexual skills. A woman's fear of rejection may be expressed in anger or withdrawal.

Gary had a long history of hypertension, treated with medication. He and his second wife had been married for 4 years, but in the last year he had gradually developed difficulty maintaining erections. Gary and Helen began to bicker about nonsexual issues. When one fight escalated into Helen threatening divorce, Gary sought medical help. Although Doppler tests suggested a vascular cause for the erection problem, the couple was also sent to the sex therapy clinic for an interview. When asked what drew them to each other, they laughed and said that they each had been rejected by their first spouses in favor of new partners who were 20 years younger. As they described their sexual interaction, Helen broke in:

"You know in my first marriage, my husband and I had no sex for 3 years. He told me he couldn't get an erection with me but he could with other women. So when Gary came up with this problem, I was afraid the whole thing was beginning again."

Sexual counseling may resolve enough anxiety for a couple like Gary and Helen that erections improve to an acceptable level. A change in antihypertensive medication or dosage can also help. Even if the husband and wife opt for a penile prosthesis, their fragile sense of trust must be explored and strengthened so that erections become an instrument of pleasure rather than a proof of love.

Limited evaluations also fail to identify the man who seeks a penile prosthesis to solve a relationship crisis, telling a story that seems, at face value, to indicate a simple, medical problem.

Thomas, a 50-year-old attorney, was referred to a sex therapy clinic because the urologist who was planning to insert a penile prosthesis was required to obtain a presurgical evaluation. The surgeon was so sure that the sexual problem was caused by Thomas's diabetes that he had not performed any specialized medical examinations. According to the urologist, Thomas reported no erections in any situation, including on waking from sleep.

Although Thomas was asked to bring his wife, he came alone for his appointment. He said his wife was not interested in receiving counseling or information on sexuality. She had not accompanied him to his urology appointment either. The urologist had noted only that the spouse was "a healthy woman of age 50."

Thomas quickly took the role of prosecuting attorney, asking the psychiatrist if he questioned the qualifications of the eminent surgeon who had referred him for this rather foolish visit. "I'm sure you won't interfere in this decision, will you—young man?" he said.

But as the interview progressed, Thomas began to drop his defenses. "My wife has metastatic cancer and is having chemotherapy," he confessed. "She's lost her hair, and she's almost down to skin and bone. I know she'll never recover." Thomas felt the only thing he could offer his wife was to make love to her "like a real man," during her brief times at home between hospitalizations. However, he was unable to get erections. Thomas did not want to discuss his wife's approaching death. When the therapist asked how he felt about being an attractive and vigorous man living with a gravely ill and often absent wife, Thomas disclosed that in fact he had a new lover, 15 years younger. He had no erection problems with her.

Thomas was offered further counseling, but he refused. The psychiatrist recommended against penile prosthesis surgery. Two years later he received a letter from the urologist:

> Dear Colleague:
>   Some time ago you saw one of my patients, Thomas, and advised against a penile prosthesis. We proceeded with surgery in any case, and I recently saw Thomas on a follow-up visit. He reports he now has a happy and satisfying family and sex life. Just for your information—we all make mistakes.
>
>   Sincerely yours,
>   Dr. Q.
>   Chief Urologist

Thomas was also contacted as part of a follow-up study in the sex therapy clinic. His wife had died and the former lover had become his new wife. Their sex life with the penile prosthesis was satisfactory, just as it had been without it.

From a rather cynical point of view, one could say that everyone felt vindicated by this story's ending. The urologist felt the surgery was justified. The psychiatrist knew it was not and that he had made the correct recommendation. Thomas got what he wanted and was apparently little the worse for wear. But what if Thomas develops a need for a revision of the prosthesis and has to undergo another unnecessary surgery? If he has to have the prosthesis removed, he will never be able to have erections again. Because every surgery is a risk to health, some guidelines and controls are needed.

Stories like this are all too common, especially in the United States where urologists in private practice are performing a growing number of operations. Until recently, most penile prosthesis surgery took place in teaching hospitals, where more complete evaluations were the rule. When the surgeon is in complete control, the goal of psychological evaluations, if performed at all, is usually to exclude men who may cause trouble, for example, by committing sex offenses, having a psychotic break, committing suicide, developing psychogenic pain, or suing the physician.

Another limitation of current evaluations is that many urologists classify all sexual problems as "impotence," paying little or no attention to dysfunctions of sexual desire or orgasm (Schover & von Eschenbach, 1985a). Sexual problems in the female partner are rarely discovered, since she is usually not included in the presurgical interview. Older women with postmenopausal vaginal atrophy often receive no counseling on avoiding dyspareunia when a couple resumes their sex life after years of no genital touching, let alone intercourse. We have personally engineered some narrow escapes from inappropriate surgery and wonder how many other patients never get the benefit of a competent evaluation:

Dr. D., a urology resident, brought Ernie, a 48-year-old recovering alcoholic, to the sex therapist, asking, "Could you tell this man about the penile prosthesis? He has an organic erection problem, probably from all his drinking."

The clinician asked Ernie to describe a typical sexual experience. He said, "Well, I get it up, and we start, and that's that. It's all over."

"Do you mean your penis gets hard and you start intercourse, and then it just gets soft?" asked the clinician.

"Yes," Ernie answered.

"Does it get soft before you can reach your climax, or after the climax?"

"Oh afterwards!"

It developed that Ernie had begun to ejaculate prematurely in the year since he stopped drinking. He had always felt shy and awkward with women. When he was drinking heavily, he met women in bars. His sexual performance was unimportant since he hardly remembered the details in the morning and rarely saw the woman again. Since joining Alcoholics Anonymous, however, he had begun a relationship with a neighbor. With her, he felt sexually inadequate. She would get angry when he ejaculated quickly, not because of his clumsiness, but because he refused to help her reach orgasm through noncoital stimulation after intercourse. Ernie agreed that surgery was a rather drastic solution for his problem and decided to bring in his partner for a couple session.

How can we, as health professionals, put the penile prosthesis in its proper perspective? In Scandinavia, detailed studies of surgical outcomes are being conducted, and a mental health professional always participates in the evaluation process (Berg, Mindus, Berg, & Gustafson, 1984). In the United States, our medical system is not centralized enough to allow such control over the availability of the prosthesis. The risk of malpractice suits, however, has led to voluntary psychological evaluation of surgical candidates. We propose a model system of presurgical assessment that we hope will be widely adopted (Schover & von Eschenbach, 1985a).

A pretreatment evaluation should follow the comprehensive format outlined in Chapter 6. We believe the man's partner should always be included if he is in a committed relationship. A few men are no longer sexually active with their wives but do have other partners. In those cases we discuss the impact that surgery could have on the marriage relationship so that if a man decides to proceed, he has considered all emotional consequences.

A number of factors besides the "cause" of the erection problem determine whether a man will be happy with his surgery. The interview may reveal that his sexual desire is low or his orgasms are reduced in intensity. If so, he must be informed that the prosthesis may not improve his sexual pleasure. His partner may have trouble getting aroused or reaching orgasm. Perhaps she fears that her husband will demand too much sexual activity if he can have erections at will, or that he will be unfaithful. The stereotype is that the wife pressures her husband to have surgery, but, in fact, we rarely see such couples. In our experience, the man is usually far more enthusiastic about surgery and discounts his partner's assurances that she is satisfied with noncoital orgasms. In fact, in a series of couples evaluated for erectile dysfunction, wives reported the problem to be far less severe than did the husbands (Jensen, Sjögren, & Meidahl, 1984). Women often worry about the surgery's effect on a man's health, especially when he already has medical problems.

Unfortunately, the men most likely to seek a penile prosthesis are those who believe that intercourse is the only "normal" way of achieving sexual satisfaction. Often they have stopped initiating any sexual activity and have even ceased showing much affection to the wife because of fears of being unable to "perform." Couples who have little sexual communication or flexibility, and consequently cease sexual activity when an erection problem begins, are less likely to be satisfied with a penile prosthesis (Gee, McRoberts, Raney, & Ansell, 1974). Men who focus on erections are also disappointed that even an inflatable prosthesis can never duplicate nature entirely. A marital power struggle over the lack of erections may be transformed after surgery to dissatisfaction with penile size or shape.

When risks for postsurgical sexual dissatisfaction are identified, sex therapy should be offered before the decision is made to implant a penile prosthesis. The goals of counseling include improving couple communication, remedying sexual dysfunctions other than the erection problem, and resolving disagreements and power struggles that focus on sex. If the clinician can build a good relationship with an individual patient or couple, the man may develop a different perspective on surgery. Currently, if a responsible urologist refuses to operate because of emotional factors, patients often find a less scrupulous surgeon.

A brief case description demonstrates the role of presurgical sexual counseling, even for a man with a clearly organic erectile dysfunction.

Phil was a 47-year-old factory foreman who had a radical prostatectomy. During his hospitalization, the sex therapist got to know him well. Phil had divorced his wife 4 years previously on discovering that she had had a string of affairs. He recently had been dating a woman of 35 but had difficulty getting along with her children. When his cancer was diagnosed, he ended their relationship, telling his girlfriend that he did not want her pity.

After surgery, Phil lived for several months with his married daughter, although his physical recovery was proceeding well and he could easily have returned to his home city and resumed work. He regained good urinary control. The daughter loved Phil, but fostered his dependency while complaining vigorously about her father's abdication of his adult responsibilities. Phil came back to the clinic from time to time. He did not try to date because he felt no woman would accept him without erections.

About a year after surgery, Phil appeared for a follow-up visit with a very attractive woman whom he introduced as his fiancée. He had finally gone back to work and they had been introduced by friends. The couple was obviously in love, and, indeed, Phil's girlfriend reported that they had a wonderful sex life. Phil could not get rigid erections, but his penis grew just firm enough for vaginal penetration. He could reach orgasm through thrusting and she was quite happy to reach orgasm afterwards with manual or oral caressing. She had never been coitally orgasmic in any case. Phil was dissatisfied, however. He felt he was failing to carry out his "duty" as a man. The jealousy and periods of emotional withdrawal sparked by his sexual insecurity created the only real conflict in the couple's relationship.

Phil had recently met a man who had a semirigid prosthesis. He wanted more detailed information on this option than he had received before. The surgery was discussed with both partners, but the therapist emphasized their good sexual communication and general happiness. She suggested they continue enjoying their lovemaking and discuss whether or not they needed a prosthesis.

Phil eventually decided to proceed with a Flexi-rod™ prosthesis. He and his fiancée, Minnie, had married and continued to be happy. She saw little reason for the surgery, but acknowledged that Phil would never feel like a whole man again unless he could have erections.

The selection of a particular type of penile prosthesis depends on a number of factors. We describe all available models to a patient or couple, discussing pros and cons. The possibility of revisions with an inflatable type must be weighed against the ease of concealment. How active is the man's lifestyle? Does he jog, play tennis, or belong to a health club? If so, an inflatable may be preferable. Does he have medical problems that make surgery more than usually risky? Perhaps a malleable or self-contained inflatable type would be better then.

Ideally, once a man opts to have surgery, the clinician should visit during the hospitalization.

While Phil was recuperating from his operation, a couple session was held. The clinician helped the partners discuss their feelings about the month's ban on sexual intercourse, how to resume sexual activity gradually by using a sensate focus format, and how to avoid putting pressure on Minnie to have coital orgasms, as well as positions for intercourse, vaginal lubricants, and their initial impressions of the appearance of his penis. The couple planned how they would initiate sex, and Phil gave himself permission to stop intercourse after his orgasm, even if his wife had not reached a climax. The couple was given a chapter to read about having sex with a penile prosthesis (Schover, 1984, pp. 130–157).

Even with adequate preparation for surgery, couples often need post-surgical sexual counseling. It is wise to schedule a follow-up visit soon after the couple resumes intercourse. Indications at that time for sex therapy include persistent sexual dysfunctions such as desire discrepancies, difficulty reaching orgasm, or prolonged penile pain with no clear organic cause. Whether or not sex therapy is needed at the initial follow-up, a second visit should take place 6 to 12 months after surgery to make sure the couple remains satisfied with their sexual relationship.

Phil and Minnie did not require postoperative sex therapy. When last seen, 6 months after surgery, both were content. Phil had no difficulty concealing his penile prosthesis but remarked that he no longer danced closely with women who were only casual acquaintances. He complained that his penis was shorter than it had been before his erectile dysfunction. He was not really distressed, however, and Minnie pointed out that although she had not known him in his original "mint" condition, she was satisfied now. She commented that Phil's increased sexual confidence made him a warmer, more relaxed husband. The couple was having daily intercourse and enjoyed the freedom to experiment with positions, which they could not manage before the prosthesis surgery. Minnie was occasionally orgasmic during intercourse but continued to enjoy noncoital orgasms.

Minnie had worried when Phil became flirtatious with other women after his surgery. The couple had discussed her fears, however, and Phil had reaffirmed his contentment with their marriage. Minnie had been afraid that her husband would stop needing her when he was fully sexually functional, but their ability to talk out their feelings helped her to resolve her anxiety.

Better follow-up data are needed on both partners' satisfaction with the penile prosthesis. Existing studies suggest that 80% to 90% of men are glad they had surgery, but methodology has been poor (Schover & von Eschenbach, 1985a). Measures of sexual satisfaction have been limited to one general, overall rating. Partners' perspectives have rarely been studied. High rates of satisfaction may reflect patients' tendencies to express gratitude to their physicians, since surveys have not been anonymous. We must also recognize the bias inherent in the classic psychological principle of cognitive dissonance: A man who has gone through the pain and expense of surgery will be likely to see it as worthwhile.

Men who choose a penile prosthesis are a special group from the start. Even among men with clearly organic erectile dysfunction, only a small percentage opt for corrective surgery. For example, 112 men undergoing radical cystectomy were educated about changes in sexual function and were given a full explanation of the penile prosthesis (Schover *et al.*, 1986). Seventy-eight percent of wives also participated in the counseling. By the time of follow-up assessment, 31 men had cancer recurrences and 5 had recovered full erections. Yet, of the remaining 76 men, only 13 (17%) had chosen to have a penile prosthesis.

Although many men expressed interest in a prosthesis, those who went through with the surgery were insecure about relationships. Four of the 13 were divorced or widowed, and several others were recently remarried or had a long history of having extramarital affairs. These men believed strongly that a woman needed intercourse with a rigid penis to be contented in a relationship. They saw the penile prosthesis, not just as a means to have intercourse again, but as a hedge against ending up alone. Such attitudes are ingrained and are difficult to change with short-term psychotherapy.

One case not only illustrates the way that a penile prosthesis is treated as a key to gaining intimacy and nurturance but also shows how little power a clinician has to prevent a patient from having surgery if he is determined to have it.

Eric was a 44-year-old engineer with recently diagnosed invasive bladder cancer. It is always worrisome when such a young patient needs radical surgery, but Eric gave more than usual cause for concern. His wife Nancy did not accompany him when he was admitted to the hospital. He described her as a beautiful and seductive woman who had had many lovers in the past. He spent a long time stressing how little he minded her reputation among his friends as "easy." Eric asked for a pass to go out to dinner 2 nights before his surgery. He became so intoxicated that the restaurant put him forcibly into a taxi and he was found by the hospital staff unconscious on the front lawn.

When Nancy did join her husband after the cystectomy, it became clear that their marriage was in trouble. Areas of conflict included Eric's extravagance in spending money, Nancy's preference for oral sex instead of intercourse, and stormy relationships with their families of origin. Both partners were alcoholics, but only Eric acknowledged that they needed help. He described a long history of affective disorder, although not of psychotic proportions. He best fit the DSM-III diagnosis of cyclothymic disorder.

We lost contact with Eric until a year after his cystectomy. At that time he called the sex therapist to say that his wife had left him and he wanted a penile prosthesis. Several months before, he had been hospitalized for depression but left against medical advice. His consulting business was in disarray, and he had been drinking heavily. He believed his cancer would soon recur because of the stress he was experiencing.

The sex therapist urged him to go back to his psychiatrist, particularly when Eric mentioned that he had been having obsessive thoughts about shooting himself and confirmed that he kept a pistol in his house. In fact, the sex therapist obtained Eric's permission to contact his psychiatrist, and the two clinicians convinced him to enter an inpatient alcohol treatment program. We told Eric that a penile prosthesis was no substitute for solving his other life problems and that he would not be a good surgical candidate until he stopped drinking.

Two months later, the sex therapist received another call from Eric, who was hospitalized in a neighboring institution, having had a penile prosthesis implanted. The sex therapist was stunned, because she had not made a referral. Eric explained that he had referred himself, using a letter written to his insurance company by the surgeon who performed his cystectomy. The letter had been intended to help him get insurance reimbursement for a penile prosthesis once he was psychologically prepared for surgery. The urologist who implanted the prosthesis had not contacted Eric's medical team or obtained a psychiatric consultation. Eric had successfully concealed his history of alcoholism and psychiatric hospitalization, which would not have escaped a trained clinician with the time to complete an in-depth assessment.

At last contact, Eric was trying to win back his estranged wife, although he claimed she was simply the most convenient sexual partner he could find. Having fulfilled his purpose, he has refused further follow-up care.

OTHER MEDICAL TREATMENTS FOR ERECTILE DYSFUNCTION

Sexual counseling has a more limited role in helping men choose other medical treatments for erectile dysfunction, including penile revascularization surgery, papaverine injections, or medications such as yohimbine or vasodilators. Since all of these treatments are experimental, the mental health clnician's role may be to educate the patient on their pros and cons. Typically, a man has read media coverage hailing a new discovery that can cure all sexual problems. He needs to have more accurate expectations. Clinicians need to stay abreast of the field to be effective educators. To evaluate miracle "cures," clinicians should read whatever reports have been published in peer-reviewed journals, looking carefully for biases in patient selection, lack of long-term follow-up, failure to conduct double-blind studies, and, most of all, lack of adequate controls for the placebo effect.

Penile Revascularization

Surgery to restore adequate blood flow to the penis holds out a hope for a "natural" cure for vascular erectile dysfunction. Thus far, however, results have been disappointing for a number of reasons:

- Many men have a combination of neurological and vascular disease. If pelvic autonomic nerves or penile neurotransmitters are malfunctioning, increasing the blood flow to the penis will not restore good erections.
- Most candidates for vascular surgery are men over age 50 with diffuse arteriosclerosis in the smallest pelvic arteries, including those inside the penis. Successful revascularization is mainly limited to men with discrete lesions in one or several of the larger, less distal arteries, for example, young men who have had a fractured pelvis (Sharlip, 1981; Shaw & Zorgniotti, 1984).
- The most successful revascularization procedures use microvascular surgical techniques (Hawatmeh *et al.*, 1983), which are technically quite difficult. Differing success rates may depend on the surgeon's experience and skill.
- Even if the surgeon can supply just the right amount of extra blood flow to the penis, achieving a delicate balance between insufficient change and priapism (Michal, Kramar, Pospichal, & Hejhal, 1977), the new connections are liable to close within a few months because of scarring or blood clots.

In one recent case series, when penile blood flow was increased in middle-aged men with diffuse arteriosclerosis by connecting the inferior epigastric artery (normally providing circulation to the stomach) to a dorsal penile artery, the rate of success was only 26% (Goldstein, Mortara, & Krane, 1985). These operations are currently advisable only in very special circumstances.

Although penile revascularization has limited applicability, surgeons have increased their success in restoring erectile function and in avoiding damage to the sympathetic nerves controlling emission when they repair aortic aneurysms or bypass or eliminate blockages in the larger iliac arteries (Dewar, Blundell, Lidstone, Herba, & Chin, 1985; Flanigan *et al.*, 1982). The major goal of such operations is not to cure erection problems, however, but to treat serious vascular disease. Using transluminal angioplasty to dilate blocked pelvic arteries may have more promise in treating erectile dysfunction as an isolated problem (Goldwasser, Carson, Braun, & McCann, 1985).

Penile Injections

Physicians in the United States and in Europe have begun advocating penile injections with drugs that cause priapism as a treatment for erectile dysfunction. The first drug tested was phenoxybenzamine (Brindley, 1983). Its use was curtailed abruptly, however, by the disclosure that, in injectable form, it is potentially mutagenic and carcinogenic (Flind, 1984).

Investigators soon switched to papaverine, often combined with phentolamine (Virag, Frydman, Legman, & Virag, 1984; Zorgniotti & Lefleur, 1985). Papaverine injections produce a prolonged, full erection unless a man has severe vascular disease in the penile circulatory system. Even if a man reaches orgasm, the erection does not detumesce for several hours. Unfortunately, even with small doses, a few men have erections that persist longer than 4 hours, necessitating emergency medical treatment for priapism. The potential for long-term side effects, such as infection, carcinogenesis, or at least local neurological damage or fibrosis, is unknown (Sidi, Cameron, Duffy, & Lange, 1986). Cases of fibrosis are already being reported, however (Larsen *et al.*, 1987).

The clinicians using papaverine say that if it fails, a man can always have a penile prosthesis, but scarring of the cavernous bodies or damage to sensory nerves can also interfere with successful surgical treatment. Some researchers have warned of the potential abuse of papaverine by sexually functional men who want to prolong erections or by clinicians treating men with psychogenic erectile dysfunction (Virag *et al.*, 1984). Urologists, however, are already using papaverine instead of sex therapy to treat men who have no organic basis for their erection problems, although Brindley (1983) is the only one who has yet advocated this in print. We fear this practice will become widespread. Until papaverine's long-term impact is known, physicians and patients must temper their enthusiasm and continue stringent monitoring of men on home injection programs.

Oral Medications for Erectile Dysfunction

The search for the magic pill never ceases. In 1984, the media heralded a study published in *Science* demonstrating that yohimbine, an alpha-adrenergic antagonist, enhanced male rats' sexual performance. Rats given yohimbine injections mounted females more often and ejaculated more quickly (Clark, Smith, & Davidson, 1984). Thus a new cure for "impotence" was born. In fact, yohimbine in oral doses has had a long history of use in men with erectile dysfunction. Despite the lack of evidence of its effectiveness, researchers continue to investigate it (Morales, Surridge, Marshall, & Fenemore, 1982). Even without a double-blind study, only 26% of men in one series reported improvement in erections, a success rate well within the range expected for a placebo. This research group repeated their studies with no better results, but, ever hopeful, they now believe they have simply not found the right way to administer the drug (Owen *et al.*, 1985).

Others have administered oral doses of vasodilators to men with erectile dysfunction. In one study (Elist, Jarman, & Edson, 1984), a third of men with previously abnormal NPT improved their erectile function when they either stopped smoking, took a vasodilator, or had both "treatments." In a few patients, objective measures such as NPT monitoring and Doppler studies also improved. The research design obviously lacks a control for the placebo effect, but at least the physicians made a contribution by encouraging men to quit smoking.

COUNSELING FOR WOMEN BEFORE BREAST OR GENITAL RECONSTRUCTION

Although there is no parallel treatment to the penile prosthesis for women, operations to alter the breasts or to repair a vaginal deformity often have the goal of improving a woman's sexual self-concept or function. Individual or couple counseling can help a woman to decide whether surgery is right for her and to gain maximum psychological benefit from the changes in her body.

Breast surgery may include breast augmentation, reduction mammaplasty, or reconstructive surgery performed after a mastectomy. Elective operations to change breast contours raise many of the same issues as the penile prosthesis. Just as our society has focused on erections as the criterion of a good lover in a man, we have regarded women's breasts as a crucial aspect of sexual attractiveness. When is surgery beneficial, and when are we encouraging women to conform to destructive sexual stereotypes? Since breast surgery does not restore reproductive "function," women who seek it are often regarded as frivolous and vain by the same physicians who believe that the penile prosthesis is the answer to all erection problems.

Women also castigate themselves for wanting to change their breasts, even when surgery would repair a true disfigurement. It is common to see guilt and self-doubt in a woman considering reconstruction after mastectomy or in a young woman who desires breast reduction after being tormented for years about her pendulous, disproportionately large breasts. Some women do not feel that the pain of surgery is necessary, but that is an individual choice, not an index of moral superiority. The clinician's job is to make sure that a woman has accurate expectations about surgery and will benefit emotionally. Women who choose breast reconstruction after cancer surgery (Schain, Jacobs, & Wellisch, 1984) or even at the time of mastectomy (Schain, Wellisch, Pasnau, & Landsverk, 1985; Stevens *et al.*, 1984) are not psychologically maladjusted. They usually want the freedom to wear a wider range of clothing styles and believe that having a breast mound will help them feel more whole and sexually attractive. In the United States, studies of women without a history of cancer who have cosmetic breast surgery also disconfirm the stereotype that patients are narcissistic or hysterical. Male partners, like wives of men considering a penile prosthesis, rarely press for breast surgery and, in fact, often feel neutral or somewhat opposed to the idea (Schain *et al.*, 1984).

Whether the operation in question is a breast augmentation or reduction in a healthy woman or a breast reconstruction in a woman who has had cancer, the needs for evaluation are similar. The clinician can conduct couple and brief individual sessions to assess each partner's beliefs and hopes about the outcome. Are they aware that visible scars will remain? Does a woman undergoing breast reconstruction after mastectomy realize that her breast mound and reconstructed nipple will have little erotic sensitivity? Does either partner expect breast surgery to cure a sexual dysfunction or repair a damaged relationship (Schlebusch & Levin, 1983)? As with men seeking a penile prosthesis, a minority of patients have severe psychopathology that could be exacerbated by an operation that cannot fulfill its function in their distorted cognitive or interpersonal system.

An assessment for breast surgery can afford an opportunity to engage a woman in much-needed psychotherapy.

Irene, a 27-year-old secretary, was first seen by the sex therapist as a research patient participating in a study of women with early breast cancer. Since Irene's tumor was small, she was able to have a segmental mastectomy that only removed a wedge of tissue from her breast. The surgery was followed by radiotherapy. One of Irene's axillary lymph nodes was positive for cancer, however, so she also received six courses of chemotherapy.

Initially, Irene seemed much younger than her age. She lived alone with her cat and had few friends. Her mother lived only a few blocks away and accompanied her to the interview with the sex therapist. Irene and her mother were both firm in wanting to be seen together.

Irene said that she had not dated at all in the 2 years since her divorce. She had been briefly married to a man who abused alcohol and street drugs. He frequently stayed out all night and taunted Irene about his other women. She did not leave, however, until he beat her one day.

The mother communicated the clear message that Irene was a fragile and naughty adolescent who needed protection from the world. Irene was very anxious at the time of her surgery. She was convinced she would die of her cancer and believed she had brought it on herself by agreeing to her husband's demand that she use oral contraceptives. She had a history of severe migraine headaches and had had rheumatic fever as a child. In her mother's presence, Irene said she had never enjoyed sex and was not orgasmic. She believed that men only wanted to exploit women for sex.

Irene had her radiotherapy and chemotherapy at home in a distant city rather than remaining at the hospital. She did return for a 6-month follow-up and filled out research questionnaires, but declined to see the sex therapist. Her Brief Symptom Inventory scores were mildly elevated on scales measuring somatic symptoms, interpersonal sensitivity, depression, phobic anxiety, and alienation (psychoticism scale). Her scores were within the normal range, however, and were not surprising given her recent illness and treatment.

A few months later, Irene returned to have partial breast reconstruction. Her segmental mastectomy had left her with a hollow in her breast and unequal breast size. A flap of skin and muscle from her back would be used to fill out the area where the breast tissue had been removed.

She complained to her medical team that her headaches were worse than ever, and she was constantly exhausted. At their urging, she kept her follow-up appointment this time to see the sex therapist. Irene presented quite a different picture when seen without her mother. She disclosed that she had been dating a man when her cancer was diagnosed, but he had rejected her when she became ill. She talked about her dissatisfaction with her boring job and the small town where she lived, which did not afford opportunities to meet compatible women friends or men to date. She wanted to move to a larger city but realized that she was overly dependent on her mother. She also seemed far more interested in exploring her sexuality than she had appeared in the first interview.

Irene responded eagerly to the suggestion that psychotherapy could help her control her headaches, separate emotionally from her family, feel more comfortable with her sexuality, and prepare herself to move away from home. She was given several referrals to clinicians in her home town and promised to contact one of them as soon as she returned there.

The psychotherapist should also be aware of the medical aspects of breast surgery. Some basic facts are as follows:

- For a complete breast reconstruction, the choice of method depends on the amount of extra skin left on the chest after mastectomy and on other physical aspects of a woman's body. If a simple mastectomy was performed with ample skin left intact, a silicone implant can be placed under the remaining chest muscle to recreate a breast mound. Many women need additional tissue, however, to cover an implant, for example after a radical or modified radical mastectomy. One new technique is to implant an inflatable "tissue expander" reservoir under the skin and gradually fill it with liquid. After several months a permanent breast implant can be substituted. In another type of surgery, skin and its underlying muscle can be moved from the back to the chest. Using microsurgical techniques, surgeons leave the flap of tissue connected to its nerve and blood supply (Figure 8-2). Some women now have breast reconstruction with a rectus abdominus flap taken from their abdominal area. This flap provides enough tissue to create a breast without a silicone implant, reducing the risks of infection or tight, scar tissue formation around a prosthesis. Women who have slightly protruding stomachs are good candidates. Surgery involving a flap creates a good deal of pain in the area where the flap was removed. Most women say that healing from the reconstruction is more painful than recovery after the original mastectomy.

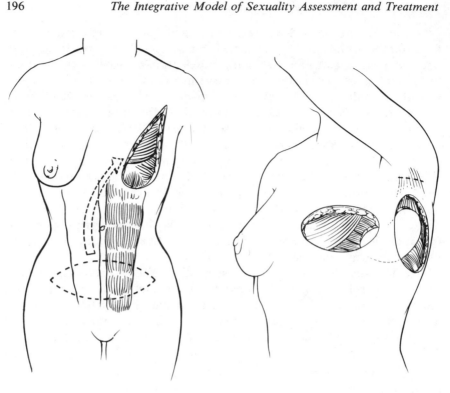

Rectus abdominus   Latissimus dorsi

Figure 8-2. Flaps used in breast reconstruction.

- Surgery that involves reconstruction with skin and muscle flaps always leaves some visible scars on the breast and on the back or stomach where tissue is removed.
- If surgery involves reconstructing the nipple, the breast mound is restored first and the nipple is usually created several weeks later in a separate procedure. The breast mound needs the time to settle into its final shape. A nipple added immediately would probably end up off center.
- After mastectomy, the remaining healthy breast may need to be slightly enlarged or reduced to match the reconstructed breast mound. This will usually be done at the time of the nipple reconstruction.
- Any breast surgery, even a breast reduction or a subcutaneous mastectomy that removes most of the breast tissue, destroys the nipple's erotic sensitivity because sensory nerves are damaged.

Some women also have genital reconstructive surgery. Such operations are most commonly performed to repair damage from cancer surgery, but they are discussed in this chapter because vaginal reconstruction is also used when women are born with genetic or hormonal anomalies. For the approximately 1 in 10,000 women born without a vagina, reconstruction usually is not recommended until late adolescence because the new vagina requires vaginal dilation or sexual activity to stay open (Poland & Evans, 1985). The condition is often not diagnosed until a young woman fails to begin menstruation.

The most common surgical procedure is to create a vaginal opening and line it with a split-thickness skin graft. During the early days of healing, a woman has to wear a *stent*, or cylindrical form, at all times to keep the vagina open (Edwards *et al.*, 1981).

Within 6 weeks after surgery, the woman can remove the stent for several hours each day and begin sexual activity. Unless she is having intercourse at least three times a week, she needs to use a vaginal dilator for several months until healing is complete. Poland and Evans (1985) found that visits every 2 weeks during this period helped the medical team monitor a woman's compliance with dilation. Since many women regard the stent or dilator as something artificial and somehow sexual, dilation can be emotionally distressing, as well as physically painful at first. Women who have never masturbated or even touched their genitals fear that dilation will be disgusting or shamefully arousing. We find that several techniques help desensitize a woman to vaginal dilation.

- We begin by using life-like genital models to illustrate the role of the vagina, vulva, clitoris, and other sexual organs in arousal, orgasm, and reproduction. We encourage a woman to go home and look at her genitals in a mirror. A physician may use a mirror in the office to teach a woman about her own anatomy, being careful not to be seductive or inappropriate. If a woman feels comfortable enough, we suggest she put a finger inside her vagina to explore its size and texture. We explain that a vagina reconstructed with skin grafts may or may not produce enough lubrication for comfortable intercourse, giving the woman a supply of lubricant to use with her dilator and to apply before intercourse.
- Women with small vaginas may need to use a series of dilators that gradually increase in size. They and their partners may benefit from viewing a film created for women with vaginismus (J. LoPiccolo, 1984). The film shows a woman using dilators to overcome her fear of penetration. A woman and her partner should be prepared emotionally for this sexually explicit film, however, and be given a chance to discuss their reactions to it.
- Emotional support is crucial from the partner, or, for young, single women, from the parents (Poland & Evans, 1985). The partner or parents should understand how dilation can help.
- A woman should begin with daily dilation, making it a routine part of her schedule. We suggest that she put dilation in a nonsexual context, for

example using the dilator while taking a bath or while lying in the bedroom and watching television or reading.

- We teach the woman to identify her pubococcygeal muscles, which are still functional after many vaginal reconstructions. We teach her to tense and relax the muscles, noting during urination how she uses them to shut off the flow of urine, and later putting a fingertip in her vagina while she squeezes so she can feel the movement. Sometimes we assign her to practice squeezing and relaxing the muscles 10 times, twice a day.
- We instruct a woman to tense her vaginal muscles and then relax them before placing the dilator in her vaginal entrance. She then can hold it there, tensing and relaxing her muscles again before pushing it a little further into her vagina. We suggest she repeat this sequence several times until she pushes the dilator as far as it will go without pain.
- For most women, keeping the dilator in the vagina for 5 or 10 minutes daily is sufficient, but a sex therapist should always consult with the surgeon and modify the instructions to fit her or his specifications.

Some vaginal reconstructions do not require postsurgical dilation. The same microsurgical techniques used in breast reconstruction can be used after radical pelvic cancer surgery to create a neovagina (or less commonly to rebuild a vulva when it is removed for vulvar cancer). Flaps of skin and underlying muscle are taken from the inner thighs and sewn together to create a vaginal tube lined with the skin (Edwards *et al.*, 1981). Since the skin is full-thickness and has a good blood supply, the vagina does not shrink appreciably during healing, and dilation is unnecessary. A woman will need to douche several times weekly to prevent odor, however, and her vaginal lining will not become a true mucosa, able to produce lubrication with sexual arousal. Women often report strange sensations when they first resume intercourse. The vagina may feel numb, or pressure may create a feeling as if the inner thighs were being touched because the vaginal walls still have their original nerve supply. Over time, intercourse often becomes more pleasurable. Clitoral sensation should remain normal unless the vulva was also removed in the initial cancer surgery.

No matter what type of vaginal reconstruction is performed, a woman may need counseling on how to become orgasmic again. Clitoral or breast stimulation becomes crucial in reaching orgasm when vaginal sensations are weak. Sex therapy techniques used for inorgasmic women, such as masturbation exercises and prolonged, sensual caressing from a partner (Barbach, 1982; L. LoPiccolo, Heiman, & LoPiccolo, 1976) can easily be adapted for the woman or couple resuming sex after a vaginal reconstruction. The woman must reassure her partner that she will tell him if any stimulation is painful. We suggest beginning couple sessions at home with noncoital caressing. If a woman is using a vaginal dilator, her partner can watch her insert it and then gently insert it himself. Some couples prefer to keep dilation separate from sexuality. In that case, the man can gently and slowly use his fingers to caress his partner's vagina, giving the couple confidence that intercourse will not be painful or difficult.

Young women who have vaginal reconstructions may not have been sexually experienced before surgery. They often can use some basic sex education.

Valerie was 17 at the time of her split-thickness skin graft procedure to create a vagina. She had a normal clitoris and vulva, but her bladder, vagina, uterus, ovaries, and tubes had been removed at age 4 to treat a genital sarcoma. She was an attractive and lively young woman who grew up in a Fundamentalist Protestant family. Valerie had a boyfriend and had tried some breast and genital caressing. Her parents, however, did not know the young couple had engaged in any sexual activity. They plainly had ambivalent thoughts about the daughter's surgery. Given that she was not yet ready to marry and could never have a child, the parents would have preferred that their daughter wait until she was engaged to have a vagina created.

Valerie herself was torn between her parent's ideals and her own readiness to become sexually active. She had never had an orgasm and wanted to find out how to experience one. She was seen for brief counseling by the sex therapist, with her parents' knowledge. Sessions focused on teaching basic facts about sexuality, giving her a self-help book on learning to reach orgasm and helping her come to terms with her own sexual attitudes and values about relationships.

Other women have to adjust to a neovagina after years of normal sexual function. A couple counseling format is the most effective way to help.

Rita was a 36-year-old homemaker with four children. She and her husband, an automobile mechanic, had been married for 15 years. After her cervical cancer had been treated with radiotherapy, it reappeared locally. She needed a total pelvic exenteration, removing her bladder, urethra, vagina, uterus, ovaries, fallopian tubes, and rectum. She was left with two ostomies, one to eliminte urine and one for stool. Her vagina was reconstructed using myocutaneous gracilis flaps.

Rita had difficulty looking at her ostomies and learning to change her pouches after surgery. She and her husband, Andy, received sexual counseling while she was still in the hospital. When they got home, even cuddling in bed was too anxiety-provoking. Before trying sensate focus exercises, the couple was assigned to exchange small acts of caring and to touch more during the day. Later they worked on cuddling comfortably while watching television. Being seen in the nude was too advanced a next step for Rita, but she did allow Andy to caress her under her nightgown. He had always felt ambivalent about the moistness and odor of a woman's genitals. Before cancer surgery the couple had showered before sexual activity and never had had intercourse during her menstrual period.

Andy's emotional reaction to his wife's altered bowel and bladder function was also more extreme than usual. One night when she accidently leaked urine onto their mattress, he stormed out of the bedroom, although he felt terribly guilty and apologetic afterward.

Over several months, the couple resumed mutual manual stimulation to orgasm. Clitoral stimulation was just as enjoyable to Rita as it had been before surgery, but she felt pain when her husband tried to penetrate her vagina. She had not followed instructions to use a lubricant, however. With adequate lubrication, the couple tried slow penetration under her control, with Andy lying quietly. The pain and anxiety subsided over several tries. The first time that intercourse finally succeeded, Andy went to sleep afterwards without saying any loving or encouraging words to his wife. She was able to express her anger in the next couple session, with the support of the therapist. Although frequency of intercourse did not return to presurgery levels, the couple functioned normally and each partner was reasonably satisfied.

Part 1 of this book has set forth the skills a clinician needs to assess and treat sexual problems in patients with chronic illnesses. Part 2 provides techniques to use with the specific medical conditions that most often interfere with good sexual function. Knowing the general principles that apply to all cases, the reader can focus on the populations most relevant to his or her practice.

PART TWO

SPECIFIC ILLNESSES AND SEXUALITY

9

Life-Threatening Crises and Sexuality: Cardiovascular Disease, Cancer, and End-Stage Renal Disease

The illnesses discussed in this chapter are those that threaten the patient's very survival. The time of diagnosis and acute treatment is a period of crisis, when sexual issues may seem of low priority. With modern medical care, however, these diseases have become chronic illnesses for many men and women. As survival time increases, quality of life, including sexual function, becomes crucial. We include separate sections on each illness, so that a clinician can use them as a quick reference resource for a particular patient. We begin by reviewing the psychosocial and physiological impact of each disease on sexuality and highlight special issues in assessment and treatment. Combined tables on assessment and treatment strategies allow the reader to compare the three illnesses. Case examples demonstrate the use either of brief sexual counseling by the primary care team or of intensive sex therapy by a specialist.

CARDIOVASCULAR DISEASE

Coronary artery disease is the number one cause of death in the United States (W. Kaplan & Kimball, 1982). This section focuses on sexuality in men and women who have hypertension or cardiac disease or have experienced a myocardial infarction, cerebrovascular accident, or coronary artery bypass surgery. Although the consensus is growing that cardiac patients need sexual counseling, our actual state of knowledge about effective sexuality assessment and treatment remains rather primitive.

It is clear that sexual problems are common in both men and women with cardiovascular disease. The frequency of sexual activity decreases in 40% to 70% of patients after MI (Papadopoulos *et al.*, 1983; Sjögren & Fugl-Meyer, 1983; Wiklund, Sanne, Elmfeldt, Vedin, & Wilhelmsson, 1984), coronary bypass operation (Althof, Coffman, & Levine, 1984; Kinchla & Weiss, 1985; Papadopoulos *et al.*, 1986; Thurer, 1982), or a CVA

(Bray *et al.*, 1981; Hawton, 1984; Sjögren, 1983; Sjögren & Fugl-Meyer, 1982). Sexual dysfunction increases, particularly loss of sexual desire in both sexes, and erectile dysfunction and difficulty reaching orgasm in men. Many patients experience angina or other cardiac symptoms during sexual activity (Jackson, 1981; Papadopoulos *et al.*, 1983; Sjögren & Fugl-Meyer, 1983).

Yet, many patients and spouses report that sexuality remains an important issue, rarely addressed by their medical team (Bray *et al.*, 1981; Papadopoulos *et al.*, 1983; Papadopoulos *et al.*, 1986; Sikorski, 1985).

Psychosocial Impact on Sexuality

The degree of emotional distress that a patient experiences on diagnosis of cardiovascular disease is related to past psychological health and coping skills (Bass, 1984; Ramshaw & Stanley, 1984; Wiklund *et al.*, 1984). Those who are older or who do not have the resources to adjust to illness have poorer psychological and social outcomes after MI, CVA, or coronary bypass. Recovery of sexual function is related to the general ability to overcome depression and anxiety and to return to work and other activities of daily life.

Depression has been commonly identified as a sequela of a cardiovascular health crisis (Goodstein, 1983; W. Kaplan & Kimball, 1982) and may account for some loss of sexual desire after MI or CVA (Sjögren & Fugl-Meyer, 1982). Herd (1984) has suggested that depression is a risk factor in cardiovascular disease because depressed patients have exaggerated cortisol release in response to stress. In a review of the literature on adjustment to coronary bypass, however, Kinchla and Weiss (1985) suggest that both depression and cognitive impairment are less common than has been believed.

Several long-term studies have linked Type A behavior, including competitiveness, a pressured attitude about time, vigilance, and hostility, to cardiovascular disease (Herd, 1984; W. Kaplan & Kimball, 1982). People who are Type A may also have an exaggerated physiological response to stress. Although the components of Type A behavior that are the crucial cardiac risk factors have been debated, Type A attitudes overlap with many features of a performance orientation to sexuality and thus may interfere with a patient's willingness to resume sex when illness has impaired sexual function even mildly (Sjögren, 1983).

Another risk factor for cardiovascular disease is life stress (Herd, 1984; W. Kaplan & Kimball, 1982), although the impact of stress probably depends not just on the number of recent life changes, but also on their meaning for the individual (Sarason, Johnson, & Siegel, 1978). One could view sexual dysfunction resulting from cardiovascular disease as a life stress in itself. For example, a man who suffers his first MI and must cope with subsequent angina, work limitations, and erectile dysfunction might be more at risk for a second MI than another man who was more successfully rehabilitated.

Sexual dysfunction in patients with cardiovascular disease correlates with feeling stigmatized by ill health (Sjögren, 1983; Sjögren & Fugl-Meyer, 1983). Men, particularly those who hold traditional beliefs about the male's directive role in sexual activity, are apt to suffer a loss of self-esteem after MI or CVA when they can no longer "perform" as effectively. In contrast, women in their 50s or 60s deny concern with physical attractiveness or body image after coronary bypass surgery (Althof *et al.*, 1984). Perhaps women are more likely to react to an illness by denying the importance of sexuality in their lives. Althof and colleagues observed that a number of women used their illness as an excuse to discontinue an unsatisfying sex life.

One special anxiety for men and women who are hypertensive, have angina pain, or have had an MI or a CVA is the fear that sexual activity will promote a heart attack or stroke. Papadopoulos *et al.* (1983) reported that 51% of women and 44% of their husbands feared the wife could die during intercourse after having had one MI. Wiklund *et al.* (1984), studying men after MI, found that fears about the safety of sexual activity were common at 2-month follow-up, although anxiety had decreased somewhat by the 1-year mark. Normal signs of sexual arousal, including increased heart rate, respiration, and sweating are often misinterpreted as cardiac symptoms (Sanders & Sprenkle, 1980). Goodstein (1983) also notes that elderly patients may regard a CVA as a punishment for engaging in sexual activity.

Fears about being sexually active, as well as anxiety about the ability to continue to function sexually, may contribute to increases in "spectatoring" (i.e., watching oneself during sexual activity rather than relaxing and enjoying arousal) in patients recovering from MI (Sjögren & Fugl-Meyer, 1983) or a CVA (Sjögren, 1983).

Cardiovascular disease also affects the marital relationship. Sikorski (1985), interviewing wives of men who had been home from the hospital for 2 to 3 weeks after coronary bypass surgery, found that most reported fatigue, anxiety, and bickering about what the husbands were allowed to do during convalescence. Bedsworth and Molen (1982) studied wives of men who were in intensive care after MI and observed that the majority were anxious about the husband's survival and future disability. Overprotectiveness on the spouse's part can encourage the patient to assume the invalid role and is also likely to interfere with resuming sex (Sjögren, 1983).

Being married promotes survival after MI for both men and women, whether during the initial hospitalization or over the long term (Chandra, Szklo, Goldberg, & Tonascia, 1983). Having good social support may reduce the risk of cardiovascular disease, as well as moderate its severity (Herd, 1984).

Can we predict which patients with cardiovascular disease will remain sexually active? Younger men and women are more like to resume sex after an MI (Papadopoulos *et al.*, 1983; Wiklund *et al.*, 1984). Kornfeld, Heller, Frank, Wilson, & Malm (1982), studying men after coronary bypass surgery, found that an increase in sexual frequency was related to improvement in cardiac symptoms, ability to return to work, and less Type A behavior. After a CVA, patients were more likely to resume sex if they had less motor impairment, retained a normal capacity to sense touch, and were more independent in their own care (Sjögren & Fugl-Meyer, 1982). Hawton (1984) also found that previous level of sexual activity, more than age, predicted resumption of sex after a CVA. Papadopoulos *et al.* (1983) found that women were more likely to be sexually active if they had had frequent activity before having an MI and had received brief, post-MI sexual counseling.

Physiological Impact on Sexuality

A salient concern for patients with cardiovascular disease has been the safety of sexual activity. Although the risk of an MI or a CVA during sex appears very minor, most advice to patients is based on one or two old and inadequate studies (Derogatis & King, 1981), for example a series of coroners' reports from Japan in the 1960s suggesting that only 0.6% of sudden deaths occurred during sexual activity. From that report, it was suggested that most coital deaths occur in unfamiliar surroundings with an extramarital partner, but of course such statistics are confounded by the likelihood that a cardiac arrest during intercourse in a man's own home during the 1960s in Japan would not be officially reported as a coital death.

The actual cardiac demands of sexual acitivity and orgasm have been studied. For middle-class Caucasian men, monitored at home during sexual activity with their wives, peak heart rates are around 120 beats per minute, similar to the demands of a mildly stressful work situation (Hellerstein & Friedman, 1970; Stein, 1980). Recently, Bohlen, Held, Sanderson, & Patterson (1984) studied cardiac requirements of sexual activity in men in healthy young couples, including the man stimulating himself, noncoital stimulation from the wife, intercourse with the husband on top, and intercourse with the wife on top. Maximum heart rates and oxygen consumption varied widely, so the researchers suggest that each cardiac patient be given individualized guidelines on resuming sex. In general, heart rate and pulse did not vary with coital position, but respiration and metabolic consumption were less if the wife took a more active role. Noncoital activities also were less demanding than intercourse.

Intercourse can be risky for patients with congestive heart failure or those whose ischemic threshold heart rate on an exercise test is under 115 beats per minute. Angina may be a problem during intercourse for those whose threshold is between 115 and 125 beats per minute, but pain can usually be minimized by a dose of nitroglycerine before sexual activity (Stein, 1980). Unfortunately, some patients respond to nitroglycerine with headaches.

The true risk of sudden coital death is probably not assessed by measures of heart rate (Derogatis & King, 1981; Herd, 1984). Such deaths result from ventricular fibrillation, an arrhythmia that occurs at moments of intense sympathetic nervous system activity, for example during orgasm. Sexual activity has been observed to provoke cardiac arrhythmia in some patients (Derogatis & King, 1981; Jackson, 1981). Hypertension patients who are not taking medication have also been found to achieve peak intraarterial blood pressures of 237/138 mm/Hg during orgasm. The higher the baseline blood pressure, the higher the peak (Mann, Craig, Gould, Melville, & Raftery, 1982).

Beta-blocking medications can significantly reduce peak heart rate, peak blood pressure, and the risk of ventricular fibrillation during sexual activity (Derogatis & King, 1981; Herd, 1984; Jackson, 1981; Mann *et al.*, 1982). Such medications also have a clear dose-related impact on erectile function (Moss & Procci, 1982; Sjögren & Fugl-Meyer, 1983), so that although they make coitus safer, they may also render it impossible. The long-term use of digoxin also causes sexual dysfunction, probably by altering hormone levels (Neri, Aygen, Zukerman, & Bahary, 1980).

Men who have cardiovascular disease are also at high risk for vascular erection problems, as discussed in Chapter 5, and for erectile dysfunction due to medications that affect autonomic neurotransmitters. In fact in one series of 131 men interviewed during hospitalization for MI, 64% had erection problems before the heart attack (Wabrek & Burchell, 1980). Dhabuwala *et al.* (1986) also found that sexual dysfunction was equally common in MI patients and a control group of urology outpatients matched in age, smoking history, and hypertension.

Assessment Issues

Sexual assessment for the cardiovascular patient follows the format outlined in Chapter 6, but some especially important issues are highlighted in Table 9-1. The interview should include a discussion of the psychological impact of the illness and whether it has promoted sexual anxieties. Since sexual rehabilitation is one aspect of general rehabilitation, specific cardiac risk factors such as Type A behavior and failure to modify unhealthy habits such as smoking or a high-fat diet should be assessed. A patient who is not complying in general cardiac rehabilitation will present a complex and difficult challenge to the sex therapist as well. The interviewer should ask the spouse about anxiety related to the illness and about his or her coping style. After a CVA, difficulty with sensation or movement can also interfere with sexual activity.

Table 9-1. Special Assessment Issues

	Cardiovascular Disease	Cancer	End-Stage Renal Disease
Interview Topics	Reaction to diagnosis	Reaction to diagnosis	Reaction to diagnosis
	Partner's coping strategies	Partner's coping strategies	Partner's coping strategies
	Beliefs about prognosis	Beliefs about prognosis	Beliefs about prognosis
	Depression and anxiety	Depression and anxiety	Depression and anxiety
	Compliance with lifestyle modifications	Compliance with modifications	Compliance with lifestyle modifications
	Fears about safety of sex and sudden death	Fears about sex and cancer contagion or recurrence	Anxiety about infertility
	Type A sexual attitudes (time pressure, performance orientation)	Feeling stigmatized	Feeling stigmatized
			Dependence on dialysis equipment or on renal transplantation
			Family attitudes about organ donation (N. B. Levy, 1986)
Questionnaires	Jenkins Activity Survey (Jenkins Zyzanski, & Rosenman, 1971)	The Cancer Inventory of Problem Situations (CIPS: Heinrich, Schag, & Ganz, 1984)	No special questionnaires available
	Life Experiences Survey (Sarason, Johnson, & Siegel, 1978)	The Functional Living Index–Cancer (FLIC) (Schipper, Clinch, McMurray, & Levitt, 1984)	
	Neuropsychological testing		

208

Medical History	Symptoms of vascular erectile dysfunction Current antihypertensive and cardiac medications	Other chronic illnesses All cancer therapies received All current medications	Underlying illness leading to renal failure Medications, especially antihypertensives or immunosuppressants Menstrual status for women
Physiological Assessment	Comprehensive evaluation for erectile dysfunction with special attention to vascular measures Assessment of neurological impairment of sensation or mobility Home EKG monitoring during sexual activity Treadmill testing	Comprehensive evaluation for erectile dysfunction with special attention to vascular measures after pelvic radiotherapy and to hormonal assays in men with testicular cancer, lymphoma, or Hodgkin's disease	Comprehensive evaluation for erectile dysfunction Symptoms of autonomic or peripheral neuropathy Special attention in men and women to prolactin levels, and for women to possible estrogen deficiency Current renal status (creatinine, proteinuria)

Questionnaires that measure Type A behavior or recent life events and their impact on the patient can be helpful in deciding whether intensive therapy is needed and in designing strategies to intervene in the relationship.

Because the safety of sexual activity is at issue, some patients benefit from portable electrocardiogram (EKG) monitoring during a typical daily schedule, including sexual intercourse (Bohlen *et al.*, 1984). Any tendency to have arrhythmias during sexual arousal or orgasm can be identified. Stein (1980) also suggests that the spouse routinely be invited to witness a full exercise EKG 10 to 12 weeks after MI. This test gives both partners a chance to see that exertion is safe. Taylor, Bandura, Ewart, Miller, and DeBusk (1985) have found that having wives actually take a treadmill test themselves at 3-week follow-up, as well as observing the husband's test, further increased their confidence in the husband's capacities. Men's and women's ratings of their psychological sense of self-efficacy after the treadmill test were good predictors of the men's peak heart rate and work load 11 and 26 weeks later. The more confident the husband and wife felt of his abilities, the more he improved.

Treatment Issues

Special treatment issues relevant to cardiovascular disease are listed in Table 9-2 and draw on techniques described in Chapters 7 and 8. The sexual counselor needs to collaborate closely with the primary care physician since many treatment decisions depend on whether intercourse is safe, on managing the patient's medication (Cooper, 1985), and on cardiac rehabilitation techniques, including modifying Type A behavior, diet, smoking, and exercise habits. Brief sexual counseling should be routinely provided in a cardiac rehabilitation program (Cole, 1979; Cole, Levin, Whitley, & Young, 1979) or as part of counseling programs for patients after CVA (Goodstein, 1983). Both partners should be included. In fact, after a 3-month cardiac rehabilitation program that encouraged spouse participation and focused on exercise and education, the frequency of sexual activity increased slightly in a group of 28 men in contrast to a decline in sexual activity in a control group given routine care (Roviaro, Holmes, & Holmsten, 1984). Table 9-3 presents guidelines on staying sexually active for patients with cardiovascular disease.

Brief Sexual Counseling Case

David was a 67-year-old veterinarian. His wife Anne, aged 63, sold real estate. The couple was interviewed by a sexual counselor in a department of cardiology. Fifteen years before, David had had an MI, followed 2 years later by triple coronary artery bypass surgery. A year before the interview he had also undergone a bilateral aortofemoral bypass operation. Currently he had congestive heart failure and had been told by his cardiologist that little improvement could be anticipated in his quality of life. David's medications included Lanoxin (digoxin) and Lasix (furosemide).

Anne was in good health, though she had had a hysterectomy 20 years before and a recent operation to remove her gallbladder. She had discontinued replacement estrogens several months before the interview because of chronic breast tenderness and fibrocystic changes. She had had three breast biopsies for lumps, all benign.

The couple had been married for 44 years and had two children. They saw their grandchildren at least weekly. Anne was an attractive, well-dressed woman who appeared younger than her age, but David was gray and frail. He was barely able to raise himself out of a sitting position and walked slowly, appearing short of breath.

Anne described her husband as a workaholic who claimed he would never retire until the year before, when ill health forced him to give up his veterinary practice. He had been a heavy smoker until quite recently and also tended to drink to excess when he felt stressed. Anne had always resented David's preoccupation with work and saw herself as having raised their children without his help. The couple did enjoy socializing at their country club, however, and both were golfers.

In the past year, David's life had changed radically. The couple no longer went to the club. During weekdays, David sat around the house or tried to do some light gardening. He complained of absent-mindedness in daily tasks and difficulty in concentrating, although a neurological work-up revealed only a mild cognitive deficit. He slept 12 hours a night and had little appetite for food or desire for sex. His mood was also depressed.

During a split therapy session, Anne complained that David would not let her out of his sight. If she went grocery shopping, he was waiting outside the house on her return, demanding to know what had taken her so long. Since David had always been a rather private or even withdrawn man, Anne was shocked and not a little dismayed by his behavior.

David said in the couple session that he felt Anne was avoiding him. Anne protested vigorously. The therapist helped them clarify that although David and Anne spent most of their waking hours together, David felt lonely and isolated much of the time.

In the past, the couple's sexual relationship had been problematic. David believed that Anne never enjoyed sex very much. He always had wanted her to be more aggressive and playful. Anne replied that David often made harsh comments about women who failed to act like "ladies," and she felt he had given her double messages. The therapist asked David if he had heard the old saying that a man wants his wife to be "a lady in public but a whore in bed." David agreed that it expressed his views, but could also see that it was a difficult agenda for Anne to follow.

Table 9-2. Special Treatment Issues

	Cardiovascular Disease	Cancer	End-Stage Renal Disease
Format	Brief counseling can be provided as part of a cardiac rehabilitation program May need to modify treatment for patients who are aphasic or cognitively impaired	Daily sessions or widely spaced sessions needed if patient lives far away Time sessions to avoid periods of acute illness, e.g., during a course of chemotherapy	Can plan support groups including sexual counseling in dialysis centers Modify treatment to accomodate limited energy levels
Brief Counseling			
Education	Safety of sex for cardiac patients	Effects of cancer therapy on sexual function	Effects of medications and disease-related factors on sexual function and fertility, protection against HPV for women after renal transplantation
Attitude Change	Reducing feelings of stigmatization, minimizing invalid role, reducing Type A sexual performance orientation	Reducing feelings of stigmatization, minimizing invalid role, improving body image, debunking myths about sex and cancer	Reducing feelings of stigmatization, minimizing invalid role, improving body image, focusing on internal locus of control for sexuality
Resuming Sex	Gradual resumption of unpressured sexual activity, minimizing shortness of breath and chest pain with medication and comfortable setting	Using noncoital stimulation when intercourse is impossible, accommodating to periods patient is more symptomatic	Planning sex for least fatigued periods or for times of maximum well-being between dialysis sessions, timing sex between CAPD exchanges, finding a setting for sex away from home dialysis equipment

212

Marital Conflict	Reducing spouse overprotectiveness, promoting changes in couple health habits such as diet, smoking, and/or exercise	Discussing emotional reactions to the cancer, renegotiating daily life tasks, teaching coping skills when illness is terminal	Encouraging patient's independence, helping spouse feel appreciated, promoting changes in couple's diet
Physical Handicaps	Coping with organic impairment of erections, compensating for aphasia, cognitive impairment, loss of sensory zones or limited mobility after CVA	Coping with organic impairment of erections, dealing with ostomies, laryngectomies, limb prostheses, loss of genital zones, indwelling catheters, vaginal irritation, chronic fatigue and pain	Coping with organic impairment of erections; overcoming fear of damaging sites of fistulae or transplanted organs; adjusting techniques for weakness, reduced vaginal lubrication, or mild sensory loss from neuropathy
Intensive Therapy	Marital conflict intensified by current disability or fear of sudden death	Marital conflict intensified by current disability or dying process	Couple is overwhelmed by the illness, especially at crises of beginning dialysis or experiencing transplant rejection

Table 9-3. Guidelines for Cardiovascular Patients on Staying Sexually Active

1. The safety of sexual activity depends on your individual health. Your doctor can give you guidelines based on your medical history, exercise testing, or a home EKG.
2. Some medications for hypertension or cardiac problems can interfere with sexual function. If you have a sexual problem, discuss it with your doctor. Do not change the dose of your medication or stop taking it without consulting your doctor.
3. An aerobic exercise program can help your sex life by reducing the amount of work your heart does during sexual activity. For those who have had a stroke, working on recovering as much mobility and independence as possible is also part of sexual rehabilitation.
4. For men with erection problems, reducing smoking and limiting drinking to small amounts of alcohol can sometimes improve sexual function.
5. If you have not had sexual activity for a while, try resuming sex in a gradual, nonpressured way. Using self-stimulation to orgasm or asking your partner to help you reach orgasm by hand or oral caressing can be a good preparation for trying intercourse.
6. When you plan to have sex, avoid heavy meals or too much alcohol, and make sure the room is at a comfortable temperature.
7. Most men and women can use any position they prefer for caressing or intercourse. If you get short of breath or tired, however, try a position that gives your partner more of the responsibility for movement.
8. It is normal to have a more rapid heart beat or to breathe heavily when you are sexually excited. If you have chest pain during sex, however, consult your doctor because such symptoms should be investigated and can usually be reduced by medication.
9. Good communication is a key to a happy sex life. If you or your partner is worried about sex, talk with each other and with your doctor. If you need to make changes in your sex life because of your illness, your willingness to share your desires and reactions with each other is crucial.

After David's original MI, the couple's frequency of sexual activity decreased, although the cardiologist had reassured them that sex was safe. David began to have intermittent erection problems, which became more severe over the years. His aortofemoral bypass surgery had little impact on his erections. Usually, if David and Anne began kissing and caressing each other, David could get a fairly full erection, but as soon as he penetrated for intercourse he would become short of breath and quickly fatigued, losing his erection long before he could reach orgasm. The couple had experimented with intercourse positions, but even if Anne held the base of David's penis in her hand, he could not maintain his erection and rarely could reach orgasm. When he did, his semen volume was reduced, as was the intensity of his pleasurable sensation.

David had not offered to help Anne reach orgasm through manual stimulation because he believed she would be disgusted by the idea. She had never been willing to try oral sex, either as giver or receiver. Anne said she felt little spontaneous desire for sex, but always was able to get aroused if David initiated. Their lovemaking had become so frustrating, however, that sexual activity only took place once every 2 or 3 months. Anne was more receptive to the idea of noncoital orgasms than David had anticipated. In fact, she disclosed that once in a great while she masturbated to orgasm because she felt it relieved tension. Anne had had some concern that sex could exacerbate her fibrocystic disease and was glad to know that there was no connection. She no longer had many hot flashes from her lack of estrogen, but was counseled to try a vaginal lubricant when the couple had sexual activity.

David and Anne were given an explanation of the effects of aging, arteriosclerosis, and cardiac medications on men's sexual function. Menopause and hysterectomy were also discussed. David's cardiologist had already been consulted and had suggested resuming sexual activity gradually, using common sense to cope with fatigue and shortness of breath. Implicit in his attitude was the knowledge that David had a limited life expectancy and might as well enjoy his time as much as possible. The therapist was not sure how David and Anne perceived David's prognosis and asked them if they feared a coital heart attack.

David smiled sadly. "I know I'm dying," he said. "Inch by inch. That's what makes it tough. Sometimes I wish I could just get it over with."

Anne responded by taking her husband's hand and saying stoutly, "Nonsense. We're all dying. After all, we could get hit by a car tomorrow. You can't just sit around, waiting to die."

The therapist turned to David. "How do you feel when Anne tells you to be cheerful?"

David began to weep. "I want to be. I want to be strong for her, but I can't. I feel so alone. I think she can't understand what it's like for me to imagine her going on after I'm gone. She'd be better off. She's still a pretty woman, and all our friends love her. She shouldn't be tied to an old invalid."

Anne also began to cry. "Do you think I want to live without you?" she asked her husband. "Don't you know that I wake up 3 or 4 times a night and check to make sure you're still warm and breathing, and each time I'm so grateful that you're still there."

The therapist suggested that Anne and David needed to find ways to feel intimate again, both sexually and emotionally. The couple began a series of sensate focus exercises and David found that he could enjoy the touching and reach orgasm without much fatigue if he sat propped up against pillows and allowed Anne to caress his penis with her hand, using lotion to make the touching more pleasurable. He had more difficulty when the couple tried intercourse in the same position, with Anne taking the more active role. Occasionally David could reach orgasm during intercourse, but often the couple ended the session with noncoital stimulation to orgasm. Anne was able to show David how to use clitoral and vaginal touch to bring her to orgasm. She had to remind him to touch her breasts only very lightly, however, because of continued tenderness. David was surprised and pleased by his wife's ability to communicate her desires.

The couple also went back to their country club for an occasional dinner, letting friends know in advance that they would be leaving early to conserve David's energy. Their friends were supportive and made David feel welcome. During the day, Anne scheduled golf, errands, or work activities at times when a housekeeper could stay with David. Both spouses were able to discuss his fear of dying alone, once the topic of death became less taboo. Anne and David planned activities they could enjoy together, such as playing cards or watching movies on their home video recorder. They also bought a small puppy for David, a lifelong dog lover, to train and enjoy. The dog gave David a sense of companionship and did not overtax his strength. Although life could never be problem-free, David and Anne felt closer than they had in their hectic, younger days and had no further need for counseling.

CANCER

Until recent years, survival rates were so poor for patients with cancer that we did not think of it as a chronic illness. Now predictions are that 30% of Americans will have some form of cancer and 49% of them will live at least 5 years beyond their diagnosis (Cancer Facts and Figures, 1986). Sexuality is an important aspect of quality of life for cancer patients, no matter what the site of their disease.

Psychosocial Impact on Sexuality

From an emotional and social point of view, cancer treatment can be devastating to sexuality (Andersen, 1985; Schover, 1986a). For younger patients or those whose treatment affects sexual attractiveness and function, sexual issues may be almost as crucial as survival. Concern about losing sexual function can even influence patients to choose a less-than-optimal cancer therapy, as when a man refuses a radical cystectomy and has radiotherapy instead. Depression is also more common in cancer patients than in the general population. The concomitant loss of sexual desire and disruption of marital roles and boundaries often presages a complete halt of sexual activity during or after cancer therapy. Several studies have shown, however, that marital separation or divorce is no more common among cancer patients than it is in the general population (Rieker, Edbril, & Garnick, 1985; Schover & von Eschenbach, 1985b; Schover et al., 1986b). Break-ups occur principally in couples who have already had high levels of marital conflict (Schover et al., 1985; Schover et al., 1986b). Cancer therapies are particularly likely to change physical appearance, often impairing body image. Surgery for cancer not only leaves scars, but may also involve removing an external body part such as a limb, breast, vulva, or penis.

Operations to treat colorectal or bladder cancer may entail creating a permanent ostomy. Radiotherapy requires temporary markings that may be publicly visible or at least obvious to a lover. Patients often cannot bathe the irradiated area for several weeks and complain of feeling dirty. Permanent changes in skin texture or loss of hair may take place within the target area. During months of chemotherapy, patients suffer hair loss, pallor, and often periodic nausea. They may gain or lose weight and must also manage indwelling catheters. Even hormonal therapy for prostate, breast, or uterine cancer can subtly alter body fat distribution, skin texture, and hair growth patterns. Patients taking steroids have to cope with the "moon face" and acne that often result.

Myths about cancer and sexuality are still fairly prevalent, including fears that cancer is contagious through sexual activity, that resuming sex will promote a recurrence, that a sexual partner can be exposed to radiation during a patient's external beam radiotherapy treatment period, or that cancer is a punishment for a past sexual misdeed. Although only a minority of patients believe these myths (Schover & von Eschenbach, 1984; Schover *et al.*, 1986b; Schover *et al.*, 1987) those who do give them credence often needlessly discontinue sexual activity.

Physiological Impact on Sexuality

Much of the physiological impact of cancer on sexual function results from the treatments rather than the tumors themselves (Schover, 1986a). Cancer and its therapies can affect all systems necessary for normal sexual function, impairing hormonal, vascular, or neurological function or damaging genital structure.

Hormonal Impact

People treated for cancer may have abnormal hormonal levels for a variety of reasons. A few rare tumors, such as adrenal or testicular cancers, can produce ectopic hormones. As soon as the malignancy is controlled, however, the hormones normalize.

More common hormonal abnormalities in women result from removal of both ovaries as part of radical pelvic surgery for gynecological malignancies, damage to ovarian function by pelvic radiotherapy or high doses of systemic chemotherapy, or use of antiestrogen compounds to treat metastatic breast or uterine cancer. Any of these treatments can produce premature menopause, with more severe symptoms than usual, as discussed in Chapter 5. The damage is usually permanent, although some young women may recover normal menstrual cycles after chemotherapy, depending on the dosage and drugs used (Chapman, 1982). Chemotherapy can also interfere with sexual pleasure by causing temporary vaginal irritation and discharge.

In men, surgical treatment for testicular cancer entails removing only one testicle (Schover & von Eschenbach, 1984). If the other is healthy, testosterone production remains adequate. Occasionally a malignancy may develop in the remaining testicle, or testosterone levels may simply be low so that replacement hormones are needed. Men with metastatic prostate cancer are usually treated by deliberately decreasing serum testosterone to prepubertal levels. Such hormonal therapy may be accomplished by removing both testicles or by prescribing estrogens, progesterones, or an LHRH-agonist drug. Men receiving hormonal therapy often have severe problems with loss of sexual desire, erectile dysfunction, and difficulty reaching orgasm (Bergman *et al.*, 1984; Schover, 1987).

Men or women taking phenothiazine antiemetic drugs or opiate pain medications may experience sexual problems related to moderate hyperprolactinemia.

Vascular Impact

Vascular erection problems are believed to result from high doses of pelvic irradiation used to treat prostate, bladder, or colon cancer (Goldstein *et al.*, 1984). Even with the lesser doses given to men with seminoma (a type of testicular cancer), dose and field of radiotherapy were predictive of erectile dysfunction and problems with orgasm (Schover *et al.*, 1986b). Other possible factors in vascular erectile dysfunction include ligation of blood vessels during pelvic cancer surgery or infusing chemotherapeutic agents through pelvic arteries. Little is known about vascular factors in sexual dysfunction in female cancer patients.

Neurological Impact

Cancer patients also are at high risk for neurological impairment of sexual function. Some types of chemotherapy or immunotherapy promote peripheral neuropathy. Tumors of the central nervous system can also destroy nerve pathways essential to sexual function. More common, however, is damage from radical pelvic surgery to the prostatic plexus in men, causing erectile dysfunction (see Chapter 5). Patients with testicular cancer who have retroperitoneal node dissections or men with colon cancer who have abdominoperineal resections may have dry orgasms (Balslev & Harling, 1983; Schover, 1987). Radical pelvic operations in women have no clear consequences for sexual arousal and orgasm (Schover & Fife, 1985). In both men and women, the pudendal nerve is rarely damaged by pelvic cancer operations, so the capacity to reach orgasm remains intact.

Cancer surgery for pelvic or genital tumors can actually damage genital structure. Tables 9-4 and 9-5 list the most common operations performed on

Table 9-4. Organs or Parts of Organs Removed During Radical Surgery for Pelvic or Genital Cancer in Men

Surgical Procedure	Organ or Part						
	Testicles	Penis	Prostate	Vasa Deferens & Seminal Vesicles	Urethra	Bladder	Rectum
Radical prostatectomy	No	No	Yes	Yes	Prostatic only	No	No
Radical cystectomy	No	No	Yes	Yes	Usually prostatic, sometimes entire	Yes	No
Abdominoperineal resection	No	No	No	No	No	No	Yes
Total pelvic exenteration	No	No	Yes	Yes	Prostatic only	Yes	Yes
Partial penectomy	No	Glans & part of shaft	No	No	Distal end only	No	No
Total penectomy	No	Corpora cavernosa, corpus spongiosum, & crus	No	No	Distal end only; perineal urethrostomy created	No	No

Source. Schover & Fife (1985).

Table 9-5. Organs or Parts of Organs Removed During Radical Surgery for Pelvic or Genital Cancer in Women

Surgical Procedure	Organ or Part							
	Labia Majora & Minora	Clitoris	Vagina	Uterus & Cervix	Ovaries & Fallopian Tubes	Bladder & Urethra	Rectum
Radical hysterectomy	No	No	Upper one third to one half	Yes	Sometimes	No	No
Radical cystectomy	No	No	Anterior wall; posterior wall used to retubularize vagina	Yes	Yes	Yes	Yes
Abdominoperineal resection	No	No	Sometimes posterior wall, repaired with skin graft	Sometimes	Sometimes	No	Yes
Total Pelvic Exenteration	Rarely, unless disease is in introitus	Rarely, unless disease is in introitus	Yes. Neovagina constructed with myocutaneous gracilis flaps	Yes	Yes	Yes	Yes
Radical vulvectomy	Yes	Yes	No	No	No	No	No

Source. Schover & Fife (1985).

men and women and the genital parts removed. Tables 9-6 and 9-7 detail the effect of each operation on sexual function (Schover & Fife, 1985). The reader can also refer to Chapter 5. Several of these operations involve creation of a colostomy, urostomy, or both. Sexual counseling for cancer patients with ostomies is discussed in detail by Schover (1986c).

Assessment Issues

Although sexuality assessment for a cancer patient follows the general outlines given in Chapter 6, some special issues are highlighted in Table 9-1. Topics to include in the interview center around the feeling of being stigmatized or helpless because of the cancer diagnosis and the effect of the illness on body image and willingness to engage in sexual activity. Although these issues are relevant to any chronic illness, cancer still is regarded with a special kind of dread, and some patients feel isolated just by the fact of having a malignancy.

Two questionnaires developed just for cancer patients may add valuable information about emotional reactions to the illness and its impact on daily life. The CIPS is a 131-item inventory that assesses 21 problem areas including sexuality. The FLIC is a shorter questionnaire that combines items on physical and emotional discomfort into a general score measuring "quality of life."

Physiological assessment covers a broad spectrum for cancer patients because each component of sexual physiology can be impaired. The clinician should be alert for noncancer risk factors that can predispose to sexual dysfunction, since cancer patients are a largely elderly population. All previous and current cancer therapies should be considered as risk factors, remembering that many patients receive multiple types of treatment. Similarly, the clinician should identify all the patient's current medications, including those unrelated to cancer and drugs prescribed to control nausea and pain. Physiological assessment is planned to evaluate all likely organic risk factors for sexual dysfunction.

Treatment Issues

Table 9-2 presents the most salient issues in treating the sexual problems of cancer patients. These techniques have been discussed in Chapters 7 and 8, so we proceed to the case examples.

Intensive Sex Therapy Case

Larry was a healthy 25-year-old wildlife biologist until a lump developed on his neck and was diagnosed as lymphoma. His wife Sandra was a medical technician, but was not working outside the home because she was taking care of the couple's 2-year-old daughter, Jenny.

Table 9-6. Effects of Surgery for Pelvic or Genital Cancer on Male Sexual Physiology

Surgical Procedure	Hormonal Basis of Sexual Desire	Capacity for Pleasure with Genital Touch	Capacity for Erection	Sensation of Orgasm	Ejaculation	Dyspareunia
Radical prostatectomy	Unchanged	Unchanged	Usually impaired.[a] Men younger than 60 are more likely to recover; full recovery takes 6 months	Unchanged, or mild loss of intensity	No semen produced; dry orgasm	Rare
Radical cystectomy	Unchanged	Unchanged	Usually impaired.[a] Men younger than 60 are more likely to recover; full recovery takes 6 months	Unchanged, or mild loss of intensity	No semen produced; dry orgasm	Rare, but is more likely after complete urethrectomy
Abdominoperineal resection	Unchanged	Unchanged	Often impaired, but recovery rates are higher than for radical prostatectomy or cystectomy	Unchanged, or mild loss of intensity	Dry orgasm is common because of damage to presacral sympathetic nerves	Rare, but some perineal pain or phantom rectal sensations
Total pelvic exenteration	Unchanged	Unchanged	Almost always permanently impaired	Unchanged, or mild loss of intensity	No semen produced; dry orgasm	Occasional
Partial penectomy	Unchanged	Erotic sensations still occur in remaining genital area	Unchanged. Penile shaft lengthens to permit coitus & (often) female orgasm	Unchanged	Unchanged	Rare; genital edema after groin dissection
Total penectomy	Unchanged	Erotic sensations still occur in remaining genital area	None	Unchanged, but need to relearn erotic zones	Unchanged, but semen is expelled through perineal urethrostomy	Occasional; genital edema after groin dissection

[a]With the development of new nerve-sparing techniques, rates of erectile recovery are higher. However, a 6-month recovery period is still necessary. Whether these procedures eradicate the cancer successfully remains controversial.

Source. Schover & Fife (1985).

Table 9-7. Effects of Surgery for Pelvic or Genital Cancer on Female Sexual Physiology

Surgical Procedure	Hormonal Basis of Sexual Desire	Capacity for Pleasure with Genital Touch	Capacity for Vaginal Lubrication	Ease of Reaching Orgasm	Sensation of Orgasm	Dyspareunia
Radical hysterectomy	Unchanged[a]	Unchanged	Unchanged[b]	Unchanged	Unchanged	Rare; must adjust to shallower vagina[c]
Radical cystectomy	Unchanged[a]	Unchanged	Reduced[b]	Unchanged, despite loss of anterior vaginal wall	Unchanged	Frequent, but can be reduced
Abdominoperineal resection	Unchanged[a]	Unchanged	Unchanged[b]	Probably unchanged; no research available	Unchanged	Frequent, but can be reduced
Total pelvic exenteration & vaginal reconstruction using myocutaneous gracilis flaps	Unchanged[a]	Some loss of erotic zones, vagina, & occasionally part of vulva. Erotic sensations still occur in remaining genital area. Neovagina can develop erotic sensitivity	Lost. Must use artificial lubricants in neovagina and daily douches to reduce odor	Often must relearn how to reach orgasm	Unchanged, or mild loss of intensity	Occasional; can be reduced
Radical vulvectomy	Unchanged	Some loss of erotic zones; erotic sensations still occur in remaining genital area	Unchanged	Often must relearn how to reach orgasm	No research data available	Frequent, because of urethral irritation or stenosis of vaginal entrance; can be reduced

[a]Even if bilateral oophorectomy is included, adrenal androgens should maintain an adequate degree of desire. Some clinicians recommend a combination of androgen and estrogen replacement therapy. "Hot flashes" from estrogen deficiency may interfere with sexual pleasure.

[b]If bilateral oophorectomy is included, vaginal lubrication is reduced unless estrogen replacement therapy is prescribed.

[c]Dyspareunia is more common when surgery is combined with pelvic irradiation, which reduces vaginal lubrication even further and can promote vaginal atrophy and stenosis.

Source. Schover & Fife (1985).

223

Larry's family had an unusual history of cancer. His father had also had lymphoma and died. His younger sister had died at age 18 of Ewing's sarcoma. Sandra did not like the way Larry's family dealt with illness, believing that he and his mother denied too much, pretending that nothing was wrong.

Sandra and Larry had some other disagreements. Sandra enjoyed cultural things while Larry was an outdoors person. Sandra had gained 15 pounds after her pregnancy, and Larry, a runner and weight-lifter, often nagged her to diet and exercise. The partners agreed, however, that Jenny was the most brilliant, beautiful, and loving child possible. They spent much of their leisure time playing with her. They had been planning a second child when Larry's cancer treatment interfered. He was receiving high doses of combination chemotherapy that might permanently impair his fertility. There had been no time to bank semen before starting cancer treatment.

When Larry and Sandra were referred for sex therapy, Larry had already been through 18 months of chemotherapy and Jenny was almost 4 years old. The presenting problem was that the couple had had no sexual activity since Larry's diagnosis. At first Larry was so ill that nobody was sure he would live. When his condition stabilized and he began to have some periods of reasonable well-being between courses of chemotherapy, his sexual desire returned. Sandra, however, had developed an aversion to sexual activity. In spite of her intelligence and background in biology, Sandra feared that she could contract cancer from Larry. She wondered why there was so much cancer in his family and read him newspaper items about wives who had gotten AIDS from their husbands. Sandra made Larry wash his hands before touching Jenny and discouraged the little girl from cuddling with her father, saying that "Daddy is too sick." Larry felt hurt and angry, stating that his wife treated him like a leper.

Larry and Sandra had both been "clean-cut kids," who met at college after growing up in middle-class families that were similar in religious beliefs and social attitudes. Sandra tended to be more psychologically minded than Larry, who was not a very introspective person. He noted that his wife had an unusually long and detailed memory, especially for slights and insults. When the couple disagreed, Sandra often won arguments by using a logical approach. Larry did not think it was worthwhile to get into a debate. The partners had always expressed affection easily, however, until Larry's cancer diagnosis. Now they rarely even kissed on the mouth or cuddled in bed, although they were still verbally loving to one another. Sandra said she missed the touching and knew her fears were illogical, but did not know how to change them.

Before the cancer diagnosis, Larry and Sandra had sexual activity about twice a week, usually at Larry's initiation. He complained that he had always had a hard time knowing if Sandra was in the mood for sex, and he wished she could be more playful in lovemaking. Larry had never had a problem with erections or with premature ejaculation and could still masturbate to orgasm without difficulty. Sandra had enjoyed sex and lubricated easily, but needed clitoral stimulation to reach orgasm. She felt defensive about not being orgasmic during intercourse, especially when Larry expressed disappointment about it. She had not masturbated before Larry's cancer or since.

Now Sandra felt no desire for sex at all. She felt she *should* give Larry sex and, in fact, had a somewhat overdeveloped sense of duty about all areas of life. Larry could ask for what he wanted during sex, but Sandra rarely communicated a sexual preference.

In individual sessions, the depth of each partner's anger and fear became apparent. Larry said that he doubted he would survive his cancer and at least wanted to have sex again before he died. He was seriously considering leaving Sandra and discontinuing his cancer treatment so that he could travel and make love with other women. He had a fantasy that Sandra would be disfigured in a car accident so that she would know how it felt to be treated like a leper. Larry had difficulty undergoing painful spinal taps and bone marrow biopsies. He sometimes felt angry at his doctors and nurses for being uncaring but never expressed his feelings to them. Instead, he would pour them out to Sandra, who then scolded the medical team. Sandra's aggressiveness made Larry feel very anxious because he felt dependent on the doctors' and nurses' good will.

Sandra talked about how frightened she felt when Larry first became ill. He was so emaciated for a few months that he reminded her of her grandfather. This antisexual image stayed with her, although Larry was currently up to a more normal weight. When Sandra had attempted to hug Larry at first or to sit close to him, he had warned her sharply to be careful of his subclavian catheter. This line for chemotherapy had been difficult and painful to insert, and Larry did not want to risk having to have it replaced. Sandra felt clumsy and alienated. She could acknowledge fears that Larry would die and wondered herself whether her phobic avoidance of sex was a way to distance herself from her husband. Sandra disclosed that Larry had hit her several times over the past few months, although never hard enough to leave a bruise. These episodes of violence occurred when Sandra refused to have sex. They were so out of character for Larry that Sandra feared he had brain metastases, although Larry's physician had assured her that he did not.

The therapist asked Sandra's permission to bring up the episodes of hitting in the couple session, since it was such an important issue. Larry agreed that he had hit Sandra, but said that she had hit him back. Although Sandra saw Larry as athletic and overpowering in his anger, Larry said he felt so weak and ill that he thought Sandra could easily hurt him. Each was frightened by the anger that was revealed on these occasions, and they agreed to stop any fights by Larry leaving the room before the situation escalated to hitting.

Because the couple lived in another state, therapy was planned to take place in daily sessions while the couple and Jenny rented a furnished apartment. Larry and Sandra were assigned to begin homework with a sensate focus exercise, but both would wear pajamas. The first exercise went smoothly, but Sandra cried for half an hour, a rare event for her. The closeness to Larry had made her aware of how lonely it would be to live without him. Larry was surprised by Sandra's tears, but was able to let her express her fears. He felt the intensity of her love more than he had for a long while.

The couple was so elated by the first sensate focus exercise that they spent 3 hours on their second session. This time Sandra began to feel tense. She had thoughts about getting cancer and feared that Larry and the therapist would push her into having sex before she was ready. During Sandra's description, Larry broke in and said that the goal of therapy was to feel more loving, not just to have intercourse. This was a reversal of his earlier statements, both in the individual and couple sessions, that intercourse was what he wanted most in life.

The therapist asked Sandra what limits would feel comfortable to her for the next sensate focus assignment. She wanted to repeat the homework at the same level of intimacy. She also developed some self-statements to use when she felt anxious about cancer contagion. One effective one for her was, "If cancer were contagious, all the wives at this hospital would have it." As Sandra talked about how vulnerable she felt during the exercise, Larry related her experience to how he felt when the doctors poked and prodded him and he did not know what to expect.

The couple soon proceeded to the step of caressing each other in the nude, with no breast or genital touching allowed. Sandra felt anxious, but said nothing to Larry because she felt obligated to finish the exercise. The therapist pointed out that engaging in touch out of a sense of duty was very counterproductive for Sandra and asked the couple what Sandra could do instead of going on silently the next time that she felt obligated during a sensate focus exercise. Sandra and Larry agreed that she should ask to stop the touching if she felt anxious and, instead, tell Larry about her feelings.

Each partner was also assigned to say "no" to two things that he or she normally would do out of obligation. Both were enthusiastic about carrying out their "no's." Sandra did not make her usual daily call to Larry's mother and also declined Larry's request that she sit in his lap while they watched television.

At the next session, Larry asked how important the limits were for the exercises. On gentle inquiry by the therapist, it developed that Larry had become so aroused during the exercise that he had masturbated to orgasm afterward while Sandra lay next to him. Sandra had told him he was cheating, but actually had enjoyed Larry's excitement because she felt no responsibility to satisfy him. She thought that allowing Larry to masturbate would make her feel less pressured. Sandra did not feel ready herself for breast or genital caressing. The therapist agreed that the innovation had worked well but cautioned Larry and Sandra in the future to build their suggestions into the homework agreement during the therapy session, rather than making a new contract at home that could potentially pressure Sandra into going further than she wanted.

Sandra began to feel sexually aroused during the touching, and then would immediately feel highly anxious. In the therapy session, Larry asked her why she was so frightened. "If we get close, and then you get sick again, I'll just feel worse," she told him.

"If Larry died and this problem in your sex lives had not been solved, how would you feel?" asked the therapist.

"Awful," answered Sandra.

"I think if we got closer than we've ever been, it would be sad if I died, but at least we would know we had shown that we love each other," Larry put in.

The therapist commented that it must have been very difficult for Sandra to ignore her sexual needs for 2 years. In fact, she had had to develop a phobia in order to keep those feelings under control. The therapist reminded Sandra and Larry that it would take time and patience for Sandra to allow herself to feel aroused again.

The next steps in the homework were for Sandra to take a more active role in helping Larry to reach orgasm. She enjoyed caressing him but still felt very tense when she allowed him to touch her vulva even lightly. She could allow the touching to continue, however, if she told herself, "I can let Larry touch me a minute longer because I know he'll stop right away if I ask him to." For several sessions, Sandra's arousal occurred only with kissing or nongenital caressing. She felt too vulnerable and embarrassed to enjoy clitoral stimulation.

At around this point, Larry's mother came into town for a few days. Sandra was very frightened by a CT scan suggesting that Larry's lymphoma might be progressing. The physicians were discussing switching to a different combination of chemotherapy drugs. Larry and his mother did not want to discuss these new developments and seemed to be taking them in stride. Sandra became very angry one afternoon when Larry's mother wanted Sandra to take her to a shopping mall while Larry had his clinic appointment. Sandra wanted to be there to see the doctors, since she felt Larry often forgot to ask important questions or did not report all that was said. Sandra did not know how to refuse, however, when Larry's mother said she needed to buy a birthday present for one of her grandchildren. Sandra felt Larry was on his mother's side and would prefer that Sandra be absent when he saw his physician.

In the next therapy session, Larry became quite angry when discussing this incident, telling Sandra that he was tired of her interfering in his medical care. Sandra, in turn, reminded her husband of times when he had begged her to make the doctors stop during a bone marrow biopsy. She told him how angry she felt when he was sweet to one of the nurses and then snapped at her. The therapist told Sandra that this was the angriest statement she had ever made in a therapy session. The therapist asked Sandra to look Larry in the eye and tell him again how angry she was. Sandra needed two tries before she was able to express herself without smiling and in a truly angry tone of voice.

Larry realized the double bind he was creating by being passive with his doctors and complaining to Sandra, but then resenting her if she took action to protect him. He made a resolution to be more assertive with the doctors instead of putting his wife in the middle. "I also would like Sandra to let me play with Jenny in my own way. She's always breathing down my neck and telling me I'm too rough," he added.

The therapist asked Sandra whether she had a concern about Larry's treatment of Jenny. Sandra told her husband that ever since he had hit her, she had feared he might harm their daughter. She told him she had even asked the doctors if Larry had brain damage from his cancer. Larry was so shocked that he began to cry. He told Sandra she was a bitch and that he would never hurt Jenny. "If you just gave me sex like a normal wife none of this would have happened!" he sobbed. "I don't need you! I know I'm going to die and I'll just go live my own life and enjoy myself until then."

The therapist asked each partner to be silent for a moment and to choose from the past few minutes the most important message that each wanted to communicate. Larry and Sandra both agreed that their most important message was their love for each other and their fear that Larry would die. This session was an important turning point in their relationship.

As Larry's medical tests continued, couple exercises progressed to the point where Sandra could allow her husband to put a finger in her vagina. At first she felt the penetration was painful, but after learning Kegel exercises, inserting her own fingers into her vagina, and using a vaginal lubricant, Sandra could accommodate two of Larry's fingers in her vagina without discomfort. The couple also was expressing affection more easily and often short-circuited quarrels by taking time to listen to each other's feelings. Twice a week, Sandra scheduled an afternoon of leisure time for herself, away from Larry and Jenny. She allowed Larry to care for their daughter during these short absences, and no untoward incidents occurred.

The couple had another quarrel, however, when they got to the step of penile–vaginal penetration and Sandra asked Larry to use a condom. Although the condom would serve as a contraceptive, Larry insisted that he was 99% likely to be infertile and that Sandra was treating him like a leper again. The therapist suggested a compromise, viewing penetration with a condom as a comfortable next step for Sandra in overcoming her phobic fear of cancer contagion but not as the final goal of treatment. Both partners agreed and couple sessions proceeded with few problems.

Larry was no longer even in partial remission with his cancer, however. His disease was advancing rapidly, and since he had already had three different chemotherapy regimens as well as local radiation, the physicians could only offer an experimental protocol, with little hope of completely controlling the cancer. Larry decided he had had enough experimental chemotherapy. He was not yet in pain and wanted to go home and live as long as he could in comfort, and then have home hospice care until his death. Sandra agreed with her husband, but Larry's mother could not accept his decision. After role playing with the therapist, the couple was able to sit down with the mother and help her see their point of view. This was one of the first times that Larry and Sandra had acted as a team in interacting with his mother.

Sandra and Larry continued couple exercises at home and maintained weekly phone contact with the therapist. They were able to have intercourse, but soon after, Larry became too ill for sexual activity. He died 2 weeks later at home, having been kept free of pain. He and Sandra felt a loving intimacy and were able to help Jenny say good-bye.

One year later, Sandra was not dating but had gone back to work. She and Jenny were coping well and had good social support. Sandra saw Larry's mother occasionally, but the two women were never close. Sandra had been able to mourn for Larry and was beginning to feel optimism about the future.

END-STAGE RENAL DISEASE

Once considered a death sentence, end-stage renal disease has become a treatable chronic illness with the advent of modern dialysis techniques and successful kidney transplants (Flechner, Novick, Braun, Popowniak, & Steinmuller, 1983; Neff *et al.*, 1983). Patients with end-stage renal disease include several groups. Some have uremia that has not yet reached a level necessitating intervention. Others are being treated with hemodialysis (HD) or continuous ambulatory peritoneal dialysis (CAPD). For hemodialysis, the patient may use equipment at home that filters impurities from the blood, or may have treatments at a dialysis center for about 4 hours, usually 3 times a week. A catheter is inserted into a fistula in the patient's arm (i.e., a surgically created connection between an artery and a vein). Peritoneal dialysis uses special fluid which is cycled into the peritoneum through a surgically implanted catheter. The patient wears a series of external bags during the day, allowing freedom of movement and activity. The dialyzing fluid attracts elements from the blood that would normally be filtered out by the kidneys. Many patients on dialysis are awaiting kidney transplants. A final group of men and women discussed in this chapter have already had successful kidney transplants. In the United States, over 65,000 patients are undergoing dialysis and in 1984, 5,000 transplants were performed (N. B. Levy, 1986).

Sexual problems are common in all of these groups of patients. In men with untreated uremia, 35% had erectile dysfunction in one study (Procci & Martin, 1985). Studies of men on dialysis suggest no difference in sexual function depending on type of treatment (HD vs. CAPD), and an incidence of erection problems ranging from 20% to 87% (Ngiem, Corry, Mendez, & Lee, 1982; Rodger et al., 1985a).

Early research suggested that sexual function deteriorated after dialysis was begun, but a careful, prospective study of 43 men by Procci and Martin (1985) showed that self-reports of erections and of the frequency of sexual activity, as well as objective measurements of NPT remained quite stable over 30 months. In fact, frequency of intercourse increased slightly when uremic men began dialysis, perhaps reflecting an increase in physical well-being. About half of men had erection problems, similar to a rate of 60% in another recent case series of 100 men on dialysis (Rodger et al., 1985a).

As in research on other chronic illnesses, attention has focused on erectile capacity, with no real study of the desire or orgasm phases of the sexual response cycle. Spouses have rarely been included as research subjects. Data on women's sexual function are sparse, although a questionnaire survey in the 1970s revealed that women with renal disease decreased their sexual activity and had more difficulty reaching orgasm during intercourse (N. B. Levy, 1983). Weizman et al. (1983) found that half of a small group of women undergoing hemodialysis had a complex of sexual dysfunction including loss of desire and arousal, and difficulty reaching orgasm. Mastrogiacomo et al. (1984) interviewed 99 Italian women treated with hemodialysis. Frequency of intercourse and the percentage of coital episodes culminating in orgasm were significantly reduced compared with a control group of gynecology patients matched in age, and in respect to the women's own pre-illness sexual function. Although many women said they continued to have sex to satisfy their husbands, even the youngest group (age 26 to 40 years) only had orgasms on 30% of occasions, compared to 75% for healthy women.

Does sexual function improve after a successful kidney transplant? The answer appears to be yes, although prospective studies are needed (Glass et al., 1987). Transplant patients are a younger, healthier group than those on long-term dialysis, so it is not surprising that rates of erectile dysfunction after successful first transplant range from 10% to 38% (Brannen et al., 1980; Ngiem et al., 1982), lower than those in other groups with renal disease. Age and previous sexual function appear to be stronger sexual function predictors than transplantation status (Brannen et al., 1980; Ngiem, Corry, Mendez, & Lee, 1983).

Two studies have retrospectively asked men and women about sexuality before and after renal transplant. Flechner *et al.* (1983) surveyed a very special group: 27 men and 22 women who had survived 10 years or more after renal allograft. None were diabetic, and the mean age at the time of surgery was 27 years. The men reported that while on dialysis only 60% had had normal erections, but all could function sexually after transplant. Of the women, only 11% had been sexually active at least monthly on dialysis and none had regular menstrual cycles, whereas all were sexually active and menstruated posttransplantation. Fourteen men and women conceived healthy children after the transplant.

Toledo-Pereyra *et al.* (1985) studied a more typical group of 106 renal transplant patients. Many were "high-risk" patients, that is, poor and in ill health. Some had histories of drug abuse. Their mean age was 38 at the time of surgery. Only 30 gave information on their sex lives. Only 17% felt they had functioned normally while on dialysis, compared with 40% after renal transplantations. A full 31% remained sexually abstinent after surgery. The researchers were also disappointed to find no increase in employment, in contrast to Flechner *et al.*'s (1983) study, although general activity levels improved.

Psychosocial Impact on Sexuality

Patients with renal disease often have difficulty in coping with their poor prognosis, limited physical energy, dependency on medical technology, and the uncertainty of transplantation (Nichols & Springford, 1984). While on dialysis, they must comply with strict dietary and fluid intake restrictions. Spouses often assume a caretaking role, suffering from pessimism and a sense of helplessness (Chowanec & Binik, 1982; Nichols & Springford, 1984). The patient's coping and even survival have been linked to the spouse's emotional adjustment.

As Chowanec and Binik (1982) have pointed out, however, research on psychological aspects of renal disease has been limited by small sample sizes, the use of unvalidated questionnaires, and dependence on the patient's own self-report. When standardized measures of depression are used, the incidence of diagnosable clinical depression is actually surprisingly low among patients with renal disease (Devins, Binik, Hollomby, Barré, & Guttmann, 1981; Procci & Martin, 1985). Perhaps patients willing to participate in research are more healthy and better able to cope than the group at large. After renal transplantation, depression or more rarely psychosis can be a side effect of high doses of steroids (N. B. Levy, 1986).

Two studies suggest that continued sexual function is correlated with overall psychological adjustment. Berkman, Katz, and Weissman (1982) evaluated 32 patients on dialysis, finding that sexual function was better in patients who considered sex important and continued to have good self-esteem. Bouchelouche, Bartram, and Jensen (1985), studying 23 couples including a spouse with renal disease, found that the 79% with sexual problems also reported many symptoms on the Disease Acceptance Scale (see Chapter 6), similar to couples with a diabetic spouse (Jensen, 1985a).

Clinical experience suggests that many of these patients are too ill to regard sexuality as a high priority. Low sexual desire is the most common complaint for both men and women. Even health professionals who work with dialysis patients are vulnerable to burn-out and disillusionment as they see the slow but steady attrition over the years.

Physiological Impact on Sexuality

Most research on physiological factors in sexual dysfunction of renal patients has focused on finding a cause for the ubiquitous erectile dysfunction. As with other chronic diseases, the search for a unidimensional cause, even in the organic realm, is fruitless. Men with end-stage renal disease are often at high risk for vascular pathology because of their underlying disease process, for example hypertension or diabetes. In addition, they commonly take antihypertensive drugs or steroids that disrupt sexual function. They often have peripheral or autonomic neuropathy as well as metabolic abnormalities such as low serum zinc levels. In addition to low serum testosterone levels, they often have moderate elevations in prolactin and are oligospermic with low sperm motility (Mahajan, Prasad, & McDonald, 1984; Waltzer, 1981).

Nevertheless, researchers continue to look for a unique cause of erectile dysfunction in men with renal disease. Vascular pathology has been assessed by Doppler penile/brachial indices. In Rodger *et al.*'s (1985a) group of 100 men on dialysis, only six had abnormally low Doppler values, and one of these men had normal erections. Billet, Dagher, and Queral (1982) suggested that vascular erectile failure was common after kidney transplantation because blood flow was diverted away from the penis, depending on the surgical technique. They reported a case of successful revascularization in a man who had had both internal iliac arteries ligated in a series of two transplants. Other researchers, however, have documented that many men continue to have good sexual function even when both hypogastric arteries have been diverted in transplant operations (Brannen *et al.*, 1980; Ngiem *et al.*, 1982, 1983). Age is a better predictor than Doppler indices of erectile function after kidney transplant (Ngiem *et al.*, 1982, 1983).

Autonomic neuropathy was evaluated in 25 uremic men by Campese *et al.* (1982). Using heart-rate response to the Valsalva maneuver as a measure of neuropathy, they found that those with erectile dysfunction (documented by NPT and reports of frequency of sex) were more likely to have abnormal test results. Another group compared men's self-reports of sexual function and the results of nerve conduction tests for peripheral neuropathy in 32 patients on hemodialysis, finding a significant correlation (Berkman *et al.*, 1982). Thus evidence for a link between neuropathy and sexual dysfunction is a little stronger than the findings on vascular pathology.

The search for a metabolic abnormality to account for erectile dysfunction zeroed in on zinc levels for a few years. Zinc deficiency can delay human sexual maturation and produces testicular atrophy in laboratory animals. Mahajan *et al.* (1984) reported several studies in which men with renal disease not only had abnormally low zinc levels on several different assays, but also benefited from a 6-month regimen of zinc replacement. They claimed that men taking zinc improved more in serum testosterone, sperm counts, and sexual function than those on placebo. Their methodology and findings have been challenged, however, by two other research groups who have been unable to replicate their studies (Rodger *et al.*, 1984; Sprenger, Schmitz, Hetzel, Bundschu, & Franz, 1984).

The most recent enthusiasm is for hyperprolactinemia as a causal factor in sexual dysfunction. It is clear that a subgroup of uremic patients on or off dialysis has moderately elevated prolactin (Muir *et al.*, 1983; Rodger *et al.*, 1985a; Ruilope *et al.*, 1985; Weizman *et al.*, 1983; Vircburger, Prelevic, Peric, Knezevic, & Djukanovic, 1985). Weizman *et al.* (1983) report a correlation between elevated levels of serum prolactin and sexual dysfunction in 38 men and 21 women on hemodialysis. Mastrogiacomo *et al.* (1984) found a similar correlation in 99 women on hemodialysis. When hyperprolactinemia is treated with a dopamine agonist, men's sexual function improves more than with placebo (Ermolenko *et al.*, 1986; Muir *et al.*, 1983; Ruilope *et al.*, 1985), although these medications also have unpleasant side effects such as nausea, weakness, and hypotension.

Although hyperprolactinemia may be one factor in sexual dysfunction in patients with renal disease, it is unlikely to be the only answer. The hormonal deficit in end-stage renal disease is highly complex. Hyperprolactinemia may result from decreased clearance of prolactin, but more likely is part of a blunting of central nervous system feedback loops. Hyperprolactinemia persists regardless of HD or CAPD, but usually normalizes after a successful renal transplant (Vircburger *et al.*, 1985). Even when bromocriptine improves sexual function, testosterone levels do not always increase from the subnormal (Ermolenko *et al.*, 1986; Ramirez *et al.*, 1985). Normalizing prolactin does not normalize blunted responses in renal patients to a wide variety of hypothalamic and pituitary stimulating challenges, including abnormal LH and FSH responses to GnRH (Ramirez *et al.*, 1985). Rodger *et al.* (1985b) have recently documented that men who are on CAPD or HD usually lose the capacity to release LH in periodic pulses every 90 to 130 minutes. Pulsatile LH release is restored after successful renal transplant, however.

Sophisticated studies of hormone release are needed in women as well as men with renal disease. Effects of estrogen deficiency in young women on dialysis have been largely ignored. Not only does the methodology for sampling hormones need improvement, but a far more precise system of specifying sexual dysfunctions should be used.

The medications, including prednisone and azathioprine, used to prevent rejection of renal allografts and to treat rejection episodes have no clear impact on sexual function or fertility (Flechner *et al.*, 1983), although more careful research is needed to rule out side effects. Women are exposed to one additional hazard, however, after renal transplantation. They have a ninefold increased risk of developing malignancies of the cervix, vulva, or anus (Halpert *et al.*, 1986). Evidence is growing that the problem results from exposure to the human papilloma virus (HPV) during immunosuppression. Although many of the cancers are noninvasive, half of malignancies occurring in 10% of a group of 105 women occurred at more than one genital site. The immunosuppression makes the malignancies more virulent, so that many women end up with radical operations that certainly affect their sexual function (Chapter 5). All women should be advised after transplant to limit their number of sexual partners and to use barrier methods of contraception to reduce exposure to HPV. They should also have yearly Pap smears and examinations of the vulva and anus.

Assessment Issues

Table 9-1 summarizes the special assessment issues for this group of men and women. Assessment of a patient with renal disease should include a thorough medical history. The clinician must understand the patient's prognosis, and recognize the emotional strain of living on dialysis or coping with the uncertainty of kidney transplantation. Partners should always be included in the interview process because they play such a crucial role in the patient's adjustment (Berkman *et al.*, 1982).

No special questionnaires are available for patients with renal disease, but the standard measures of depression or coping with illness that are described in Chapter 6 can be helpful.

Treatment Issues

Special treatment issues are presented in Table 9-2. Clinicians can take advantage of centralized dialysis centers in planning groups for education and counseling of patients and families. When patients are undergoing the stress of dialysis or are awaiting kidney transplantation and its results, sex therapy must often be combined with supportive couple counseling and work on sharing marital responsibilities. As Michalski (1986) points out in discussing the case of a homosexual man who was almost refused CAPD because of fear of infection via anal intercourse, staff's prejudices about sexuality and its possible interference with treatment are often exaggerated. Flechner *et al.* (1983) make a similar observation about discouraging young patients from having children. This group of patients includes some men and women with very limited physical vigor, but nevertheless, sexuality and intimacy issues must not be ignored.

Brief Counseling Case

Jeremy was a 35-year-old social worker who had been married for 13 years to his wife, Beth. They had a 10-year-old daughter. At the age of 25, Jeremy was diagnosed as having chronic pyelonephritis. His renal function gradually deteriorated until at age 34, he was placed on maintenance hemodialysis while awaiting a renal transplant.

During a periodic visit with his nephrologist at the dialysis center, Jeremy disclosed that he and Beth were having severe problems in their sexual relationship. Although Jeremy still felt a desire for sex, the frequency of lovemaking had dropped gradually over the past 3 years to once every few weeks. Beth had always been the initiator of sex, but somehow no longer was giving her husband cues. He was afraid to reach out to her, feeling like his illness had already subjected Beth to too many demands.

The nephrologist and his nurse-clinician asked Jeremy and Beth to come in together for a visit. The partners sat at opposite ends of the couch, turned away from each other. Both Jeremy and Beth talked to the doctor and nurse, making no eye contact with each other.

Beth soon became tearful as she described her struggle to teach a class of second graders, keep up with the housework, give attention to her daughter, and nurse Jeremy as well. She hated the dialysis clinic, and had nightmares in which she and Jeremy were both hooked to a dialyzer, with her blood gradually draining out to nourish her husband. She confessed that his fatigue, as evidenced in his motor slowness and gray complexion, was a sexual turn-off for her.

When the couple did attempt lovemaking, Jeremy often lost his erection before he could penetrate and was unable to regain it. If he did manage to enter his wife's vagina, he ejaculated almost immediately, in contrast to his good ability to delay orgasm before his illness. The couple then would give up on sex for a few weeks. Although Beth would have liked Jeremy to give her oral stimulation to orgasm, she was afraid to ask him, believing he was too weak for such efforts. Instead, she masturbated to orgasm in private.

Jeremy looked very upset as his wife described her frustration. "Why didn't you tell me?" he asked. "I thought you were just so disgusted with me that you didn't want me to touch you after intercourse."

"I was afraid I'd hurt your feelings," Beth replied. For the first time in the session, the partners turned toward each other. Beth reached out and put her hand over Jeremy's. The nurse and nephrologist just listened, letting their patients communicate with each other.

Jeremy broke the silence by telling the nephrologist that he had noticed swelling and tenderness of his breast area. "I feel like I'm turning into a woman or something," he complained. The nephrologist ordered serum prolactin and testosterone assays, but the team also counseled Beth and Jeremy to enjoy cuddling and touching, and to help each other reach orgasm in any way possible.

Jeremy's prolactin was twice the upper limit of the normal range and testosterone was a little below normal. His nephrologist prescribed a dopamine agonist medication, which after several weeks lowered prolactin to a normal level. Jeremy's serum testosterone rose to the midrange. Although Jeremy was nauseated at first by the medication, he was determined to keep taking it. After 2 or 3 weeks, the side effects lessened. Jeremy's sexual desire improved, as did his ability to maintain a firm erection.

Jeremy and Beth decided to make love in the den, after their children were asleep. They found they now viewed the bedroom as Jeremy's sickroom. It was no longer a sensual setting. They also learned to plan sexual activity when Jeremy was off dialysis for a day, but not yet ready for his next session on the machine. This was the time of his maximal energy level. On a follow-up visit, the couple reported that they were much more satisfied now with their sex life. The combination of medication and brief counseling had met their needs.

10

Insidious Illness and Sexuality: Diabetes, Chronic Obstructive Pulmonary Disease, and Chronic Pain

A number of chronic illnesses have an insidious course, sometimes staying well under control, but often gradually interfering more and more with a person's normal daily life. Sexual dysfunction related to these illnesses may begin at diagnosis or can occur as part of the gradual progression of symptoms. This chapter includes sections on diabetes, chronic obstructive pulmonary disease (COPD), and chronic pain.

DIABETES

Since the introduction of insulin to clinical practice (Banting & Best, 1922), diabetes has been used as a model for studying the psychosocial impact of chronic illness. Sexuality has been more extensively investigated in diabetics than in any other group of medical patients. The earliest mention of erectile dysfunction in a diabetic man was in the writings of the Scottish physician, John Rollo (1798). He described a 30-year-old patient who had fathered several children but could no longer obtain firm erections after being "seized with diabetes."

Rubin and Babbot (1958) conducted the first modern study of sexual function in diabetic men, finding erectile dysfunction in 55% of a group of 198. Despite methodological flaws, most subsequent research has shown that about half of diabetic men experience sexual problems (Ellenberg, 1971; Kolodny, Kahn, Goldstein, & Barnett, 1974; Montenero & Donatone, 1962). Kolodny (1971) published the first study of sexuality in female diabetics. Comparing a hospitalized group with women hospitalized for other medical illnesses, he found a significantly higher rate of orgasmic problems in the diabetic women (35% vs. 6%). All subsequent studies, however, have failed to replicate this finding (Ellenberg, 1977; Jensen, 1981a, 1986; Newman & Bertelson, 1986; Schreiner-Engel et al., 1985).

237

Several issues complicate research on the incidence and causes of sexual problems in diabetics. Few studies have distinguished between type I diabetics, who have a juvenile onset of the disease and depend on insulin, and type II diabetics who have an adult onset and can often manage the disease with diet alone or oral hypoglycemic drugs (Wagner, Hilsted, & Jensen, 1981). Within the group of older diabetics, sexual problems may also result from other chronic illnesses, particularly from hypertension and its treatment (Newman & Marcus, 1985). Few researchers have specified medications or illnesses other than diabetes that affected their subjects. Many studies in the literature also fail to inform the reader about the severity of subjects' diabetic complications.

Nevertheless, some estimates of rates of the various sexual dysfunctions can be made from the recent studies that separate type I and type II diabetics. Most data have been gathered on type I diabetics. Jensen (1981a) compared 80 men whose mean age was 36 years with healthy, age-matched controls. Diabetic men had a significantly higher rate of erectile dysfunction (34% vs. 12%). Low sexual desire was almost as common a problem for the diabetic men (31%). The same study included 80 type I diabetic women. Their sexual function was not significantly different from that of healthy controls, although diabetic women did have an unusual incidence of reduced vaginal lubrication (24%). Jensen (1986) found rates of sexual dysfunction to be unchanged 6 years later in a follow-up study of 101 of the original 160 subjects.

Two other researchers have studied type I diabetic women. Tyrer *et al.* (1983), interviewing a group of 82 women, agreed with Jensen that vaginal lubrication was reduced compared with healthy controls (34% incidence). They also noted a trend to more desire problems in the diabetic group. Schreiner-Engel *et al.* (1987) found no differences at all in sexual function or satisfaction between 32 type I diabetic women and a matched group of healthy controls.

For type II diabetic women, however, the picture in this latter study was grim. Compared with age-matched controls, the type II women were significantly less sexually satisfied and functional, with more desire problems, a 29% rate of inadequate lubrication, and a 32% rate of difficulty reaching orgasm. The mean age of the 23 type II diabetic women was 46, older than the mean age in the early 30s of the three type I groups already described. Schreiner-Engel and colleagues are not sure whether type II diabetes is more damaging to sexuality than type I diabetes, or if the differences reflect more negative attitudes about sexuality and illness in this older cohort of women. Perhaps the younger women grew up in a social climate that encouraged them to live as normally as possible, despite having a chronic illness, whereas the older women saw the diabetes diagnosis as an end to sexual attractiveness.

Only one recent study restricted its sample to type II diabetic men. Miccoli *et al.* (1985) interviewed 77 men aged 40 to 64 years. Sexual problems were present in 52%, including low sexual desire in 28% and erectile dysfunction in 31%. Although men taking medications that impair sexual function were excluded, the researchers correctly observe that some of the sexual problems may be influenced by diseases of aging other than diabetes. The rates of sexual dysfunction were surprisingly similar, however, to those in Jensen's (1981a) younger, type I sample.

Psychosocial Impact on Sexuality

As discussed in Chapters 2 and 4, Jensen (1985a, 1985b) found that both a clinician's rating of a couple's disease acceptance and the number of psychological symptoms reported by the diabetic patient and spouse were good predictors of the diabetic's sexual function. Newman and Bertelson (1986) also found a higher incidence of depression and psychological distress in diabetic women with sexual dysfunction compared to a functional group. Although physiological damage is usually considered the cause of impaired sexual responsiveness in diabetics, Jensen's (1986) 6-year follow-up study demonstrated that spontaneous remission of sexual problems can occur even in patients with diabetic neuropathy, usually when they form a new relationship or marital conflict decreases in an ongoing one. Rates of spontaneous remission of dysfunction in men were 36% in Jensen's (1986) study and 9% in another 5-year prospective survey of 466 diabetic men including older subjects with type II diabetes (McCulloch *et al.*, 1984).

The danger of assuming that erectile dysfunction in diabetics is an irreversible result of organic damage is underscored by a recent study of NPT in diabetic and healthy men (Schiavi *et al.*, 1985). In general, whether they had erectile dysfunction or not, all young type I diabetics had abnormal REM sleep and reduced penile circumference changes during episodes of tumescence. Thus, diabetics may be misdiagnosed by NPT as being organically impaired.

Psychological factors common in diabetic sexual dysfunction include depression, anxiety about future health, and a negative body image (Jensen, 1985a). Schreiner-Engel *et al.* (1987) observe that type I diabetic women often find caretaking husbands who see their wife's fragility as part of her feminine role. The disability of an older woman who develops type II diabetes may interfere, however, with her usual role as family nurturer. Issues are similar for the aging man who loses some of his sexual capacity and his wage-earning ability because of diabetes. Thus, the illness may foster more marital conflict when it appears in a long-term relationship than when one spouse has been diabetic since childhood.

Physicians can unwittingly promote sexual dysfunction by warning patients that problems are inevitable. We have seen one patient who was told his erectile function would last only another 5 years after he became dependent on insulin. Five years later, he duly developed a psychogenic erection problem that, fortunately, was reversed by short-term sex therapy. Some physicians also caution diabetics that intercourse can bring on a hypoglycemic episode and advise them to eat a carbohydrate snack before sex. Yet a recent study of 16 patients who monitored their blood glucose before and after sex revealed only mild, nonsignificant drops in glucose levels (Moses & Colagiuri, 1985). Sexual activity, then, appears to be quite safe for insulin-dependent diabetics whose disease is well-controlled.

Physiological Impact on Sexuality

Physiological aspects of diabetes that have been studied in relation to sexual function include hormonal abnormalities, microvascular pathology, neuropathy, and the severity and duration of the illness.

Hormonal Abnormalities

Modern studies have not found an increased incidence of abnormal levels of testosterone or gonadotropins in diabetic men (Buvat et al., 1985b; Ficher et al., 1984; Jensen, Hagen, Frøland, & Pedersen, 1979; Kolodny, Kahn, Goldstein, & Barnett, 1974; Lester, Grant, & Woodroffe, 1980). Not only are baseline hormonal levels normal in diabetics with sexual dysfunction, but hormonal responses to stimulation with GnRH and thyrotropin-releasing hormone are also unimpaired (Pierini & Nusimovich, 1981; Zeidler et al., 1982).

Unfortunately, no data exist on hormonal levels in diabetic women either before or after menopause. It is unlikely, however, that differences would be found between diabetic and healthy groups.

Diabetic Neuropathy

Peripheral neuropathy has been proposed to explain erectile dysfunction in diabetic men. Several studies have found correlations between diabetic neuropathy and erectile dysfunction in men (Ellenberg, 1971; Jensen, 1981a, 1986; Jensen et al., 1979; Kolodny et al., 1974), but the evidence for a neurological factor in diabetic women's sexual problems is unconvincing (Ellenberg, 1977; Jensen, 1981a, 1986; Newman & Bertelson, 1986; Tyrer et al., 1983).

To disrupt erectile function, the neuropathy would have to involve the autonomic nervous system. It is clear that diabetic men can develop disturbances of emission, with reductions in semen volume or dry orgasms (Ellenberg, 1971; Fairburn et al., 1982; Jensen, 1986). Such symptoms suggest that the short adrenergic neurons are impaired but do not reveal anything about the nerves involved in erection.

Some researchers have tried to correlate the findings of gross, clinical tests of autonomic neuropathy in diabetics with sexual function. Jensen

(1981a, 1986) found beat-to-beat variation (respiration sinus arrhythmia) was not a helpful test. Fairburn *et al.* (1982) were also disappointed with results from five tests indicating cardiovascular reflex function.

No direct method of measuring autonomic neuropathy in pelvic nerves is available. Several researchers have reported that a subgroup of diabetic men with erection problems has prolonged bulbocavernosus reflex latencies (Buvat *et al.*, 1985b; Jevtich *et al.*, 1982; Lehman & Jacobs, 1983). Samples have been small, however, and the rate of abnormal tests suggests that neuropathy is not the entire explanation for the sexual problems. Buvat *et al.* (1985b) also observed prolonged reflex latencies in 4 out of 7 normally functioning diabetic men. They found urine-flow rates to be the only neurologic test showing consistent differences between diabetic men with and without good erections. Lin and Bradley (1985) found bulbocavernosus reflex latency and pudendal evoked potentials to be useless in distinguishing between healthy men with normal erections and diabetics with erectile dysfunction. They advocate measuring the nerve conduction velocity in the penis, a parameter that was abnormal in half of their 20 diabetic subjects. Of course, the dorsal nerve belongs to the sensory nervous system, and thus the test still does not measure autonomic disruption.

Recently, researchers have begun to look for abnormalities in neurotransmitters or cell structure in tissue removed from the corpora cavernosa of diabetic men, usually as a byproduct of surgery to implant a penile prosthesis. Melman and Maayani (1985) have been unable to identify a deficit in the response of diabetics' erectile tissue to various nerve-stimulating drugs. Crowe *et al.* (1983) believe that diabetic men lack adequate VIP immunoreactive nerves in their corpora cavernosa. Thus far, however, their hypothesis is based on a rat model for diabetes and on data from one human subject. Jevtich, Kass, and Khawand (1985) examined tissue from 10 diabetic men and found extensive fibrous changes in the cavernous bodies resulting, they believe, from inadequate blood flow to the penis. They suggest that any neurological contribution to diabetics' erectile dysfunction occurs when fibrosis entraps the nerve fibers in the penis, interfering with their function.

Vascular Pathology

With the advent of noninvasive measures of penile blood flow, researchers began looking for evidence that diabetic erectile dysfunction was caused by arteriosclerotic changes related to the disease process. Several studies concluded that retinopathy, a measure of vascular changes not specific to the genital area, was not correlated with sexual function in diabetics (Fairburn *et al.*, 1982; Jensen, 1981a, 1986; Jensen *et al.*, 1979; Kolodny *et al.*, 1974). McCulloch *et al.* (1984), however, found that diabetic men with erection problems were more likely to develop retinopathy over the next 5 years than were sexually functional diabetics.

Diabetic men with erectile dysfunction have high rates of abnormal findings in noninvasive Doppler examinations, suggesting inadequate penile blood flow (Jevtich *et al.*, 1982; Lehman & Jacobs, 1983). Sexually functional diabetics, however, have an equal rate of abnormal vascular examinations (Buvat *et al.*, 1985b). Thus, the role vascular pathology plays in diabetic erectile dysfunction is still in question. Larger samples of functional versus dysfunctional men must be studied, using not only the Doppler techniques described in Chapter 6, but also the newer diagnostic papaverine injections. Research on vaginal blood flow in diabetic women is also long overdue.

Factors Related to Diabetes

Researchers have not been able to demonstrate a relationship between sexual function and age at diabetes onset, duration of diabetes, or need for insulin or oral hypoglycemic drugs (Jensen, 1986; Miccoli *et al.*, 1985; Newman & Bertelson, 1986; Schreiner-Engel *et al.*, 1987). Measures of metabolic control are also poor predictors of sexual capacity (Jensen, 1981a, 1986; Miccoli *et al.*, 1985), although McCulloch *et al.* (1984) found a correlation between degree of metabolic control at the time of initial assessment and subsequent erection problems. Indeed, erectile dysfunction has been proposed as a common initial symptom of diabetes that has not yet been diagnosed (Goldman, Schechter, & Eckerling, 1970). Melman *et al.*, (1984) diagnosed 15 new cases of impaired glucose tolerance or overt diabetes in a series of 70 men referred for evaluation of erectile dysfunction.

Diabetics who abuse alcohol (McCulloch *et al.*, 1984) or are heavy smokers (Jensen, 1986) have a higher incidence of erection problems. Diabetics are also at high risk for hypertension and for the iatrogenic effects of antihypertensives on sexual function (Lipson, 1984).

Assessment Issues

Table 10-1 details areas of assessment that are particularly relevant for the diabetic patient. The interview should include questions on the impact of diabetes on close relationships, emotions, and self-image. The Disease Acceptance Scale presented in Chapter 6 was designed especially for couples with a diabetic partner and scores are predictive of sexual function (Jensen, 1986).

Physiological assessment of sexual function has focused on men with erection problems. In fact, one recent survey found that few physicians even attempt to assess sexual function in women with diabetes (House & Pendleton, 1986). A comprehensive workup is needed, perhaps including special attention to metabolic control and tests of diabetic neuropathy.

Table 10-1. Special Assessment Techniques

	Diabetes	COPD	Chronic Pain
Interview Topics	Impact of illness on daily life Ability to make lifestyle changes in diet, exercise, insulin management Illness-related depression Use of diabetes to manipulate spouse Impact on plans for parenthood	Impact of illness on daily life Ability to make lifestyle changes in smoking Illness-related depression Assumption of invalid role Coping strategies for breathlessness during sex	Impact of illness on daily life Pain behavior, its antecedents and consequences Illness-related depression Secondary gains from spouse Coping strategies to manage pain during sex
Questionnaires	Disease Acceptance Scale (Chapter 6, Table 6-1)	Battery of Asthma Illness Behavior (Dirks *et al.*, 1982) Neuropsychological testing	Patient Pain Questionnaire (Turk *et al.*, 1983) Significant Others' Pain Questionnaire (Turk *et al.*, 1983)
Medical History	Other chronic illnesses Substance abuse and smoking Age at onset of diabetes Metabolic control and medications used Diabetic complications Frequency of hypoglycemic episodes	Other chronic illnesses Substance abuse and smoking Current medications	Substance abuse Current medications Adequacy of vaginal lubrication in women with rheumatic disease
Physiological Assessment	Comprehensive evaluation of erectile dysfunction, with special attention to vibratory sensation on the penis, urine flow, orthostatic hypotension, or abnormal sweating patterns Measures of metabolic control	Comprehensive evaluation of erectile dysfunction Evaluation of general pulmonary function	Comprehensive evaluation of erectile dysfunction, with special attention in men with back pain to penile sensory thresholds, sacral electromyogram, full-scale NPT monitoring, and sexual stimulation in the laboratory to evaluate neurogenic factors

Treatment Issues

Table 10-2 highlights treatment techniques useful for diabetics with sexual problems. Many hospitals and specialized clinics offer patient education programs or support groups to help diabetics and their families adjust to the disease and make healthy changes in diet and lifestyle. Brief sexual counseling should be offered routinely as a part of such programs. Table 10-3 lists some of the educational information that could be provided. Patients who need intensive sex therapy could also be identified. Such counseling may be most effective when offered early in the course of disease, before sexual problems become chronic (McCulloch, Hosking, & Tobert, 1986).

Because diabetes often impairs erectile function, the penile prosthesis has become a popular option for diabetic men (Beaser, Van der Hoek, Jacobson, Flood, & Desautels, 1982; Peterson *et al.*, 1985). All of the information presented in this chapter suggests that specialized medical examinations are as crucial in determining the cause of a diabetic's erection problems as they are in evaluating any other surgical candidate (Chapter 8). The mere diagnosis of diabetes is not an adequate rationale for choosing a medical or surgical therapy over sex therapy.

Intensive Sex Therapy Case

Christine and Frank had been married for 17 years when they were referred for sex therapy. She had been diabetic since the age of 7 and was now aged 37. She had a slight sensory peripheral neuropathy and mild retinopathy but no signs of autonomic neuropathy or renal impairment. Frank had undergone a vasectomy 3 years before. The couple's children were 14 and 16, and both parents worked. Frank was a schoolteacher; his wife had recently finished a program to become a practical nurse and worked in a hospital part-time.

The presenting complaint was Christine's lack of sexual desire. Frank's ideal was to have sex five times weekly, but his wife found once a month to be sufficient. "I know no one else our age has sex as often as Frank wants it," Christine asserted. "I wouldn't say that," her husband replied with a slightly mysterious air. Christine wanted the therapists to make her husband see that, as she put it, "I just am not in the mood most of the time—even though I think he's sexy and I love him." Frank wanted treatment to spark some of the desire that his wife had shown earlier in their marriage. He also wanted her to reach orgasm more often—a problem Christine did not mention.

When the couple filled out assessment questionnaires, some discrepancies in their perceptions became apparent. Both agreed that Christine's mood fluctuated often, but Frank also saw this problem in himself, whereas his wife saw him as rather stable in his moods. Frank found his wife quite beautiful and appealing, but she saw herself as sexually unattractive. On the other hand, both agreed that Frank was not particularly good-looking. Frank and Christine each saw the other using diabetes as an excuse: "You're so bitchy tonight, you must have low blood sugar." "I think I'll go to bed early. My sugar is high and I have a headache." Their attitudes about sexual variety revealed Frank was more adventurous. He masturbated twice a week, whereas Christine had never masturbated, believing it was only for men.

Their couple time lines were also discrepant. Christine noted a postpartum depression for several months after the birth of their youngest child. Frank had not even noticed or had forgotten about it. Frank currently saw their relationship as less happy than his wife did, but expected that therapy would put them back near the top of the scale. Christine only predicted a mild improvement from current, somewhat unhappy functioning.

The second session was a split, with the cotherapists taking individual sexual histories. Frank revealed that he was currently involved in an extramarital affair. He often thought about leaving Christine. "But how can you desert a sick wife?" he asked. The therapist had Frank role play being himself and his wife, using two chairs to set the stage. "Christine" heard the message: "I stay with you only out of pity. If you didn't have diabetes, I would leave." Back in his own role, Frank realized that he would never accept such a message himself. He went on to consider his own ambivalence and whether he was just staying in his marriage out of guilt or if, in fact, he received some payoffs. Frank spoke about his fear of abandonment if Christine became disabled or died young and acknowledged that his girlfriend was a hedge against loneliness. The therapist was supportive but told Frank that in order to continue couple therapy, Frank would have to stop seeing his girlfriend. Otherwise, progress would be severely hindered. Frank decided to stop the affair but never to mention its existence to Christine.

In Christine's individual session, she emphasized that Frank had reacted in a typical "macho" fashion to his vasectomy. "He has to prove he's still a real man. Even after 17 years, if we don't have sex every 3 or 4 days he's impossible to live with. The worst is when he's extra nice, doing chores or being sweet to the kids, and I know he's just running up brownie points to trade in for sex. I can just about feel my vagina tense up."

Since both partners had expressed a wish for more affectionate touch of a nonsexual nature, the therapist assigned sensate focus exercises. The couple agreed to try them, but with some skepticism, especially from Frank when the ban on intercourse was introduced. "That's crazy! I thought we were here to have more sex, not less!"

"I think it sounds nice," said Christine, with a glint of triumph in her eyes. At the next session, life was paradise. They had tried the sensate focus exercise twice and both vied to tell how much they had enjoyed it. They had discussed how much energy they wasted fighting about sex, and one night

Table 10-2. Special Treatment Issues

	Diabetes	COPD	Chronic Pain
Format	Brief counseling can be offered routinely in educational and support groups	Brief counseling can be offered as part of a COPD rehabilitation program	Brief counseling can be offered routinely as a component of chronic pain treatment programs
Brief Counseling			
Education	Effect of diabetes on erections and vaginal lubrication, with emphasis on coping strategies	Need to reduce smoking and drinking and to improve exercise tolerance as part of sexual rehabilitation	Effects on sexual function of pain medication, chronic pain itself, and any underlying disease process
Attitude Change	Reducing feelings of stigmatization, maintaining a healthy lifestyle	Reducing feelings of stigmatization, avoiding invalid role, rejecting performance orientation to sex	Avoiding invalid role, reducing fear that sex will trigger pain, focusing on pleasurable sensations or fantasies instead of on painful zones
Resuming Sex	Using varied ways to reach orgasm when intercourse is difficult	Using varied ways to reach orgasm when intercourse is difficult, choosing time of day when least fatigued, finding positions that allow comfortable breathing	Using varied ways to reach orgasm when intercourse is difficult, choosing time of day when pain is least restricting, taking advantage of medication or pain reduction techniques, using positions that minimize low back pain or allow for limited hip mobility

Marital Conflict	Avoiding use of illness as excuse or alibi, encouraging patient to manage own care	Minimizing dependency on spouse, promoting positive changes in couple health habits	Reducing spouse overprotectiveness, encouraging assertive expression of anger, involving spouse in program to increase patient's activity level
Physical Handicaps	Coping with organic impairment of erections, using vaginal lubricants, suggesting positions for amputees, teaching sexual communication skills to the blind	Coping with organic impairment of erections, learning to make love wearing an oxygen mask, proper use of inhalers	Coping with organic impairment of erections, using pillows in positioning back pain patients or amputees, using vaginal lubricants when needed, using vibrator for self or partner when arthritis limits hand dexterity, exploring hip replacement as option for debilitating arthritis
Intensive Therapy	Guilt over having diabetic child, marital conflict intensified by manipulation of diabetic control	Poor body image and reduced self-efficacy in patients with history of childhood respiratory disease	History of sexual trauma or inactivity in patient with chronic pelvic pain

Table 10-3. Guidelines on Sexuality for Diabetic Patients

1. About 50% of diabetic men experience sexual problems. The most frequent dysfunctions are low sexual desire and erection problems.

2. Diabetic women are not at higher risk than healthy women for any sexual problem except reduced vaginal lubrication. A water-based lubricant can compensate for this difficulty and prevent vaginal dryness during sexual activity.

3. Although couples often blame a sexual problem on the diabetes, a combination of medical and emotional factors is usually present. Even men with peripheral neuropathy often have good sexual function or can recover from an erection problem without a medical "cure."

4. The changes in sexual function that normally occur with aging are accelerated in diabetic men. Diabetics may be younger than most men when they notice a slowing of the erection response, a need for more penile caressing to achieve full erection, and a longer refractory period between orgasms. These changes are not a reason to panic, however, but rather are a signal to take a more relaxed attitude to lovemaking.

5. Even if an organic erection problem develops, most diabetic men continue to be able to reach a satisfying orgasm.

6. Semen volume decreases gradually in some diabetic men, so that eventually they have "dry orgasms." The sensation of orgasm is still pleasurable, but this symptom can interfere with fertility.

7. A sexual problem may be a sign that a couple needs to work on accepting the diagnosis of diabetes and feeling more comfortable with the effects of illness on their relationship. Professional help is available.

8. Set aside some time each day to talk about your feelings. It is important to schedule "adult time" together that is just for you as a couple.

9. Make a special effort to express affection through touch. Not every session of kissing and cuddling has to end in intercourse.

10. Share some of your preferences for caressing during sex and think about how your fantasies could be translated into more sexual variety. Instead of worrying about intercourse and orgasm, enjoy the process of lovemaking.

11. Are there any bad health habits (eg., smoking, heavy alcohol use, use of tranquilizers) that could be causing the sexual problem? You can work on reducing those habits and building more healthy ones such as getting enough rest, increasing your physical exercise, and improving your diet.

12. Medical examinations can be performed to find out whether physical damage from the diabetes is likely to be the cause of your erection problem. If so, you can consider penile prosthesis surgery. If surgery becomes an option, you and your wife will be asked to see a sex therapist who will help you decide together if the prosthesis is right for you.

had even gone out on a "date," out to dinner and a movie. Frank and Christine did agree that it felt a bit artificial to do the exercises on a schedule, but they had chosen not to be impromptu so they would be sure to finish the homework. "After all a teacher should practice what he preaches," said Frank.

Subsequent sessions focused on the role of diabetes in the couple's relationship. By using diabetes to shape their lives, Frank and Christine had developed a very indirect style of communication. "You know my sugar's low before lunch," Christine would say. "I think your sugar's low when it's convenient," Frank might reply. In the sessions, Christine and Frank were taught communication skills: to frame a message as an I-statement that includes a feeling, for example, "I feel annoyed when it's your turn to cook and you get out of it by blaming your blood sugar"; and to reflect back the meaning of the partner's message, in this case, "You mean you get angry if you think I'm using my blood sugar to avoid a chore."

Both partners began to perceive their own responsibility in maintaining conflict. Frank was aware of what he called his "broom syndrome." He felt his role in life was to sweep obstacles out of Christine's path so that all would be smooth. He enjoyed sweeping much of the time, and Christine liked it too. They decided, however, that Christine was going to have to start sweeping her own doorstep, and Frank needed to hand over the broom to her more of the time.

By the seventh session the partners were feeling much more satisfied with their communication, but were beginning to get impatient with the sensate focus exercises. Frank felt more and more frustrated by the ban on sexual activity, while Christine was not ready to proceed. Frank felt that the therapists were in league with his wife. He had been good for 6 weeks, and now he wanted his reward. Christine reacted by pitying her husband as she had in earlier sessions. "Poor Frank. It's not easy being married to a diabetic."

The therapists pointed out that the same game they had been playing with sex was now being applied to the sensate focus exercises. Frank put the pressure on and Christine felt guilty. She was just about ready to say yes, even though she did not want to go further, and would just become resentful if she did.

For the next assignment, Christine was instructed to spend at least 15 minutes looking at herself in the mirror, to be followed by looking at her genital area and lightly exploring its various parts with touch. When Christine reported her emotional reactions to the exercise, she focused on her feelings that her body was defective and asexual. Frank was astonished because he had always seen his wife as a beautiful woman. He told her that he often feared that she was not attracted to him because he was not as physically perfect as she. Christine judged Frank just as harshly as she viewed herself. She told him that he needed to lose 20 pounds and that she often saw him as an older and heavier "blurred copy" of the man she married. "And I know you too well, I think," she continued. "When we have sex I can guess how you want to be touched before you even give me a clue."

Frank looked hurt and remained silent for several moments. The therapists asked him to share his feelings on hearing Christine's remarks. "I guess I mostly feel sad," he said, slowly. "I feel like I've been the one hoping that things would change for the better from this therapy. Right now, though, I don't think anything will change. She'll just keep on rejecting me."

Frank and Christine were asked to role play a typical sexual initiation in their relationship, but with the roles reversed. Christine played Frank, demanding sex. Frank acted out Christine's martyred way of saying no. The role play helped to break the impasse, because each partner saw the humor in the habitual struggle and could share feelings about the experience of asking for sex and of saying no, increasing their mutual empathy. "I think you must feel you have to be ready for sex at any moment." Christine told her husband.

"Yeah, and I guess that makes you feel like I'm always breathing down your neck," he responded. "No wonder you don't come up and give me a hug very often."

"You'd just take it as an invitation," Christine told him.

The therapists noticed that the couple came in holding hands for their next session. They both requested that the next sensate focus include genital caressing, and the therapists agreed. During the week, Christine had had a hypoglycemic episode. She expected Frank to bring her some juice, but did not ask. He assumed she was able to take care of hereslf, in keeping with the new "broom policy." Suddenly, however, Christine was lying on the floor in a faint. Frank rushed her to the hospital, where she was kept overnight. In the therapy session, Christine told Frank she was angry at his failure to see to her needs. Frank obviously felt guilty, but was angry too. "You see? If I don't sweep her path clear, she'll spend her life in the hospital." The therapists allowed Frank to go on, just reflecting back his anger until Christine broke in.

"I would not spend my life in the hospital! Sometimes I just start to feel so weak and heavy that I don't think clearly. Once in a while I may need your help, but most of the time I could handle it myself."

"You could?" the therapist asked.

"I will," said Christine.

Frank told his wife that her hypoglycemic episodes triggered his anxiety that she might die. "When I pick up that broom," he said, " I start to feel in control again." Christine told Frank that he made her feel like a naughty child being scolded by her mother. This led into a discussion of how Christine's mother had taken over all diabetes care until Christine was 15 or 16 years old, giving her daily insulin injections and planning her entire diet. Christine's mother even scheduled her after-school time.

"I could always get to her by going off my diet or skipping a meal," Christine recalled. "That's what I did when I got angry."

The therapist said, "You could punish her by letting your disease get out of control. Does that remind you of anything now?"

Christine and Frank laughed ruefully. Frank recalled from his own childhood that his father was in the merchant marines and would be away for weeks at a time. His mother had severe migraines, and he remembered her often lying in bed, being grateful when he brought her tea and kept the other children quiet. "It's really too much," commented Christine. "The naughty little girl found Mama's good boy to take care of her. Maybe it's time for both of us to grow up, hmm?"

By Session 12, homework was proceeding well. Christine complained that although she was getting sexually aroused, her vagina remained dry. The therapists reminded her that some diabetic women needed to use an extra lubricant to make intercourse comfortable. Christine bought the recommended lubrication and the problem was reduced. Although neither partner was yet allowed to reach orgasm during the sensate focus exercise, Frank had masturbated to ejaculation while lying next to his wife after the last one. Christine told him he was breaking the rules but actually had found it exciting.

At the next session, the couple appeared a bit anxious. They soon confessed that they had broken the ban on intercourse but had really enjoyed the experience. Christine took the initiative and suggested that the couple "cheat" after a romantic dinner. A week later she tried to tempt Frank again, but to her surprise he told her that he was too tired from gardening. She turned over in a huff and went to sleep, and the couple did not discuss the incident until their therapy session. Christine was able to articulate her fear that Frank no longer desired her. He told her that he had felt pressured to have sex when he really just wanted to cuddle and talk.

Christine and Frank wondered if they needed more therapy, but the therapists pointed out that they were still playing the same game, even if the roles had been switched. They agreed to have two more sessions in order to reach a more complete sense of closure on their problems. Christine had no further hypoglycemic episodes during the next several weeks and Frank felt he had put his broom away. On the day of scheduled termination, however, the couple came in with long faces. They had had a celebration dinner the night before, planning to crown the evening with a session of lovemaking. However, by the time the teenagers got to bed and the dishes were washed, Christine felt too tired for sex. Frank turned his back on her, and that morning she had a hypoglycemic episode, with Frank bringing her juice as usual.

The therapists pointed out that separation is often difficult, and perhaps the couple had been anxious about trying life on their own. They reviewed the process of the therapy with the couple, reassuring them that although the symptoms often did not disappear entirely, the couple now had the skills to deal with them when they did crop up. Sometimes they might avoid an episode of conflict entirely, and other times they might at least realize what was happening before the feelings got so out of control. Frank and Christine left feeling encouraged. At 3-month and 1-year follow-ups, they continued to have an active sex life and to use more direct marital communication styles. Hypoglycemic episodes were rare, and Christine had been hospitalized only once.

CHRONIC OBSTRUCTIVE PULMONARY DISEASE

Approximately 14% of all physician office visits for any condition involve respiratory disease and one fifth of these are for COPD (Brashear, 1980). COPD has been defined as "a disease of uncertain etiology characterized by persistent slowing of air-flow during forced expiration" (Burrows, 1976).

The three most common subtypes of COPD are chronic bronchitis, emphysema, and asthma. In this chapter, we also discuss sexuality in patients with cystic fibrosis, a genetic disease that used to be a childhood killer but now can be treated effectively enough that survivors face the challenge of adulthood (Orenstein & Wachnowsky, 1985).

Not only is COPD an illness that restricts many daily activities, including sexuality, but its incidence is increasing (R. M. Kaplan, Reis, & Atkins, 1985). Since the disease process may take 20 to 30 years to run its course, COPD is a major source of disability in the United States.

Patients with COPD are vulnerable to sexual dysfunction, not only because breathlessness limits physical exertion, but also because perceptual and motor skills are impaired (Prigatano, Wright, Levin, & Hawryluk, 1983). Like other chronic illnesses we discuss, COPD becomes more common with age. Many patients with COPD take medications that can impair sexual function, or have other risk factors for organic sexual problems.

Few studies examine the incidence of sexual dysfunction in patients with COPD. In one series of 90 men (average age 57 years), only 19% had sexual problems (Kass, Updegraff, & Muffly, 1972). In a more recent survey of 128 men and women with COPD, however, 67% reported that their illness had a negative impact on physical aspects of sexuality (Hanson, 1982). In a smaller sample (20 men), 30% had erectile dysfunction (Fletcher & Martin, 1982). The rates of actual sexual dysfunction in young adults with cystic fibrosis are lower, and problems seem more closely related to self-esteem and body image than to the severity of the disease (Coffman, Levine, Althof, & Stern, 1984). Loss of sexual desire seems to be a common complaint for men and women. Many older men with COPD also have erectile dysfunction.

Psychosocial Impact on Sexuality

For any patient with COPD, the exertion of sexual activity can promote breathlessness and fatigue. For asthmatics, in particular, emotional arousal has been linked to bronchospasm (Cluss & Fireman, 1985; Felstein, 1977). Thus, lovemaking can become associated with fear and anxiety, evoking a panic–dyspnea cycle (R. M. Kaplan et al., 1985).

Progressive disability and chronic fatigue also can lead to clinical depression, further decreasing sexual desire. Dependence on the spouse, financially and for daily care, can spark marital conflict or foster a shift to parent–child roles. A significant subgroup of COPD patients have unhealthy habits, especially smoking and alcohol abuse. The spouse's frustration with the patient's self-destructive behavior may create further distance in the marital relationship.

For young adults with cystic fibrosis, especially young women, feelings of being sexually unattractive or stigmatized by short stature, thinness, stained teeth, and clubbed fingers interfere with dating and becoming sexually active (Coffman *et al.*, 1984). The impact of a genetic disease on reproductive plans also may reduce sexual self-esteem.

In our clinical experience, childhood diseases like cystic fibrosis and asthma that entail frequent hospitalization often delay psychosexual maturation. We agree with Coffman *et al.* (1984) that it is the experience of being chronically ill, rather than the specific disease process, that affects sexuality. These patients may get lost in the system when they outgrow pediatric care and can best be given psychological support in a setting that involves the whole family in the medical care (Doherty & Baird, 1983).

Physiological Impact on Sexuality

At least for adults with COPD, the severity of hypoxia may predict sexual function (Fletcher & Martin, 1982; Semple, Beastall, & Hume, 1980). The only studies of physiological factors in sexual dysfunction focus on men's erectile problems. Semple and colleagues (Semple *et al.*, 1980; Semple *et al.*, 1984) maintain that serum testosterone decreases in hypoxic men because of suppression at either the hypothalamic or pituitary level. In contrast, Fletcher & Martin (1982) observed normal hormonal levels but abnormal bulbocavernosus reflex latencies in men with COPD and erectile dysfunction. The small sample sizes used in both studies make the controversy difficult to resolve. Risk factors for erectile dysfunction, including diabetes, cardiovascular disease, heavy smoking, alcoholism, and medications such as steroids, antihypertensives, and psychotropic drugs, are so common in COPD patients that most erection problems must have complex causes.

Assessment Issues

The interview with a COPD patient should address the impact of the illness on daily life relationships and on sexual routines and function (Table 10-1). Questionnaires thus far have only been developed for asthmatics. One research group has developed a Battery of Asthma Illness Behavior (Dirks, Brown, & Robinson, 1982), which uses questions about locus of control, asthma symptoms, and attitude toward illness to predict coping and compliance. In general, neuropsychological testing should be included if the patient seems cognitively impaired.

Because COPD patients often have other medical problems, assessment should always include a thorough medical history and examination, including specific diagnostic tests, such as glucose tolerance or liver function assays, when another disease is suspected. Men with erectile dysfunction need a comprehensive workup, including studies of hormones, pelvic vascular parameters, and neuropathy.

Treatment Issues

Rehabilitation programs for COPD patients are becoming more common
(R. M. Kaplan *et al.*, 1985). A module of sexual counseling should be added
to education on exercise tolerance, lifestyle changes, and increasing self-
efficacy. Brief counseling issues resemble those in other chronic illnesses
such as cancer, cardiovascular disease, or diabetes (Table 10-2).

Patients who have histories of childhood COPD may need intensive
therapy if they have not yet negotiated the transition to a fully adult,
intimate relationship.

Brief Counseling Case

Douglas, a 65-year-old retired factory foreman, had emphysema and
chronic bronchitis. Although his COPD had been diagnosed 10 years previously and his shortness of breath limited his ability to enjoy pastimes such
as bicycling and bowling, he continued to smoke a pack of cigarettes and to
drink six to eight beers daily. He was mildly hypertensive, treated with a
thiazide diuretic. Other medications included theophylline and a selective,
bronchodilating beta-blocker. His wife, Mary, was 63. Although she was in
good health, she had retired early from her job as an accounting clerk. She
continued to earn extra money by part-time housekeeping jobs.

The assessment began with specialized medical examinations. Douglas'
serum testosterone level was normal, and vascular examination using
Doppler techniques also demonstrated no pathology. He broke one out of
three snaps on a Dacomed snap-gauge, and then two out of three the next
night. The one clearly abnormal finding was a delayed bulbocavernosus
reflex latency. Because Douglas's wife complained that his memory was
deteriorating, and he himself seemed a poor historian, a neuropsychological examination was performed, revealing mild, diffuse cognitive impairment.

As usual, the evaluation included an interview with Douglas and Mary.
Until 6 months previously, the couple had had sexual activity about every
2 weeks. Douglas always initiated, usually by stroking Mary's breast after
the couple had gotten into bed for the night. Mary rarely refused her
husband. Foreplay lasted less than 5 minutes, and then each partner
reached orgasm during intercourse. When asked about their use of positions, Mary blushed and Douglas answered, "Oh, I think I always lie on top.
That's our favorite, isn't it, Mary?"

"Yes," his wife said. "And we keep the lights off."

Within the past several months, Douglas began to get short of breath
during intercourse, at which time he would lose his erection. Both Douglas
and Mary felt very anxious when he began to wheeze and gasp. Douglas
would turn over and lie back on the pillows his wife piled up for him. Mary

would hold his hand and stroke his hair until his breathing calmed. There was no question of resuming sexual activity after such an episode. Douglas and Mary had not considered trying a position for intercourse that would require less exertion on Douglas's part. "Old dogs can't learn new tricks," he told the therapist. He responded the same way to a question about switching the lovemaking to a morning or afternoon time when he might be less fatigued.

The therapist met a second time with the couple to give them feedback on the evaluation. He stressed that the medical examination did not demonstrate a severe impairment of erections. Douglas still woke up with erections and could achieve them during foreplay. It was the breathlessness that seemed most crucial in interfering with sexual function.

Mary then said firmly that she agreed that Douglas could function better if he was willing to be more flexible in their sexual routine. "You listen to the doctor," she told her husband, "and we'll go home and try what he says." She patted her husband's hand and he shrugged, looking embarrassed but also pleased by her resolve.

The therapist suggested having sexual activity earlier in the day. As a position for intercourse, Douglas could lean against several pillows, in a semi-sitting posture. Mary would then kneel above her husband, assuming most of the work of thrusting. Douglas and Mary were also given a handout illustrating other intercourse positions that COPD patients had found comfortable, for example, the husband seated against a pile of pillows with the wife sitting astride him, or both partners lying on their sides, spoon fashion. The therapist recommended that Douglas quit smoking and cut his daily alcohol intake to two beers. Douglas refused a referral to a stop-smoking program, however. "I'll do it myself, if I decide to," he said mutinously.

One month later, the couple returned for a follow-up. They had had three experiences of lovemaking, trying a different intercourse position each time. Mary had actually initiated two of the sessions, taking advantage of weekend mornings when she could wake her husband with a caress. "I kind of liked her showing me she was interested," Douglas said.

"Old dogs *can* learn something," Mary answered with a wink.

Douglas's erections were more lasting when he could stay relaxed during intercourse. If he began to get breathless, Mary would slow her movement and let Douglas sit up higher on his pillows. Mary also noted that her husband was being more affectionate in general, which she appreciated. The day before, he had asked her to come to bed in the afternoon, just to cuddle and talk. The couple did not feel a need for further counseling. Douglas was still smoking and drinking his full complement of beer. "I *am* an old dog," he maintained. "And if I've got to die, I'll die happy." Mary glared at her husband as if she had other plans, and the therapist decided to leave this aspect of lifestyle change to Douglas's in-house expert.

CHRONIC PAIN

Chronic pain is a health problem of surprisingly large dimensions. Turk, Meichenbaum, and Genest (1983), reviewing the literature on chronic pain, estimate that there are 20 to 50 million Americans (9% to 23%) with arthritis, 25 million (12%) who suffer from migraine headaches, and 7 million (3%) with disabling lower back pain. In 1980, over 800 pain clinics were operating within the United States. Although clinicians have observed a high incidence of sexual dysfunction and marital distress in patients with chronic pain (Infante, 1981; Roy, 1985; Turk *et al.*, 1983, p. 235), research data on sexuality and chronic pain are few.

Arthritis patients and those with other rheumatic diseases have been the most frequently studied groups. Ferguson and Figley (1979) found that 54% of a group of 70 arthritic women and 56% of a group of 30 male patients experienced sexual problems. Concerns included pain, weakness, fatigue, and limited range of motion during sexual activity. Patients in their mid-30s to mid-40s had the highest incidence of sexual problems. Herstein, Hill, and Walters (1977) reported that 63% of young adults with juvenile rheumatoid arthritis complained of similar limitations on their sexual pleasure. Elst *et al.* (1984) found that both men and women with rheumatoid arthritis scored significantly worse than normal controls on a scale measuring sexual enjoyment versus avoidance. Few researchers asked about sexual function in detail, but Ferguson and Figley reported 18% of men in their sample had erectile dysfunction and 13% of women had reduced vaginal lubrication.

In the only recent study of back pain and sexuality (Sjögren & Fugl-Meyer, 1981), 54% of men ($N = 35$) and 52% of women ($N = 25$) reported a decrease in sexual satisfaction since their pain began. Women in the sample already had had a high incidence (20%) of difficulty in reaching orgasm before the back pain started, but such problems increased (28%) after the onset of pain. Men reported both erectile dysfunction (37%) and difficulty reaching orgasm (23%) beginning after the disability. The most common reasons for decreased sexual activity were pain, fear of pain, and fatigue. Both men and women began to assume a "spectator" role during lovemaking.

Even higher rates of sexual dissatisfaction were reported by patients and spouses participating in two programs that treat chronic pain (Flor, Turk, & Scholz, 1987; Maruta, Osborne, Swanson, & Halling, 1981). The frequency of sex had decreased since the onset of pain for 77% of couples in one case series and 78% in the other, with sexual dissatisfaction ranging from 50% (Maruta *et al.*, 1981) to 67% (Flor *et al.*, 1987). In Maruta *et al.*'s sample, 28% of male patients had erectile dysfunction and 32% reported premature ejaculation. For women, problems included a 36% rate of low sexual desire and a 40% incidence of difficulty reaching orgasm.

A group of Italian researchers has studied sexuality in men and women with chronic headaches (Del Bene, Conti, Poggioni, & Sicuteri, 1982). They found that 9% of women and 14% of men ($N = 362$) experienced sexual arousal as part of a headache episode. The headache patients were similar to healthy, age-matched controls, however, in the frequency of sexual activity with a partner. Sexual dysfunction was not directly assessed.

Besides nongenital pain syndromes, sexual pleasure may also be impaired by genital pain. Women with chronic pelvic pain are a particularly difficult group to assess and treat (Charles & Glover, 1985). Pelvic pain usually includes pain during sexual activity but also entails pain in the genital or abdominal area at other times. A clinical observation is that many such women have histories of incest, sexual molestation as a child, or rape. The pain provides an acceptable way of avoiding sexual activity. Some of these women have undergone multiple gynecological operations for pain relief, including hysterectomy, unilateral or bilateral oophorectomy, lysis of pelvic adhesions, or even sacral neurectomy, a procedure that risks damaging bowel or bladder function.

Men with atypical, chronic genital pain also present a challenge to the clinician. Psychogenic factors seem to play an important role in such syndromes as pain with ejaculation or chronic prostatitis when an organic cause cannot be diagnosed (Mimoun, 1984).

Psychosocial Impact on Sexuality

As Roy (1985) points out, chronic pain is a family issue. Not only may the patient be unable to work outside the home or to carry out household chores, but chronic pain sufferers are often angry and depressed as well. Because chronic pain interferes with such a range of activities, the patient is often fatigued. Loss of ability to work and the disfigurement accompanying diseases such as severe arthritis contribute to a loss of self-esteem.

Pain can be viewed as a communication. People who cannot reveal their anger or vulnerability may feel justified in eliciting attention or nurturance with pain. Many exhibit characteristic "pain behaviors": nonverbal signals such as grimaces or postural cues, failure to perform normal tasks, or ostentatious use of pain medication (Steger & Fordyce, 1982; Turk *et al.*, 1983). Spouses or other family members unwittingly reinforce such behavior by being sympathetic or assuming the patient's responsibilities. At the same time, since pain is such a subjective phenomenon, the family may doubt whether the patient is really so disabled. An angry spouse may also become an overprotective one, out of guilt over feeling resentful (Roy, 1985). Thus, although chronic pain is very unpleasant, it also has reinforcing properties (Steger & Fordyce, 1982), allowing the patient to avoid disliked activities (which may include sexual activity for some), and eliciting caring from the family (Roy, 1985; Sjögren & Fugl-Meyer, 1981). In cases where pain has come to rule the patient's life, the physical symptom may need to be reframed (see Chapter 6) as an emotional and relationship issue.

Of course pain, fatigue, and limited range of motion distract from pleasurable sensations during sexual activity. Low self-esteem, an impaired sense of physical attractiveness, and clinical depression are common factors that interfere with sexual desire in patients with chronic pain.

Physiological Impact on Sexuality

Pain has been defined as "an unpleasant sensory and emotional experience associated with actual or potential tissue damage, or described in terms of such damage" (International Association for the Study of Pain Subcommittee on Taxonomy, 1979, p. 250). Chronic pain may be periodic, occurring intermittently; intractable but benign; or progressive, often associated with cancer (Turk et al., 1983).

According to the gate-control model of pain, the subjective sensation represents an interaction between somatic stimuli, emotion, and cognition (Turk et al., 1983). When peripheral nerve fibers reach a certain threshold of activity, a neural "gate" in the spinal cord is opened, allowing the brain to register pain. The brain can modulate painful sensation, however, by influencing spinal cord centers. Thus feelings and thoughts can either minimize or exacerbate the perceived intensity of painful stimuli. For example, if a woman fears that intercourse will set off an episode of lower back pain, she may focus on any back sensations she feels during sexual activity. The more tense she becomes, perhaps in anger at her husband for demanding sex, the more her back will hurt. On the other hand, preliminary evidence suggests that if a woman becomes highly aroused by vaginal stimulation, she perceives a painful stimulus as less intense, even though her threshold to touch is unchanged (Whipple & Komisaruk, 1985). Perhaps sexual arousal "closes the gate" (Del Bene et al., 1982).

Unfortunately, many pain patients are too distracted by their pain to reach high levels of sexual arousal. Furthermore, a temporary insensitivity to pain during sexual activity could lead to overexertion, exacerbating pain after sexual activity and perpetuating the vicious cycle of sexual avoidance out of fear of pain.

The relationship between pain and sexual arousal is complex. Del Bene et al. (1982) believe that migraine headaches are accompanied by hyperreactivity of the "mating centers" of the brain and a decrease in enkephalins in the cerebrospinal fluid. They suggest that the sexual arousal seen in a minority of headache patients during a pain episode results from an imbalance of neurotransmitters. It has also been clinically observed that some patients have headaches triggered by orgasm, but little is known about this phenomenon. Most benign sexual headaches are of a vascular type and are probably a variant of migraine headaches. Although the clinical course is unpredictable, the headaches often respond to treatment with beta-blocking drugs (Johns, 1986).

Conditions that lead to chronic pain can also directly impair the physiological systems involved in sexual function. In women, Sjögren's syndrome, a form of rheumatoid arthritis, and scleroderma, a connective tissue disease, can reduce vaginal lubrication (Buckwalter, Wernimont, & Buckwalter, 1982; Ferguson & Figley, 1979). Scleroderma is associated with erection problems in men, probably because of lesions in the pelvic arteries (Nowlin *et al.*, 1986). Erectile dysfunction can of course be caused by neurological damage from a back injury, although careful assessment of the relative contribution of organic and psychological factors is crucial in such men (Sjögren & Fugl-Meyer, 1981). In the United States, erectile dysfunction may be an alleged result of an occupational injury when a workmen's compensation suit is filed. Even using objective tests of erectile capacity, untangling the threads of causality in such cases can be difficult because of the patient's investment in proving an organic etiology.

Medications used to treat pain are a double-edged sword in regard to sexuality. Pain relief promotes sexual activity, but many drugs also can impair sexual function. Autoimmune diseases such as rheumatoid arthritis are treated with corticosteroids. These drugs not only impair physical attractiveness but may diminish erectile function (Richards, 1980). Opiate pain medications reduce sexual desire, as reviewed in Chapter 3. Patients with chronic pain also frequently take tricyclic antidepressants and benzodiazepines or muscle relaxants, which can impair neurological regulation of sexual desire, arousal, and orgasm.

Assessment Issues

Because chronic pain is a pervasive problem, sexual dysfunction should not be assessed in isolation. If the patient and spouse have already been evaluated by a clinician who specializes in treating chronic pain, the assessment can focus more narrowly on the impact of the illness on sexuality and intimacy. Otherwise, a full assessment of the antecedents of the pain (when, where, and with whom it occurs), pain behaviors, and their consequences for the patient should be completed (Steger & Fordyce, 1982). Thoughts and feelings associated with the pain are also important. Turk *et al.* (1983) provide a practical review of assessment strategies for pain patients. Their questionnaires for patients and significant others are also useful (Table 10-1).

Specific sexual interview questions should address whether pain has led to sexual dysfunction or reduced the frequency of sexual activity. How have the partners coped with pain during sex? Have they tried changing coital positions, varying medication schedules, or communicating their reactions to each other? Has depression or resentment over role shifts impaired marital intimacy?

    Medical assessment follows the outline given in Chapter 6, but a careful evaluation of the patient's use of alcohol, opiate pain medications, and of the many other medications often prescribed for pain patients is especially important. For women with arthritis, the adequacy of vaginal lubrication should be assessed. For men with erectile dysfunction subsequent to a back injury, a thorough neurological and sleep laboratory evaluation can be helpful in making treatment decisions.

Treatment Issues

Table 10-2 outlines special treatment techniques relevant to patients with chronic pain and sexual problems. Sexual counseling should be provided within the context of a broader, medical and cognitive-behavioral program to treat the pain itself (Steger & Fordyce, 1982; Turk *et al.*, 1983). Many of the brief sexual counseling techniques focus on minimizing pain by planning sexual activity at times of day that are optimal, using methods of pain control such as moist heat or analgesic medication before lovemaking, and finding comfortable positions. Cognitive techniques include focusing on genital pleasure or on an arousing erotic image to distract from pain. Hip replacement surgery for men and women with severe arthritis often reduces arthritic pain during sexual activity (Buckwalter *et al.*, 1982), but patients need information on the coital positions that minimize the risk of a hip dislocation and reassurance about the ability of the hip replacement joint to withstand the movements of intercourse.

Brief Sexual Counseling Case

Lee, a 39-year-old oil field worker, and his wife, 37-year-old Tammy, were referred for sexual counseling by the pain clinic where Lee had just completed treatment. A year previously, he had ruptured several discs in his back when he slipped on some logs in his wood pile. He had been in severe pain since that time, and the family had been living on his disability insurance plus his wife's pay as a secretary for the local school. The couple had been married for 18 years. Their older son had recently married, but they also had a younger boy, age 11.

    Lee's medical history included a splenectomy and compound fracture of one arm from an auto accident. All of his adult life he had smoked two packs of cigarettes a day and averaged a six-pack of beer daily as well. Lee and Tammy both denied that Lee's alcohol intake was a problem at work or at home. He had never been arrested for drunk driving and was not the driver of the car in which he had been injured. He denied blackouts, and his liver enzymes were within the normal range.

    The report from the psychologist at the pain clinic was confirmed by the sex therapist's interview. Lee and Tammy had a stable marriage but without a great deal of intimacy. They enjoyed fishing and camping together, but rarely discussed feelings. Although Tammy was supportive of her husband, she became irritated when he forgot to run errands or acted sullen and withdrawn. He disliked her nagging. Both partners had quick tempers, but arguments blew over rapidly as well. There was no history of spouse abuse.

Since his accident, Lee had told Tammy many times that he felt like "half a man." After he became disabled, the couple attempted to resume sex, but Lee could not maintain his erection when he tried to penetrate for intercourse. On these occasions, Lee would become very upset, but refused to discuss the sexual problem with Tammy. Initiation of lovemaking had always been Lee's role, and he was no longer willing to try. The couple had not substituted noncoital stimulation for intercourse. Tammy had offered to bring Lee to orgasm by oral stimulation. Even though Lee usually enjoyed this activity he refused because he felt Tammy was offering out of pity. Lee occasionally told his wife that she should leave him and find a man who could satisfy her sexual needs.

Lee had some minor sleep disturbance related to his back pain but had not been diagnosed as clinically depressed by the pain clinic. He admitted to occasional thoughts about suicide but had no suicidal plan and said that he intended to be around to watch his younger son grow up. Lee was close to both sons, and they had often accompanied him on hunting trips until his injury interfered.

The pain clinic had treated Lee with a combination of behavior therapy, physical therapy, and use of a transcutaneous nerve stimulator. Lee had returned to work in a supervisory job that involved less physical labor than he usually performed. He was also able to go fishing for the first time in a year. He no longer needed to take Percodan (oxycodone hydrochloride and terephthalate, aspirin) and instead used aspirin as needed. Lee had agreed to take responsibility for certain household chores, and, in return, Tammy had stopped reminding him of all he left undone. Going back to work had significantly increased Lee's self-esteem, although he complained that he missed the physical effort of his former job and made fun of his new role as boss.

One of the most important aspects of sexual counseling was improving Lee and Tammy's communication. Tammy was better able to ask for what she wanted, both in lovemaking and in other situations. When Lee felt anxious or needy he reacted with silence or an outburst of anger. Lee's sense of helplessness during his period of disability was discussed. Communicating his desires for touch to Tammy was reframed from being a sign of weakness ("A real man shouldn't have to say anything during sex") to taking control ("A real man is not afraid to ask for what he wants and also finds out what his wife would like best").

The couple was also given sensate focus exercises. One early assignment was for each partner to give the other a back massage, but the giver was instructed to caress the receiver by following the receiver's directions as closely as possible. If the receiver failed to give an instruction, the giver would stay still. The structured exercise helped Tammy and Lee be more verbally assertive during sex.

Lee believed that his back injury had damaged his erectile capacity, but he still had full and lasting waking erections. Partly to reassure him, his penile blood pressures were assessed and found to be normal. He also took home snap-gauges to monitor his erections during sleep and broke all three snaps on 2 consecutive nights. After three sessions of sensate focus exercises, Lee could maintain an erection until he ejaculated with Tammy's oral and manual stimulation. Soon after, the couple had successful intercourse. They found that having Lee lie on his back with a pillow supporting his lower spine was the most comfortable position. Both enjoyed Tammy's taking a more active role in thrusting during intercourse. Not only sexual frequency and satisfaction, but overall marital happiness returned almost to preinjury levels, and sexual counseling was considered complete.

11

Stigmatizing Conditions and Sexuality: Major Psychiatric Disorders, Alcoholism, and Infertility

This chapter focuses on three conditions that are not always regarded as illnesses. Psychiatric disorders and alcoholism are problems that have historically been blamed on the patient's lack of willpower. In recent years, however, the contribution of genetic factors has become clearer and schizophrenia, major affective disorders, and alcoholism have come to be viewed as medical rather than moral problems. Infertility, too, was often regarded as a shameful secret until modern technology uncovered a number of previously unsuspected physical abnormalities that prevent conception. Although the conditions discussed in this chapter vary widely in causing physical debilitation, all are commonly accompanied by sexual dysfunction.

MAJOR PSYCHIATRIC DISORDERS

This section reviews our knowledge of sexual function and behavior in men and women with schizophrenia and unipolar and bipolar major affective disorders. Despite clinical reports that divorce rates are increased for psychiatric patients (Merikangas, Prusoff, Kupfer, & Frank, 1985) and that elevated rates of psychiatric problems are observed in the spouses of those with schizophrenia or affective disorders (Merikangas, 1982), little effort has been expended on studying sexuality in this group.

One handicap is that acutely psychotic or severely depressed patients live lives of such turmoil that sexuality seems a minor issue. Patients are difficult to interview until their symptoms are in remission. By that time, their psychotropic medications have often disrupted sexual function so that the clinician cannot separate the impact of the disease from the treatment. Given that neuroleptics are a permanent necessity for many schizophrenics, and that lithium or antidepressant drugs are administered on a long-term basis to many patients with major affective disorders, it may be futile to worry about the incidence of sexual problems in unmedicated patients. Of course, better understanding of medication side effects may help us improve drug therapy, but primarily we must study sexual aspects of quality of life in men and women stabilized on medication and coping with chronic psychiatric disorders. In fact, as Nestoros, Lehmann, and Ban (1981) point out, schizophrenics' reproductive success in terms of fertility seems to have increased in recent years as medication and deinstitutionalization have promoted more normal lives for many patients.

Another handicap has been ignorance about sexuality on the part of the treatment team. Freud's original theory was that schizophrenia was caused by the withdrawal of libido from all human relationships. He viewed schizophrenics as unable to experience pleasure. Krafft-Ebing, in contrast, theorized that insanity was the result of sexual excesses (Nestoros *et al.*, 1981). Thus although sexuality was an important construct in early psychiatric theories, few psychiatrists asked patients about their sexual feelings or function.

In 1972, Pinderhughes, Grace, and Reyna surveyed 18 psychiatrists in a Boston Veterans Administration hospital. Not only did physicians believe that the great majority of psychiatric disorders could be caused by sexual anxiety, but two thirds agreed that sexual activity could slow recovery from an acute episode of psychiatric illness. In the same hospital, however, only 40% of patients surveyed recalled discussing sexual issues with their psychiatrists.

In fact, staff have been more concerned with limiting patients' sexual behavior than with treating sexual dysfunctions. On one inpatient unit, a mere 34 incidents of sexual "acting out" occurring across 1086 admissions were grist for a paper suggesting that psychiatric patients should be saved from their own inappropriate sexual desires. Limits were believed particularly important for patients with character disorders who formed intense relationships too quickly and women on psychotropic medications, since it was "well known" that such drugs increased libido. The authors concluded that many instances of sexual activity betweeen psychiatric inpatients were mere substitutes for the patients' real wishes: to have sex with their therapists (Akhtar, Crocker, Dickey, Helfrich, & Rheuban, 1977).

What do we know about sexual function in psychiatric patients? In schizophrenics, it is striking that more information is available about women than about men. In contrast to patients with other chronic illnesses, physicians do not see schizophrenics as a potential group for medical and surgical treatment of erectile dysfunction. Thus the usual case series with NPT and Doppler studies are missing. Verhulst and Schneidman (1981) concluded that schizophrenic men do not appear to have an unusual rate of sexual dysfunction, but are handicapped by poor social skills in forming relationships. Nestoros *et al.* (1981) compared 50 medicated, male schizophrenics who had been hospitalized on a chronic basis with 36 normal control men. They were asked retrospectively about sexual development and about current function. About a third of schizophrenic men reported a history of low sexual desire and infrequent erections in adolescence. More of them than the controls had restricted their sexual experience to masturbation during that era. Their current sexual function diverged even more strongly from that of the controls. A full 34% of schizophrenics reported no sexual activity or feelings in the past year. During this time period, 42% had erections only rarely, 10% experienced delayed ejaculation, and 32% said they could not reach orgasm at all. Only 2% had had sex with a partner in the past year.

Although type and dose of neuroleptic medication had no clear correlation with sexual function, many of these problems may have been the result of medication side effects. In a study by Blair and Simpson (1966), 35 schizophrenic men were asked to masturbate to orgasm using a vibrator. When the men were not medicated, they reached orgasm on 98% of trials. On neuroleptics, however, they ejaculated on 0% to 36% of trials. Orgasmic capacity returned to normal when the medications were withdrawn. Unfortunately, the researchers did not specify clearly whether the medication delayed orgasm, prevented orgasm, or caused dry ejaculation (Chapter 5). Few data on medication effects exist, and the specification of sexual function is so primitive that it is hard to interpret the results.

Two studies have compared schizophrenic women to normal controls with findings that agree in many respects, although one researcher surveyed 51 young inpatients in Czechoslovakia (Raboch, 1984) and the other group interviewed 20 urban patients in the United States (Friedman & Harrison, 1984). Schizophrenic women are more likely than normal controls to have low sexual desire and difficulty becoming aroused or reaching orgasm. These sexual dysfunctions show no clear relationship to dosage of neuroleptics (Raboch, 1986). Schizophrenic women in close relationships are more likely to have normal sexual function, a pattern that is probably also true for men (Nestoros et al., 1981).

Raboch (1984), however, found that schizophrenic women were delayed in their development of adolescent sexual feelings and behavior. In contrast, Friedman and Harrison (1984), observed schizophrenic women to be early in menstruating and in "learning about sex," with a 60% incidence of childhood sexual abuse and 50% incidence of being raped as an adult, rates far in excess of those for matched healthy controls. The social skills deficits of schizophrenia may well interfere with normal courtship and make a woman vulnerable to sexual exploitation.

Affective disorders also have an impact on sexuality. Clinically, a loss of sexual desire is common during a major depressive episode and hypersexuality is often part of acute manic behavior (Kolodny, Masters, & Johnson, 1979). Mathew and Weinman (1982) compared 35 women and 16 men referred to a psychiatric clinic for depression to healthy controls matched in age and gender. The depressed group were more likely to experience low sexual desire (31% vs. 6% of controls) and also excessive desire (22% vs.

0%). Other aspects of sexual function did not differ significantly from normal levels. Merikangas *et al.* (1985) found that 45 patients with recurrent unipolar depression reported more marital conflict and sexual dissatisfaction than controls. Types of sexual problems were not specified. Crowther (1985) also observed that severity of depression and marital conflict were directly correlated within a sample of psychiatric inpatients. For unipolar disorders, then, the major impact is on the desire phase. Marital relationships are often disrupted, or perhaps have been conflicted from the start because patients with depression choose equally maladjusted spouses (Merikangas, 1982).

Erection problems for men and difficulty reaching orgasm for men and women are fairly common side effects of antidepressant medication (Chapter 5). However, even in depressed men who are drug-free, erections during sexual activity and nocturnal penile tumescence may simultaneously decrease, returning to normal when the depression lifts (Roose, Glassman, Walsh, & Cullen, 1982; Thase *et al.*, 1986).

Sexuality has rarely been assessed in patients with bipolar disorders. The only reports of low sexual desire or erectile dysfunction in manic-depressive men have been related to lithium. Blay, Ferraz, and Calil (1982) described two cases of sexual dysfunction that only occurred during lithium therapy, and Raboch, Smolik, and Soucek (1983) found that 4 out of 25 men on lithium had decreased desire and erections. In a French study, half of men surveyed noted less sexual desire on lithium, but no problems with erection or orgasm (Lorimy, Loo, & Deniker, 1977).

Raboch (1986) did assess sexuality in 50 hospitalized manic-depressive women. When mania was no longer acute, the women did not differ in sexual function or behavior from healthy age-matched controls.

Psychosocial Impact on Sexuality

It is impossible to discuss the impact of major psychiatric disorders on sexuality without considering their impact on close relationships. One important factor is whether a man or woman developed normal friendships and dating relationships in adolescence before the onset of the disorder. The patients who are most impaired sexually are the ones who lacked the skills to engage in close relationships from the start, often reflecting a combination of genetic vulnerability and a disturbed family of origin that could not model appropriate social and intimate behavior. Living a life of repeated institutionalization also restricts economic and social opportunities, and can foster the type of disastrous pairings of two disordered people that has been observed by Merikangas (1982).

Even if a man or woman has formed a relationship, thought disorder, social withdrawal, and bizarre behavior during an acute psychiatric episode can frighten and alienate a spouse or dating partner. The mate may lose desire for the patient, seeing him or her as suddenly unfamiliar. Fears that a psychosis will become chronic or will be transmitted to children can break up a new relationship.

When patients are on medication, issues of body image and physical attractiveness are salient. Many antidepressants promote weight gain. Tardive dyskinesia and other visible side effects of neuroleptics are also common. Some chronic psychiatric patients are unkempt or adopt unusual styles of dress.

During institutionalization, patients have a right to sexual freedom, but must also be protected from sexual exploitation (Wasow, 1980). Thorny ethical issues are raised, for example, in helping a psychotic woman choose a method of contraception. If she is sexually active but does not have good reality testing, should she be treated with injectable or implantable hormones to prevent pregnancy? If two inpatients are having sex in a private corner, do staff have the right to interfere? Should hospitals provide private areas so that patients can masturbate or engage in partner activity? The answers often depend on the individual's capacity to take responsibility for decisions. All too often, staff err on the side of unnecessary moralizing, at the same time ignoring sexual exploitation of patients by attendants or even by family members.

Physiological Impact on Sexuality

We know little or nothing about physiological impairment of sexual function in unmedicated psychiatric patients. Despite speculation that increased brain dopamine in schizophrenia would cause hypersexuality, few schizophrenic men or women have such symptoms (Raboch, 1984). The cause of the increased levels of desire and sexual behavior that accompany manic episodes is not understood.

Depression disrupts sexual desire and diminishes NPT, but the complex effects of depressive episodes on diurnal hormone cycling and on brain neurotransmitters are still being unraveled. Simultaneous recording of NPT and hormonal levels in depressed men might yield interesting data (Schiavi et al., 1984).

Even the mechanisms by which psychotropic drugs impair sexual function remain mysterious (Chapter 5). It is almost impossible to separate the effects of the underlying psychiatric disorder from medication effects, particularly since healthy men and women rarely take psychotropic drugs on a chronic basis. After medication, the researcher is confronted both with physiological impairment of desire, arousal, and orgasm, and with improvement in mood and social skills that could facilitate sexual functioning. In most of these chapters we call for further research. Here it may be more accurate to call for the most basic studies of the causes and incidence of sexual problems.

Assessment Issues

As suggested in Table 11-1, the interview with a psychiatric patient should focus on his or her skills for communicating and responding appropriately in a close relationship, historically and currently. Because this group of patients often experiences family turmoil and includes vulnerable individuals, getting a history of sexual trauma is important. The clinician needs to understand how acute psychiatric symptoms and psychotropic medications affect the patient's sexual functioning.

Just because a man or woman has a major psychiatric disorder, the clinician must not overlook other medical illnesses relevant to sexual functioning. We know so little about the physiological impact of psychiatric disorders on sexual function that we can merely offer the guidelines from Chapter 6 as an organizing principal for medical assessment.

Treatment Issues

Brief sexual counseling or intensive sex therapy can be helpful to psychiatric patients, but the therapist must proceed carefully. Making changes in a close relationship can be stressful and some sex therapy homework assignments are potentially overwhelming to a patient newly in remission. We advocate beginning any intensive therapy only when a man or woman is stabilized and an optimal dose of medication has been prescribed, if necessary. Even sensate focus exercises can be broken into smaller steps, for example, starting with a hand, foot, or face massage. Instructions should be as simple and structured as possible. Medical interventions, such as the implantation of a penile prosthesis, should be performed with great caution and with concurrent psychological support from a mental health professional.

Including the partner is important when a close relationship exists. Partners need a clear understanding of the patient's psychiatric condition and its effect on the ability to be sensitive to social cues. Partners often have their own problems that contribute to marital conflict or poor communication. Substance abuse is common in the families of psychiatric patients. Many couples spend their lives in almost continual crisis, but could benefit from simple, structured training in solving problems and negotiating disagreements.

Single patients often need advice on grooming, how to approach a potential dating partner, and how to respond appropriately to casual conversation. In the sexual realm, some lack basic knowledge of anatomy, function, and contraception, let alone skills in lovemaking. This is particularly apt when psychiatric disorder began in adolescence.

Although patients with psychiatric disorders are a challenge to the sexuality specialist, their needs for counseling should not be overlooked.

Brief Counseling Cases

Because the problems of the institutionalized chronic psychiatric patient are often so different from those of the man or woman who is well enough to live in the community, we present two rather different brief counseling cases.

Jens, age 29, had been hospitalized in a large, county psychiatric unit in Scandinavia since age 15. His diagnosis was paranoid schizophrenia, and he was taking both perphenazine, a neuroleptic, and cyproterone acetate, an anti-androgen that is not approved for use in the United States (Cooper, 1986). A young psychiatric resident became interested in Jens's case, and asked if the use of cyproterone acetate could be reevaluated.

The resident reviewed the case with his supervisor. When Jens was 17, he was described as having sexually attacked the nurses. Episodes that were actually documented in the chart seemed to be clumsy attempts to hug or kiss a nurse. He also occasionally would explode with anger unexpectedly, for example when he was sitting in a corner with some busy work. It was obvious from the chart that the staff had debated about prescribing hormonal treatment. Jens had no close family and was not considered capable even of living in a halfway house. He was a tall man, weighing around 250 pounds, and although he was usually shy and gentle, was intimidating just in terms of his physical size. Over the years, occasionally a psychiatrist proposed discontinuing the cyproterone acetate, but each time the nursing staff would become incensed, often reporting semen spots on Jens's sheets and observing that he seemed to be masturbating alone in his room.

The resident had been working with Jens, and asked his supervisor to sit in on a session. He asked Jens about women. Jens said that he really liked them, "But they are always so scared of me! I just want to talk and they run away, or sometimes even yell at me." Jens had never had a sexual experience with a woman, but did like to look at men's magazines. He denied ever masturbating, and was ashamed that he sometimes had "wet dreams." "I wish I had a girlfriend to be nice to," he said.

Laboratory blood chemistries were normal with the exception of a reduced serum testosterone, as would be expected on his medication regimen. Although Jens had some mild gynecomastia, it was difficult to distinguish between the effects of hormonal therapy and his obesity. The supervisor agreed to put Jens on a placebo instead of cyproterone acetate, continuing his neuroleptic. He was also scheduled to move to a kind of halfway house that was on the hospital grounds. When he had been in his new quarters for 2 days, an incident occurred in which he was alone in an office with an unfamiliar nurse who knew his history and reputation. She suddenly felt threatened just by his proximity and called for help. Although everyone agreed that Jens had behaved appropriately, the cyproterone acetate was resumed.

Table 11-1. Special Assessment Issues

Interview Topics	Psychiatric Disorders	Alcoholism	Infertility
	History of dating and sexual relationships	History of close relationships, with special attention to couple communication, deviant sexual behavior, or family violence	Current life stress
	History of sexual trauma (e.g., incest, molestation, rape, exploitive caretakers)	History of drinking and other substance abuse	Reactions to infertility
	Fears of a link between sexuality and psychiatric disorder	Stressors that promote drinking	Each partner's wish for children
	Impact of acute episodes of disorder on close relationships and sexual function	Reaction of the family to patient's drinking	Effects of infertility and its treatment on sexual frequency, variety, and emotional tone
	Current living situation and opportunities for sexual intimacy	Substance abuse or emotional problems in the partner	Emotional ups and downs with menstrual cycle
	Sexual side effects of medication	Reason for seeking help with the sexual problem at this point	Sexual problems that could contribute to infertility (erectile dysfunction, male difficulty reaching orgasm, vaginismus, infrequent intercourse, etc.)
		Sexual function when intoxicated versus abstinent	
		Beliefs about effect of alcohol on sexual pleasure and function	

Questionnaires	No special questionnaire is relevant	Michigan Alcoholism Screening Test (Selzer, Vinokur, & Van Rooijen, 1975) Neuropsychological testing	The Infertility Questionnaire (Bernstein et al., 1985)
Medical History	Other chronic illnesses Current medications Patterns of acute psychiatric symptoms and history of hospitalizations	Other chronic illnesses Current medications Complications of alcoholism (liver disease, neuropathy, injuries in accidents)	Sexually transmitted diseases Contraception used in past Current hormonal therapy Elective abortions Substance abuse Nutrition
Physiological Assessment	Comprehensive evaluation of erectile dysfunction with repeat NPT testing after depressive episode in men with affective disorder	Comprehensive evaluation of erectile dysfunction Hormonal assays, male and female Neurological examination Liver function tests and clinical signs of cirrhosis	Pelvic examination for dyspareunia Search for varicoceles Hormonal profiles

Two months later, one of the young male nurses, Peter, approached the resident, knowing of his interest in Jens. He wanted to discuss Jens, but feared he would lose his job if he tried to talk to his nursing supervisor. Peter had been taking Jens out to jog, and over time the two had built a relationship. Jens had brought up his wish to have a girlfriend, and Peter had given him some advice on how to approach a woman and some information about sexuality. The head nurse had taken Peter aside, however, and warned him not to get too attached to Jens. Peter was afraid that his efforts at sex education would be seen as misguided if they became known. Peter had given Jens some basic facts about how babies were conceived, what intercourse was like, contraception, and the normalcy of masturbation. Jens had been fascinated and surprised by these revelations, and had finally asked Peter to teach him how to masturbate. This had thrown Peter into a small panic. "What would my girlfriend think, let alone the other nurses?" he asked the resident. "Maybe they were right and I shouldn't talk to Jens about this stuff."

The resident promised to intervene himself in the problem. He still saw Jens occasionally for therapy sessions, and in the next one, brought up the topic of sexuality. Jens repeated, with some frustration, his wish to learn to masturbate. "If it's normal, why won't anyone tell me how?" he asked. The resident arranged a consultation with the sexual dysfunction clinic at a neighboring university. He accompanied Jens to watch a film on masturbation, and discussed it with Jens afterwards. The resident also enlisted a female social worker to do some role playing with Jens on how to approach women in an acceptable way.

After several sessions, Jens told the resident that he now could masturbate to orgasm, and felt more like a "real man." He was still on both medications, but the nurses agreed not to disturb Jens's privacy when he wanted to masturbate. His new social skills helped them to feel more comfortable. He began to attend dances held for the hospital patients, and developed a romantic relationship with a young woman who was developmentally disabled. Two years later, Jens was living happily in the halfway house unit. He had not frightened the nurses for many months, and they ignored the small collection of erotic magazines that he kept in his trunk. He continued on the cyproterone acetate, but it was clearly prescribed more to allay the staff's anxiety than to control any deviant behavior on Jens's part.

Vic was an example of a less severe psychiatric picture. He was a 42-year-old postal clerk, retired on disability for 9 years because of chronic paranoid schizophrenia. After his initial hospitalization, he was maintained on Thorazine and Cogentin. With the support of his wife, Lynn, he was able to live at home without hospitalization except for one brief stay the year before the couple presented themselves for evaluation of a sexual problem. During that time his medication dose was adjusted, with Loxitane added to his regimen.

Vic and Lynn wanted help for an erection problem. Lynn had grown up in foster homes, but had no psychiatric history herself. The couple had a stable marriage, with few conflicts. They spent their days together, doing chores or watching television. Twelve years before, Lynn had given birth to their daughter. She had severe perineal lacerations during the birth, and when the couple tried to resume intercourse, Vic complained that his wife's vagina was too large. Lynn agreed that she no longer felt any friction during intercourse, and neither partner could reach orgasm.

The couple adjusted to the sexual problem by bringing each other to orgasm daily, using manual and oral caressing. Vic continued to have normal erections. Perhaps three or four times a year they would try intercourse, but always remained disappointed. Vic could also masturbate to orgasm with a firm erection, although at one point when his dose of Thorazine was at its peak, he had dry orgasms.

Finally Lynn found a gynecologist who said he could repair her vagina by a perineoplasty, making the vaginal entrance smaller. Lynn felt the surgery would be worthwhile if the couple could enjoy intercourse again. After she was healed, the couple eagerly tried intercourse. Both felt more sensation on penetration, but Vic suddenly lost his erection. Each time the couple tried intercourse, Vic's penis would become flaccid. Soon he also began to have intermittent difficulties in achieving and maintaining erections with other types of sexual stimulation.

The therapist, a social worker who had been providing supportive psychotherapy to Vic, noted that fear of getting Lynn pregnant was not a factor, since Vic had had a vasectomy. Both parents were proud of their daughter, who was pretty and a good student. One possible psychological stress, however, was that Lynn had never gotten along with Vic's mother, who lived just down the block. A couple of months before Lynn's operation, her elderly mother-in-law had died suddenly of a stroke. Although the bereavement removed a source of family conflict, Vic resented his wife's lack of mourning.

Vic and Lynn had a session of sex education, including an explanation of the sexual response cycle and a discussion about vaginal size and expansion with arousal. Although the therapist suspected that Lynn's perineoplasty had not been necessary, he simply encouraged the couple to think of her vagina as normal in size now. He gave them instructions for a sensate focus exercise, including genital touch but not orgasms. During the first week, Vic had normal erections with manual caressing of his penis. He explored his wife's vagina with his finger, noticing how it lubricated and deepened as she became more aroused. The second week the couple tried penetration with Lynn on top and without any thrusting. Vic was able to maintain his erection for a minute or 2 and indeed wanted to have intercourse, but Lynn reminded him of the guidelines and instead, used noncoital stimulation to help her husband reach orgasm. By the third week, both partners were enjoying intercourse, and were coitally orgasmic.

One of the counseling sessions included a discussion of the impact of Vic's mother's death on the household. Vic became tearful for a moment, remembering times as a child when his mother had been loving to him. He was also able to say, however, that his mother's interference in his marriage had made him very angry, and that he could see why Lynn was relieved by her death. Lynn herself recalled some pleasant memories of her mother-in-law, and acknowledged her husband's right to mourn. The therapist did not attempt to interpret the relationship between the bereavement and the upheavals in Vic and Lynn's sexual relationship to the couple. Symptomatic relief was a sufficient goal for the treatment.

ALCOHOLISM

Alcoholism is the most common type of chemical dependency in the United States or Western Europe, accounting for a tragic degree of waste, in terms of early deaths, medical expenses, and lost productivity. A Gallup poll in 1982 reported that a third of American families included a member who was a problem drinker (Peele, 1984). Criteria for defining problem drinking or addiction to alcohol remain somewhat controversial (Zucker & Gomberg, 1986). Most systems include some of the following: daily use of alcohol, morning drinking, at least occasional large or "critical" doses (i.e., a fifth of hard liquor), blackouts, development of tolerance to alcohol, withdrawal symptoms with abstinence, and impaired social or cognitive function (American Psychiatric Association, 1980; Royal College of Psychiatrists, 1979).

In the United States, most clinicians view alcoholism as a disease, that is, a loss of control over drinking that occurs in genetically vulnerable individuals. Cross-cultural and longitudinal studies, however, suggest that a biopsychosocial model of alcoholism is more useful, since social learning and early childhood environment clearly have a role in determining drinking behavior (Peele, 1984; Zucker & Goldberg, 1986).

Alcohol has long enjoyed a reputation as an aphrodisiac, and in many cultures is an integral part of celebrations and rites of passage. In a survey of readers of *Psychology Today*, 45% of men and 68% of women said that alcohol enhanced sexual pleasure (Psychology Today, 1970). A group of 69 college women concurred, despite reporting no advantage of alcohol use when logging daily sexual experiences (Harvey & Beckman, 1986). In a group of Danish alcoholic men, 45% also believed that drinking increased sexual enjoyment (Jensen, 1979a).

Yet, a group of healthy young men said that too much alcohol consumption sometimes caused sexual problems, including erectile dysfunction and disturbances of ejaculation (Jensen et al., 1980). This negative side of intoxication is also well known in Western societies.

Sexual dysfunction has been studied more thoroughly in male alcoholics than in women, but a few researchers have tried to document the incidence of problems in both genders. Lemere and Smith (1973) surveyed 17,000 alcoholics and reported an 8% rate of erection problems, dropping to 4% in men who had been sober for several years. Clinical observations suggest a far higher rate of low sexual desire and erectile dysfunction, confirmed in samples of men currently in treatment at inpatient or outpatient clinics. Jensen (1979a) found that in a group of 100 alcoholic men aged 30 to 45, 63% had at least one sexual dysfunction. Erection problems were present in 24%, low desire in 57%, and delayed orgasm in 25%. All men were taking disulfiram (Antabuse). Similar rates of dysfunction were observed by Fahrner (1987), in 116 alcoholic inpatients of comparable age. At least one sexual problem was reported by 75%, with erectile dysfunction in 42%, low desire in 46% and delayed orgasm in 23%. In that series, premature ejaculation was also a problem for 43% of the men.

A common belief is that alcoholic women are sexually promiscuous, but in fact, no evidence exists for such a supposition (Abel, 1985). A pilot study comparing 13 alcoholic women, 18 wives of alcoholic men, and 28 normal controls found that both former groups had reduced levels of sexual satisfaction (Peterson, Hartsock, & Lawson, 1984). A much more careful and detailed comparison of 30 young, married alcoholic women with age-matched healthy controls found no differences in rates of sexual dysfunction (Jensen, 1984b). Twenty percent of the alcoholic women and 23% of controls had at least one sexual problem, usually reduced sexual desire. Of course, it is possible that selecting a married sample underestimates the incidence of sexual dysfunction in alcoholic women as a group.

Psychosocial Impact on Sexuality

At least in the United States, alcohol is seen as a disinhibitor of sexual arousal. Adolescents learn that intoxication leads to promiscuity, and so in time, they use alcohol as an "excuse" to engage in sex outside of moral restrictions (Critchlow, 1986; Lang, 1985). A person with high levels of guilt about sexuality or shaky self-esteem may risk sexual failure, knowing that it can be blamed in retrospect on intoxication. Our attitudes about alcohol and sexuality have been tested in the laboratory, where experiments show that young men or women who believed they just drank alcohol became more subjectively aroused by erotic stimuli, regardless of whether they actually received alcohol or a cleverly disguised "placebo cocktail" (Lang, 1985). Effects of alcohol on men's sexual arousal in the laboratory suggest that interference with erections occurs when drinking is combined with cognitive distractors (Wilson, Niaura, & Adler, 1985). Thus intoxication combined with sexual anxiety may be a recipe for dysfunction.

With chronic alcohol abuse, other psychosocial factors come into play. The alcoholic may lose the capacity to work, to participate in family decisions, and to respond empathetically to a partner. The alcoholic feels powerless to stop drinking and the spouse is helpless to intervene. Either the relationship breaks up or the partners stay locked in a cycle of turmoil and pain. Male alcoholics in particular are often unmarried (Jensen, 1979b). Even when alcoholics have close relationships, the ability to communicate feelings and enjoy intimacy are often impaired. Evidence is mounting that marital violence is linked to alcohol abuse in husbands, but not in wives (Van Hasselt, Morrison, & Bellack, 1985). Incest has also been linked with alcoholism (Renshaw, 1982).

In a longitudinal study of marital stability in 31 middle-class alcoholics who were followed for 2 years after treatment, home observation was used at the time of initial assessment to classify patterns of family interaction (Steinglass, Tislenko, & Reiss, 1985). One finding was that marriages were more likely to remain intact if the alcoholic spouse became consistently sober or alternated between drinking and sobriety. The most divorces occurred in couples where one spouse was stable in continuing to drink. The researchers speculate that some families adjust to the turmoil of an alcoholic who cannot stay abstinent, but the slow, progressive decline of the consistent drinker is unbearable. Couples who broke up also were more psychologically distressed at initial assessment. The alcoholic partner was more likely to have health complications from drinking. Another strong predictor of divorce was that the alcoholic was disengaged from the family, with few daily periods of contact.

In the sexual realm, alcoholics generally lose desire for sex during periods of intoxication. If the clinician compares reports of the patient and partner, the partner often identifies a sexual dysfunction that the patient does not report, for example erectile dysfunction or a woman's not reaching orgasm. Partners also complain that they have become turned off, not only because of the alcoholic's lack of caring or poor sexual performance, but because they are haunted by ugly images of the drunken spouse, passed out or nauseated (Burton & Kaplan, 1968). This is a special example of the way that being a caretaker spouse reduces sexual desire.

The effects of alcohol abuse on relationships do not disappear with sobriety. It can take months or years of effort to rebuild trust. Sometimes when the alcoholic spouse improves, the partner leaves the relationship because the marital system depended on playing the roles of victim and rescuer.

Physiological Impact on Sexuality

Again, we must separate the effects of acute intoxication and chronic alcohol abuse on the sexual response. Laboratory studies demonstrate that alcohol produces a dose-related decrease in penile tumescence and vaginal pulse amplitude in response to erotic stimuli (Abel, 1985; Malatesta, Pollack, Crotty, & Peacock, 1982; Wilson *et al.*, 1985). For both men and women, there is also a dose-related increase in latency to orgasm by masturbation. At high blood levels of alcohol (100 mg%), men may not be able to reach orgasm at all (Malatesta, Pollack, Wilbanks, & Adams, 1979; Malatesta *et al.*, 1982).

As usual, no data is available on chronic alcoholism and women's physiological sexual functioning. In alcoholic men, Jensen has found an age effect in several studies such that sexual dysfunction is more common in men over 40 (Jensen 1979a; Jensen 1984b). Recently Bansal, Wincze, Nirenberg, Liepman, and Engle-Friedman (1986) replicated this finding. They studied alcoholics longitudinally during and after treatment to see whether sexual dysfunction involved organic factors and could be reversed with abstinence from alcohol. They included assessment of NPT and visual sexual stimulation in the laboratory. They believe two distinct groups of alcoholics exist; the younger men who experience loss of desire and erectile dysfunction while drinking but revert to normal function when sober, and men over age 40 who often evidence liver damage and have organic impairment of erection. Both Jensen and Bansal and colleagues observed that duration of alcohol abuse was not predictive of sexual dysfunction but age was important.

One probable culprit in causing sexual dysfunction in alcoholic men is abnormal hormone levels. Chronic alcohol abuse directly damages the Leydig cells of the testes and may also interfere at the hypothalamic level with the feedback loop controlling production of testosterone. In addition, damage to liver function leads to increased clearance of testosterone from the blood and decreased clearance of estrogen (Abel, 1985; Van Thiel & Gavaler, 1986). One would expect that men with cirrhotic liver disease would be the most impaired in terms of hormone levels and sexual dysfunction. Jensen and Gluud (1985), however, compared 18 cirrhotic alcoholics with an age-matched sample of healthier alcoholics. Samples were small because entrance criteria included having a sexual partner and being free of chronic illnesses other than cirrhosis. Although the cirrhotic group had abnormally low levels of free serum testosterone, their sexual function was no worse than that of other alcoholic men. Within the cirrhotic group, testosterone levels were no different for sexually functional versus dysfunctional men. Fahrner (1983) reported normal levels of testosterone in all 116 alcoholic men assessed before and after participating in an inpatient treatment program. Research on hormone–behavior relationships is needed using large and carefully defined groups of subjects.

Autonomic neuropathy has also been suggested as a factor in alcoholics' erectile dysfunction. As Jensen (1981b) points out, no data exist to substantiate this hypothesis. In fact, in a series of men who had been alcoholic for at least 5 years, neuropathy of any sort was a rare finding

(Lindenberg *et al.*, 1981). In the study of cirrhotic alcoholics, 7 out of 11 men with sexual dysfunction had clinical signs of dementia, however, (Jensen & Gluud, 1985). Damage from alcohol abuse to the central nervous system may be a more crucial factor than peripheral neuropathy in promoting sexual problems. Even in alcoholic men under age 35, CT scanning has revealed a high incidence of cortical atrophy (Lee, Hardt, Møller, Haubek, & Jensen, 1979). Not only does dementia impair social skills, but it may be relevant to sexuality that an early symptom is reduced fingertip sensitivity.

In Denmark, where disulfiram (Antabuse) is a standard part of treatment for alcoholism, Jensen (1979b; 1984b) found that half of the men claimed their sexual problem had begun on the day that disulfiram was prescribed, although women did not report sexual side effects from the medication. Reported frequency of sexual activity did not change for the alcoholic men from 1 month prior to beginning alcoholism treatment to 1 month posttreatment, however. Double-blind studies of disulfiram and sexual function have found a higher rate of problems in men on placebo than in men taking the medication (Kristensen, 1973; Krinstensen, Rønsted, & Vaag, 1984). Thus disulfiram seems to provide a convenient alibi for sexual problems but is doubtful as an etiological factor.

Assessment Issues

An interview can be helpful in assessing the impact of alcoholism on the patient's ability to sustain intimate relationships (Table 11-1). Because families with an alcoholic member may be at risk for family violence or sexual abuse, these topics should be addressed, once an atmosphere of trust has been established. Of course, assessment of sexual function should include the patient's beliefs about alcohol and sex, as well as his or her beliefs about ability to function when intoxicated versus abstinent. The partner's input is especially important, given the potential for distorted memories and disturbed family systems. Remember to assess the couple's strengths for coping, rather than focusing only on family turmoil.

No questionnaires have been designed to asssess sexuality in alcoholics, but the Michigan Alcoholism Screening Test (MAST) may be helpful in determining the severity of the patient's drinking. The spouse can also fill out the MAST to report on the patient's drinking (Van Hasselt *et al.*, 1985). If a patient shows signs of dementia, neuropsychological testing can be valuable.

Many alcoholics are heavy smokers, have poor nutrition and other health habits, and take psychotropic medications. The effects of general health as well as those of complications of alcoholism on sexual function should be assessed. A neurological exam and assays for prolactin, testosterone, and estrogen should be part of the work-up in men. In women, the neurological exam is also valuable, and if menstrual irregularities exist, hormonal studies may be helpful (Abel, 1985).

Treatment Issues

Table 11-2 summarizes the special issues in treating alcoholics' sexual dysfunctions. Sex therapy in intensive cases must be combined with marital work to change the family system that allowed alcohol abuse to continue. Couple therapy is not a substitute for comprehensive treatment of alcoholism. Currently, therapy for chemical dependency is in a state of flux. In the United States, almost all programs have abstinence as their goal, but in Europe, controlled drinking is considered an appropriate outcome for less severe alcoholics (Peele, 1984). The advantages of intensive inpatient programs as compared to less expensive outpatient clinics are being questioned (Miller & Hester, 1986). With relapse rates of 50% to 90%, new therapeutic techniques to prevent relapse are being proposed (Brownell, Marlatt, Lichtenstein, & Wilson, 1986).

Only one pilot study has examined the smaller issue of efficacy of sex therapy for alcoholics. Fahrner (1987) gave 16 dysfunctional alcoholic men 10 sessions of individual sexual counseling. Three months later, two thirds were free of sexual problems as opposed to only a quarter of men who received one hour of nonspecific supportive counseling. Such results are encouraging, but far more work is needed.

Besides the usual issues mentioned in Table 11-2, in the United States the couple therapist often encounters recovered alcoholics active in Alcoholics Anonymous (AA). Dealing with AA members is akin to working with people of a certain ethnic or religious group. Not only do AA members share a certain language and set of concepts in discussing alcoholism, but they have a sponsor who takes the role of confidante and peer therapist. Despite the great effectiveness of AA as a program, and the helpfulness of most sponsors, a sponsor who gives different messages than the therapist can present a problem. For example, we have seen an AA member whose sponsor knew he was molesting his stepdaughter, but did nothing to intervene, and in another case, a sponsor who suggested the member just forget about sex. The therapist must decide whether it would be helpful to get the patient's permission to include the sponsor in a session or at least in a phone discussion, or whether a gentle rebuttal of the sponsor's advice might be less intrusive.

Intensive Sex Therapy Case

Tony was a 72-year-old man who went through a complete medical evaluation for erectile dysfunction. Tony had drunk 4 to 6 ounces of bourbon a day for most of his adult life, and became an even heavier drinker for several years at age 62, when his wife of 42 years died from breast cancer. Tony's children persuaded him to get help, however, and he became sober after spending 3 weeks in the hospital. He was suffering from a severe hearing loss

Table 11-2. Special Treatment Issues

	Psychiatric Disorders	Alcoholism	Infertility
Format	Sexual counseling or intensive therapy should begin only when the patient is stable without acute psychosis Homework exercises may need to be simple and very structured Pace of therapy may be slowed to minimize stress of trying new behaviors	Brief counseling can be offered as part of support groups in substance abuse clinics Marital and sex therapy do not replace alcoholism treatment Alcohol-related activities never suggested in homework (i.e., share a glass of wine before sensate focus or have an evening out at a nightclub)	Brief sexual counseling should be routine, perhaps as part of an infertility support group for couples
Brief Counseling			
Education	Safety of sexual activity for psychiatric patients, sexual side effects of medications, impact of the disorder on intimacy	Acute and chronic effects of alcohol on sexual function	How to promote conception by timing of intercourse, information on the stress of infertility treatment
Attitude Change	Reducing feelings of stigmatization, increasing self-esteem and sense of own attractiveness	Reducing feelings of stigmatization, learning not to use alcohol as crutch to overcome shyness or become sexually aroused, block out images of patient as drunk and unappealing by having spouse focus on patient's positive attributes, viewing sexual problems as having complex causes instead of seeing them as side effects of medications used in treatment	Reducing feelings of stigmatization, viewing sexual pleasure as distinct from reproduction, exploring how a child would change couple's lifestyle, considering alternatives such as adoption or childlessness

Resuming Sex	Social skills training, overcoming loss of sexual desire by gradual resumption of sex, learning skills of sexual communication and stimulation, learning to enjoy masturbation as a sexual outlet	Social skills training, learning skills of sexual communication	Planning some lovemaking for infertile periods, promoting sexual variety, playfulness, and eroticism
Marital Conflict	Helping the patient take responsibility in the family, teaching communication and problem-solving skills, defusing family crises	Helping the patient take responsibility in the family, teaching spouse not to be a victim or rescuer	Resolving issues of blame, examining any ambivalence about having a child, considering relationship goals if the couple were to remain childless
Physical Handicaps	Learning to cope with sexual side effects of medication, practicing good grooming	Learning to cope with side effects of psychotropic medication, coping with dementia or loss of erectile capacity	Learning to minimize dyspareunia, using sexual fantasy and a variety of stimulation to decrease performance anxiety when sex is "on demand"
Intensive Therapy	Resolving feelings about sexual trauma, stabilizing relationships full of conflict and turmoil	Resolving resentment generated during time of alcohol abuse, especially related to family violence or extramarital affairs	Resolving mourning for lost fertility if treatment is unsuccessful, exploring choices about alternatives

that made socializing difficult, especially since he hated wearing a hearing aid. He also had had a grand mal seizure and phenytoin (Dilantin) was prescribed. A CT scan revealed a moderate degree of cerebellar atrophy, believed to be related to his alcohol abuse. In his younger years Tony had built a successful business. Now he used his determination and energy to reintegrate himself into life despite his handicaps, managing his real estate investments and spending time each day exercising at a health club.

At age 67, Tony married a divorced woman 10 years his junior. Georgia had been a friend of Tony's first wife. She was patient with his hearing loss, and surrounded him with her congenial social circle. Tony often resisted her suggestions that they go out for dinner or travel, but once they tried an activity, he always enjoyed it. Although Georgia had never reached Tony's financial bracket, she had been a competent business manager in her own right, retiring shortly after the couple married.

Tony's erectile problems developed after the couple had enjoyed several years of a good sex life. They usually had intercourse twice a week, initiated mutually. Over several months, however, Tony's erections became less firm, and he began to lose them after a few minutes of thrusting, without ejaculating. Although he could use manual stimulation to bring Georgia to orgasm after an unsuccessful attempt at intercourse, he could not regain his erection or ejaculate. He had not masturbated since he was a young man.

Tony's medical examinations were equivocal. He had a penile/brachial systolic blood pressure ratio of 0.78, basically in the normal range, with no change after exercise. He had a normal hyperemic response to penile ischemia and normal genital reflexes. His serum testosterone and prolactin were normal too, but he only broke 2 out of 3 snaps on a penile snap-gauge on 2 consecutive nights of NPT screening. A test injection of papaverine produced an erection that was not completely rigid. Based on these results, Tony was given the option of having a penile prosthesis, but he and Georgia decided to try sex therapy first, since surgery seemed like such a drastic solution.

The therapist was a female psychologist. Her first task was to forge an alliance with Tony. He wanted help for the sexual problem but was dubious about psychologists. He also complained about the expense of the sessions. Georgia tended to speak for her husband, sometimes taking advantage of his hearing loss to complain about him to the therapist.

Georgia had a number of grievances about the marriage relationship. She had not known about Tony's history of alcoholism until after the couple married. Tony's children had collaborated with him in hiding his former drinking, thinking that Georgia would make a good wife and caretaker for their father. Although Tony made Georgia sign a prenuptial agreement relinquishing all claims to his estate, his children genuinely would not have minded if Georgia inherited some of Tony's money. They were wealthy in their own right. Georgia felt, however, that Tony treated her more like a paid companion than a wife. His complaints about small household expenses, such as buying a new toaster, hurt Georgia's feelings. She devoted all of her retirement income to the couple's budget and Tony only paid expenses exceeding her monthy pension. Nevertheless, the more his sexual prowess decreased, the more he accused his wife of marrying him for his money, and the less affection he showed her.

Again, the therapist felt challenged not to take sides. As a woman, she sympathized with Georgia's anger and felt Georgia should be more assertive about her own financial rights. As a marital therapist, however, she knew she had to make Tony feel understood. She focused her comments on Tony's high need for control and mastery, praising him for remaining so active and independent. At the same time, she asked him how it felt to have some mild memory loss, and to have to strain to hear in social situations. Tony was able to talk about his feelings of helplessness and frustration. The therapist asked Georgia to join her in imagining how sexual "impotence" must add to Tony's fears of becoming powerless. Each time that Tony complained that he was getting old, the therapist turned to Georgia and reminded her that she was the only safe object for Tony's fear and anger, and commented on the difficult job of being an understanding wife.

Over the course of several sessions, the couple discussed Tony's rigid refusals to give Georgia even a small degree of control over the family budget or social schedule. Each incident during the week was analyzed in session, and inevitably Tony and Georgia could see that his stubbornness occurred in reaction to his fear that he was becoming incompetent and losing control over his life. Gradually he began to allow Georgia small privileges, such as making purchases under fifty dollars without his approval, or using the family car to visit a friend in the hospital without asking his permission. The therapist was often surprised by Tony's willingness to ease up on his previous restrictions during the week, whereas he continued to show an almost perseverative, paranoid distrust of Georgia in session.

At the same time, the couple worked on expressing affection more openly and on performing sensate focus exercises. Tony found the touching exciting, and tried some new types of caressing, including kissing Georgia's inner thighs. The partners took turns initiating the exercises. By the second week, Tony was getting firm erections. Georgia reported that her husband also was reaching out with affection during the day. Tony practiced losing and regaining erections during the sensate focus exercises. Both partners were able to have orgasms from manual stimulation as soon as that step was permitted.

During the therapy sessions, conflict continued, however. Each spouse accused the other of marrying for convenience. Georgia feared that Tony had married her to have an unpaid housekeeper. Tony believed Georgia was only interested in his money. The therapist was able to point out that Tony loved his wife. His biggest fear was that she would leave him. The therapist

also supported Georgia's statement that she had been financially independent before marrying Tony, and in fact had never tried to obtain control of
his money or to buy luxury items. Every time that Tony did acknowledge
her worth, however, Georgia seemed determined to spoil the moment by
bringing up his drinking. She feared he would begin to drink again some
day, and lamented that Tony's first wife had never told Georgia the truth
about him, and later that Tony's children had also kept his secret. Tony
became indignant, pointing out to his wife that he had been sober for many
years. The therapist suggested that Georgia was a little frightened by Tony's
new appreciation, and was more comfortable when she could feel martyred.
Georgia discussed how her own children had taken advantage of her kind-
ness and lenience.

The sensate focus exercise was not a big success the week that Tony was
assigned to "stuff" his flaccid penis into Georgia's vagina. He found this step
frustrating and difficult. He wanted to be free to use his firm erections in
penetration. The next week he did penetrate his wife with a firm erection, and
she had to remind him to disengage as instructed rather than begin thrusting.

In the therapy session, Georgia brought up her fear that Tony visited
friends in rough neighborhoods. She felt he was too old and frail for these
excursions. Recently, a mutual friend had told her that two youths had
attacked Tony and tried to snatch his wallet.

"What did you do?" the therapist asked Tony.

"I'm not even going to talk about this. Who told you anyway?" Tony
asked his wife.

"What did your friend say Tony did?" the therapist asked Georgia.

"He punched and kicked the boys and they ran away," Georgia answered.

"Really!" the therapist exclaimed. Tony stayed silent but looked proud.
He then began to castigate Georgia for driving to visit an ill friend on an icy,
winter day. The therapist pointed out how frightened each partner was of
losing the other, and how in their anxiety, they tried to limit each other's
autonomy. Tony said he wanted all limits taken off the sensate focus
exercises now. He felt ready for intercourse. The therapist was doubtful, but
saw this as an assertion of Tony's independence and so agreed.

The next week was portrayed by the couple as a total disaster. Tony
had lost his erection both times the couple tried lovemaking. On further
questioning, however, the therapist discovered that Tony had been able to
keep his erection for several minutes after penetration. When his penis
became soft, he wanted to stop the touching, but Georgia persuaded him to
continue, and both partners had orgasms through manual stimulation.

The therapist emphasized the progress they had made, and asked Tony
to focus on positive sensations or a sexual fantasy the next time the couple
made love. Georgia helped her husband by cueing him to pay attention to
his good feelings whenever she noticed him getting distracted during sex.

Although he continued to lose erections during the next three sensate focus sessions, Tony spontaneously told Georgia, "I love you and even if sex never gets better than this, I'm really enjoying it." The couple asked to take a month's break from therapy sessions because they were feeling pressured. When they returned, Tony reported he was having firm and lasting erections. Both partners were reaching orgasm during intercourse. At 3-month follow-up, both the sexual and marital gains were maintained. Tony still grumbled a little about the expense of the therapy, but Georgia told him it was the best investment they had ever made.

INFERTILITY

Infertility has been defined as the failure to conceive after 1 year of attempts. It has been estimated that 15% of American couples of childbearing age have a problem with fertility (Keye, 1984). In samples of patients treated for infertility, at least half of couples report sexual dysfunctions, usually with an onset after the infertility diagnosis (Keye, 1984; Schinfeld, 1985). The incidence of infertility is probably rising as couples delay childbearing and with increased rates of sexually transmitted diseases, such as chlamydia and gonorrhea, associated with pelvic inflammatory disease. The use of intrauterine contraceptive devices may also contribute (Link & Darling, 1986). Thus infertility-related sexual problems are a significant issue for many patients.

Research on the types of sexual dysfunctions experienced by couples treated for infertility has been minimal. Some clinicians believe that a high incidence of erectile dysfunction and difficulty reaching orgasm exists in male partners (Walker, 1983), but surveys suggest that most of these problems are episodic, occurring when men feel pressured to perform at the wife's midcycle fertile period, to provide semen samples, or to participate in the "postcoital test," an examination of the number of viable sperm cells in a woman's cervical mucus after sexual intercourse (DeVries *et al.*, 1984; Keye, 1984).

For women, dyspareunia is common when infertility is caused by endometriosis or pelvic adhesions (Keye, 1984). Women also are more likely to report decreased sexual satisfaction when the man is the infertile partner (Schinfeld, 1985). In a sample of infertile women in Italy, the frequency of reported sexual activity and desire had both decreased after the diagnosis of infertility, but sexual satisfaction was unchanged (Battaglia, Graziano, & Fonti, 1983). Link and Darling (1986) also found that only 16% of women and 12% of men in a group of 43 infertile couples were sexually dissatisfied. Interviews of 45 couples accepted for *in vitro* fertilization revealed a similar 16% rate of sexual dysfunction (Fagan *et al.*, 1986).

Researchers need to ask detailed questions about sexual function, interviewing consecutive patients treated for infertility in a range of settings. Prospective studies may not be feasible, but the sexual history should at least be obtained at the beginning of an infertility evaluation, followed by reassessment at a standard time interval. Both partners should be involved in the sexual assessment.

Psychosocial Impact on Sexuality

Early studies of psychological aspects of infertility sought to explain the failure to conceive by invoking emotional factors. With better medical technology, however, physiological causes of infertility are found in over 90% of cases (Mazor, 1984; Schinfeld, 1985). The focus has shifted to identifying psychological reactions secondary to a diagnosis of infertility.

Depression appears to be a common problem that potentially influences sexual desire and satisfaction in infertile couples. As treatment fails to promote conception, many patients begin to feel hopeless and helpless. Such emotions are particularly common in women at each onset of menstruation (Mazor, 1984; Schinfeld, 1985). Link and Darling (1986) found that 40% of wives and 16% of husbands scored in the depressed range on a questionnaire sent to infertile couples. Of course patients who were psychologically distressed might be more likely to participate in a research study, inflating the results. In assessment interviews of couples seeking *in vitro* fertilization, only 14% of participants had a diagnosable DSM-III disorder (Fagan *et al.*, 1986).

Some patients feel damaged or stigmatized by infertility so that they see themselves as sexually unattractive (Keye, 1984). Although some react by having extramarital affairs to prove that they are desirable or even to demonstrate that the infertility is the spouse's fault, a more common response is a decrease in sexual activity (Mazor, 1984; Schinfeld, 1985). Guilt is a frequent reaction when infertility may be traced to damage from a sexually transmitted disease or when a woman has had an elective abortion (Schinfeld, 1985).

If one partner is more interested than the other in having a child, the more involved one may blame the problem on the ambivalent spouse. In fact the incidence of anger is striking clinically in infertile couples. One study suggested that wives of men who refused to participate in research on emotional aspects of infertility were more distressed than the partners of men who did participate (Link & Darling, 1986). Presumably a lack of participation reflected less emotional involvement or concern about the problem.

In fact, spouse support may enhance the results of treatment for infertility. Results of a postcoital test were more likely to be favorable when the couple reported feeling close to each other while they were having intercourse (DeVries *et al.*, 1984). When the wife is inseminated with semen from an anonymous donor, more pregnancies occur if the husband is not only emotionally supportive, but is present during the procedure (Schinfeld, 1985).

Since treatment for infertility often involves instructions on when to have sex, optimal positioning, and what to do after intercourse, couples come to see lovemaking as mechanical and goal-oriented (Mazor, 1984;

Schinfeld, 1985). Their sexual routine may become constricted (Keye, 1984) and frequency of lovemaking decreases except during fertile periods. The partner who most wants the pregnancy may be perceived as demanding sex when conception would be likely.

Physiological Impact on Sexuality

Some of the organic causes of infertility can also impair sexual function. As mentioned above, women with pelvic pathology may experience dyspareunia. Infertility therapy using progesterone or progestins in women can reduce sexual desire (Keye, 1984). In men, low testosterone or hyperprolactinemia can affect both fertility and sexual function, although more often spermatogenesis is impaired by nonhormonal factors. Varicoceles, in addition to causing oligospermia, may occasionally be associated with abnormalities of venous outflow in the penis, impairing erections (Nahoum & Freire, 1985).

The physiological impact of infertility on sexuality may be mediated by behavioral factors. For example, both ovulation and spermatogenesis can be inhibited by severe emotional stress, malnutrition, or substance abuse (Walker, 1983). The mechanism is disruption of the hormonal feedback systems, affecting both fertility and sexuality.

Assessment Issues

Although taking a sexual history should be part of every infertility workup, timing is important. Many patients are not prepared to be asked detailed sexual questions in the context of a physician visit focused on conception. Given the intrusive nature of the physiological examinations that are performed, including the postcoital test, providing semen samples, and keeping diaries of sexual activity, an atmosphere of trust should be established quickly between clinician and couple. Before taking a sexual history, its purpose, and that of the medical tests, should be clarified. The clinician should give the couple as much control as possible in choosing the timing and order of the tests (Schinfeld, 1985).

Table 11-1 highlights special assessment issues relevant to infertility and sexuality. The Infertility Questionnaire (Bernstein, Potts, & Mattox, 1985) is still in the early stages of validation but includes scales measuring self-esteem, blame or guilt, and sexual distress in men and women being evaluated for infertility. The inventory is designed to identify couples who need more intensive counseling.

Treatment Issues

All couples treated for infertility should at least be offered brief sexual counseling as outlined in Table 11-2. Peer support groups for couples are one promising format for providing sexual education and advice. Intensive therapy may be required by patients who cannot resolve their grief over the loss of the chance to have a child, or who are confused about choosing between alternatives such as adoption, remaining childless, or undergoing sophisticated techniques such as *in vitro* fertilization and artificial insemination by an anonymous donor (Mazor, 1984).

Mazor states that the major goal of psychotherapy is to help couples cope with emotional aspects of infertility. She does not believe that conception can be promoted by alleviating emotional distress. Sarrel and DeCherney (1985), however, reported that 6 out of 10 couples who had no discernible organic cause for their infertility conceived after participating in a 2-hour psychiatric evaluation and counseling session, in contrast to only 1 out of 9 couples who received no counseling. The role of psychotherapy in facilitating conception remains to be explored now that the group of couples without a clear medical deficit can be better selected.

Brief Sexual Counseling Case

Sally was an unusually attractive and vivacious woman of 37. Her social skills had contributed to her success in starting her own travel agency. She had been married for 3 years to Vic, a 32-year-old marketing executive. Sally had been divorced and had a 12-year-old daughter who lived with the couple, but the marriage was Vic's first. Sally had felt reluctant to have a second child, but Vic wanted so much to be a father that Sally agreed to try to get pregnant. The couple stopped using contraception a year after their marriage, but Sally did not conceive, despite their frequent and satisfying lovemaking. By this time, Sally was just as enthusiastic as Vic about having a baby. Even Sally's daughter was disappointed with the couple's lack of success.

Sally and Vic went through an infertility workup. Vic's sperm count and motility were normal. Sally had some mild symptoms of endometriosis, and the gynecologist suggested a hysterosalpingogram (a radiograph with contrast material injected into the uterus and fallopian tubes) and a laparoscopy to make sure her fallopian tubes were not blocked. Sally was apprehensive about the operation, but Vic was supportive, bringing her to the hospital and staying with her until the last possible minute. The surgery did not reveal any abnormalities, but Sally's basal body temperature record and her hormonal profile suggested that she was not ovulating as regularly as would be optimal. Clomid (clomiphene citrate) was prescribed to stimulate ovulation.

During the second month of this hormonal therapy, Sally requested a visit with her gynecologist. She told him that she had gained 15 pounds and was feeling blue. During the session, Sally began to cry as she described her disappointment each time she began to menstruate. Sally knew that depression and weight gain were common side effects of Clomid. She also had recently stopped smoking at her husband's request. Even though it was easy to see why Sally felt stressed, she blamed herself for not being more upbeat. Her friends were getting impatient with her constant talk about pregnancy, and she felt as if her world were falling apart. Her worst fear was that Vic would leave her and find a younger woman if she did not conceive. Sometimes she felt so angry with him that she considered divorce herself.

The gynecologist asked Sally whether she had shared these feelings with Vic. Sally said she had tried to hide her depression and anger from her husband, although he noticed her decreased activities and had expressed concern about her mood.

A couple session was scheduled for the next week. The gynecologist asked Sally to tell Vic some of her reactions to her infertility therapy. She talked about her impatience to get pregnant and her frustration about gaining weight. Vic protested that he still found her attractive and, in fact, thought she had been a little too thin before. "Then why don't you ever suggest that we make love, except right around my fertile days?" asked Sally.

"Have I been doing that?" Vic responded.

"Yes," answered Sally. "I've been watching."

"Well I guess I thought I should save my strength or something. It is silly when I think about it."

The gynecologist told Sally and Vic that many couples become goal-oriented about sexuality during treatment for infertility. He suggested that Sally and Vic each take responsibility for initiating sex at least once a week no matter what the period of the menstrual cycle. He also helped the couple to identify ways to make sex more playful or erotic. Sally suggested starting lovemaking by rubbing each other with scented oil. Vic wanted to go away together for a weekend and let Sally's mother take care of their 12-year-old.

Sally also mentioned feeling "bulldozed" sometimes by Vic. She had spent 7 years as a single woman, setting her own schedule and taking care of finances and household tasks. Vic was a highly competent and organized person, however, who sometimes doubted Sally's ability to cope without his help, or ignored his wife's opinions on family decisions. In fact, choosing to have a child was a good example of Sally allowing Vic to override her initial judgment, although she felt comfortable now with their mutual decision. Vic promised to listen more carefully to Sally's opinions in the future.

The gynecologist pointed out that childrearing would require good couple communication and an ability to compromise on disagreements. Sally and Vic had already had experience in this area with her daughter and had worked out a comfortable style of parenting.

After the couple session, Sally's mood lifted. In two more cycles she became pregnant. Although both partners were excited, Sally was frightened by the prospect of amniocentesis. She and Vic watched the ultrasound image as the procedure was done. Sally later felt this had been a mistake. A fetal hand had been clearly visible, making the baby that much more real to her. The fear that evidence of Down's syndrome would be found and she would have to decide whether to have an abortion haunted her during the 3 weeks of waiting for results. The genetic counselor gave the couple good news, however, and Vic and Sally prepared for the arrival of a son.

The couple continued to enjoy sex until late in the third trimester of Sally's pregnancy. Sally had a normal delivery, and the couple eased smoothly into parenthood.

PART THREE

TRAINING AND ETHICAL ISSUES

12

Training Providers of Sexual Health Care

Throughout this book, we have stressed the complementary roles of the primary care clinician in providing brief sexual counseling and the specialist in offering intensive sex therapy or medical treatment. This chapter suggests a format for training each category of clinician.

TRAINING THE PRIMARY CARE CLINICIAN

Physicians, nurses, medical social workers, or other members of the primary care team can benefit from special training in assessing sexual problems and providing education and brief sexual counseling. Since only a minority of primary care professionals have the time and motivation to take a full-scale seminar on sexual health care, we have designed a 1-day workshop on sexuality and chronic illness. We find that the most common request is for brief training, even though a more intensive course would be optimal. The material we present here is designed for the interdisciplinary staff of a specialty department, but could easily be modified to be more relevant to a group of nurses, social workers, medical students, or psychologists.

Goals of the 1-Day Workshop

We cannot train sexuality specialists or even provide up-to-date knowledge about all aspects of sexuality and illness in 1 day. What we can do is increase clinicians' awareness of the importance of sexual health care and give them basic skills in discussing sex with patients and in making appropriate referrals. Thus, the emphasis is divided between presenting didactic material and stimulating attitude change. Experiential learning through role playing and small group exercises is the most crucial part of the workshop. If we motivate clinicians to participate in sexual health care, they can learn more facts about the topic through reading or further coursework.

After taking this workshop, a clinician should be able to:

• bring up the topic of sexuality with patients and assess their current sexual function;
• provide basic facts to patients about the sexual response cycle and the impact of illness;
• involve the partner in education and brief counseling;
• gauge his or her ability to deal with a sexual problem and know when and how to refer patients to a sexuality specialist.

In our experience, the sexuality specialist has endless opportunities to teach other health professionals. Sexuality is always a popular topic for workshops and lectures. To avoid burn-out as a teacher, we suggest a model in Chapter 19 for training students and colleagues to lead their own workshops. We also have found one of the most rewarding workshop audiences to be the specialty team, for example the staff of a multidisciplinary clinic who work together to treat diabetics or cancer patients. The workshop can not only improve patient care but also enhance team members' respect for each other's special skills. When teaching specialists, the workshop leader should become as expert as possible in research and clinical knowledge on sexuality relevant to the audience's particular area of patient care. Only by meeting clinicians on their own ground will the sexuality specialist gain their respect.

Outline for a Workshop on Sexuality and Illness

We describe the workshop in enough detail so that a specialist in sexuality could teach the course after reading this book. Of course, each clinician will modify the format to suit his or her particular audience and setting, but the essential elements are provided.

We suggest an audience of 24 to 32 participants, taught by a team of two workshop leaders. The ideal setting is a conference center where participants share meals together without distractions. The workshop can be held without an evening session, but in our experience that time adds significant emotional intensity.

At the beginning of the workshop, each participant is assigned to a small group of eight. The leaders structure the groups to be as varied as possible in terms of members' ages and professions and as balanced as possible in gender. A trefoil (three-leafed clover) seating arrangement can be used for sessions in which the entire group meets. The trefoil allows maximum interaction with the workshop leaders while preserving the cohesiveness of the small groups. If four small groups are used, the trefoil can become a four-leafed clover. The workshop area should also include a smaller room for each small group.

The workshop leaders will need a slide projector for lectures and perhaps an overhead projector, flipchart, or blackboard for recording themes during group discussions. A detailed outline of each session follows.

MORNING SESSION
  Schedule
  9:00– 9:30   Introductions
  9:30–10:00   Lecture: The Integrative Model of Sexual Health
                      Care
  10:00–10:20   Role Play: Counseling Skills
  10:20–10:35   Break
  10:35–11:00   Lecture: The Couple Approach to Health Care
  11:00–11:15   Guided Fantasy: Sexuality and Illness
  11:15–11:45   Small Group Exercise: Influence of Illness on My
                      Sexuality
  11:45–12:00   Large Group Interviews and Fact-Finding

Introductions. Workshop leaders and participants take turns standing up in the large group and stating their names, profession, current job description, and one or two goals they have in attending the course. Each participant has been given a name tag with their small group number on it as well and has been asked to sit in the section reserved for each group.

Lecture: The Integrative Model of Sexual Health Care. This lecture should review the material from Chapter 1 of this book on the importance of an integrative model of sexual health care. The patient's first contact with the sexual health care system is also described, using material from Chapter 6.

Role Play: Counseling Skills. Remaining in the large group, participants are instructed to pair up, choosing a partner they do not know well. One partner will play a person of their own age and gender seeking help for a sexual problem. The "patient" can choose a problem observed in his or her clinical practice, an imagined problem, or one from personal experience, but is not to disclose the source of inspiration. The "patient" begins by stating the problem. The other partner is the "therapist" and has 5 minutes to counsel the patient. At the end of the time, all dyads are asked to freeze, to identify in silence what they were feeling at the moment they were stopped, and to contemplate what the "therapist" did well.

The patient then has 3 minutes to give the therapist feedback before switching roles. We emphasize giving constructive feedback, including noting skills and suggesting how the therapist could have been even more helpful. The advantage of this role playing format is that the tight structure and positive feedback reduce participants' anxiety. It is obvious that the time allotted is only enough to provide a vignette, rather than testing advanced counseling skills. Clinicians of varying experience can thus role play together on an equal basis, with the more advanced participant perhaps using the role play to work on an area of difficulty in his or her clinical experience. The role playing keeps participants actively involved in new learning.

Lecture: The Couple Approach to Health Care. This lecture covers material from Chapter 2 on relationships and coping with illness, and Chapter 6 on reframing the problem as a dyadic issue.

Guided Fantasy: Sexuality and Illness. Before beginning the session, each participant receives a sign to hang around his or her neck with one of the following labels:

- I'm a diabetic.
- I'm married to a diabetic.
- I have just had my first heart attack.
- My spouse just had a heart attack.
- I'm an alcoholic.
- I'm married to an alcoholic.
- I've had a radical vulvectomy.
- My wife has had a radical vulvectomy.

In the large group, the leaders ask participants to relax and close their eyes and to imagine how they would feel if their labels were real. The fantasy begins with reactions to the diagnosis and crisis of illness and proceeds to how the couple would communicate about it. What would happen at work? How would it feel to look in the mirror? How would friends and children react? What would sex be like? What would happen to the marriage or close relationship? If the audience are the staff of a specialty clinic, several clinical syndromes from their setting can be substituted for the illnesses we choose here.

Small Group Exercise: Influence of Illness on My Sexuality. Participants divide into their small groups, which should each include a range of diagnoses. The participants take turns telling the group, in the first person, how their illness, or their partner's illness, has changed their lives. Leaders circulate to make sure that each participant takes 2 or 3 minutes for their presentation and stays within their role. Leaders also answer questions about the illness and sexual function, as if participants were patients in an educational group for couples.

Large Group Interviews and Fact Finding. Back in the large group room, participants are seated according to the four disease categories. They are asked to stay within their roles and to list the most important psychosexual problems presented by their disease. After each group has had a chance to speak, the other participants can ask questions. The leader then interviews individuals at random, asking thought-provoking questions such as, "As a blind diabetic, how do you know when your spouse is in the mood for sex?" or "What did you see the first time you looked at your wife's genitals after her vulvectomy?" The leader then takes about 5 minutes to summarize current knowledge about sexual function and the particular disease.

This segment closes with a brief body awareness exercise. Participants take off their labels and focus on their physical sensations and on a relaxing scene. Otherwise, some participants have difficulty putting aside the vivid experience of the disease roles.

AFTERNOON SESSION
Schedule

2:00–3:00	Lecture: The Sexual Response Cycle and Medical Aspects of Sexual Dysfunction
3:00–3:15	Role Play: Assessment Interview
3:15–3:30	Break
3:30–4:30	Lecture: Brief Sexual Counseling
4:30–5:00	Role Plays: Sex Education and Brief Sexual Counseling
5:00–6:30	Dinner
6:30–8:00	EVENING SESSION

Lecture: The Sexual Response Cycle and Medical Aspects of Sexual Dysfunction. Material from Chapter 3 on the diagnosis of sexual dysfunction is presented. The lecture also outlines medical causes of sexual problems, using material from Chapter 5. If the audience treats a certain type of illness, the impact of that disease is highlighted.

Role Play: Assessment Interview. Participants remain in the large group. Leaders ask for volunteers for a role play, including two cotherapists and two patients. Two more members of the audience are designated as "radio listeners" and two as "television watchers." The radio listeners will focus only on the verbal interaction, sitting with their backs to the role players. The television watchers concentrate on nonverbal cues, as if the sound were turned off.

The patient couple is given a few moments to prepare, with private instructions that the wife has dyspareunia and the husband wants intercourse much more frequently than she does. The leaders use this time to tell the cotherapists and audience how to set up an office to allow comfortable eye contact between all participants. As the role play begins, the leaders "freeze" the action at interesting points, asking the television and radio commentators to point out what is going on. If the therapists are in trouble, the leaders may ask for an "instant replay," going back a few moments and allowing the therapists to try a different tack. Feedback is kept on a constructive level, with an accent on the positive and on specific suggestions for improvement.

Lecture: Brief Sexual Counseling. This lecture includes a brief overview of levels of therapeutic intervention (Chapter 7) and then describes techniques of sex education and brief sexual counseling (Chapter 7). Criteria for referral to a sexuality specialist are also given.

Role Play: Sex Education. Participants divide again into dyads. One partner role plays a sexual counselor. If the other is a woman, she takes the role of a patient about to have an abdominal hysterectomy to treat uterine fibroid tumors. Men take the role of a patient scheduled for a transurethral prostatectomy. Again, the health problems can be tailored to fit the interests of the audience. Counselors are given a brief fact sheet about sexual function after each operation and are given 15 minutes to educate the patient. The patient gives constructive feedback to the counselor as in earlier role plays.

Within each small group, a cotherapy team and a patient couple are chosen, using the hysterectomy as the symptom, and the same role play is performed in front of the other members, followed by a discussion of helpful education techniques.

Role Play: Brief Sexual Counseling. Again dyads role play a counselor and a patient, this time reversing their roles from the last exercise. This time the patient has had the hysterectomy or the TURP 6 months previously but has developed a sexual dysfunction (inorgasmia for the women and erectile dysfunction for the men) in the interim. The counselor is given 15 minutes to offer some brief counseling, followed by feedback from the patient.

This time the role play is repeated in front of the small group by four volunteers, but the husband in the patient couple has had a TURP. Group leaders circulate to make sure the small groups provide helpful feedback to the role players and have a stimulating discussion of counseling techniques.

Evening Session. Using index cards and pencils to preserve anonymity, leaders give participants three tasks. Cards are collected after each.

• Describe briefly the last time you experienced any sort of problem in your sex life.
• Give a brief description of your favorite sexual fantasy.
• Write down the most daring or limit-pushing sexual experience you have had. What new sexual experience would you most like to try in the future?

Group leaders read the cards from each task aloud to the group. After all three sets have been heard, participants break into their small groups for discussion. Issues about judging others' behavior will usually be raised, and respect for personal boundaries should be a focus. If the group is small or the participants know each other well, this exercise may not be truly anonymous. The leaders can modify the instructions so that the written descriptions are of one's own experience or of something one has heard from a friend or patient. Participants are asked not to identify the source of the material.

Continuing Education

Primary care clinicians need continued support and encouragement to make good use of the skills taught in a beginning-level workshop. In fact, we believe that a 5-day seminar is the best introduction to this area, but rarely have the luxury of presenting one. After any initial training, the ideal is to have a sexuality specialist available in a clinical setting to provide supervision and be a resource for difficult cases. If a specialist is not available, we encourage clinicians to form their own peer supervision networks, perhaps meeting once every several weeks to discuss clinical work.

In Denmark, such groups have become local chapters of the Danish Association of Clinical Sexology, an organization with 400 members that offers frequent weekend workshops on special topics of interest. The association has also sponsored a 2-year sexology workshop for primary care clinicians (family physicians, nurses, social workers, etc.), consisting of 12 weekend seminars as well as twice-monthly supervision meetings (Jensen, 1983). In the United States, such community networking has rarely been attempted, but it should be feasible.

TRAINING THE SEXUAL HEALTH CARE SPECIALIST

In providing education and brief sexual counseling to patients, any clinician with good listening skills, a modicum of interpersonal sensitivity, and a willingness to suspend judgment about sexual issues can learn to be of help. Sexual health care specialists, however, need a higher level of psychotherapeutic skill to provide intensive therapy.

We believe that a sex therapist should be a mental health professional: a clinical psychologist, social worker, or psychiatrist who is already proficient at least in individual and group therapy techniques. Experience with behavioral and cognitive-behavioral interventions and with couple therapy is definitely helpful as well. The clinician who provides intensive sex therapy to patients with chronic illnesses needs a wide array of skills, including the following:

- Ability to screen for cognitive impairments and major psychiatric disorders;
- Skill in evaluating not only individual psychological function but also dyadic communication, ability to share intimacy, and expression of affection and anger;

- Enough knowledge about the medical causes and assessment of sexual dysfunction to make appropriate referrals and to understand the results of diagnostic tests;
- A thorough understanding of sexual physiology, behavior, and dysfunction;
- Skill in conducting interview and questionnaire evaluations of past and present sexual function;
- Comfort in applying sex therapy treatment programs for specific sexual dysfunctions, including a commitment to keep current with new developments in the field;
- Ability to use other relevant therapeutic interventions, which may include behavioral marital therapy strategies, systematic desensitization, psychodynamic or humanistic techniques, or cognitive-behavioral treatments for depression and phobic anxiety;
- Comfort in working with physicians to coordinate medical and psychological aspects of a comprehensive treatment plan;
- Ability to supervise and enlist help from members of the primary care team who refer patients to provide brief sexual counseling;
- Knowledge of legal and ethical issues in treating sexual dysfunction.

Ideally, to train a clinician to function independently at this level and to be a supervisor for others, we recommend a course lasting for an academic year and meeting at least twice weekly. One session would be didactic, and the other would involve group supervision of clinical work. A third weekly session of individual supervision would begin as soon as the therapists were prepared to begin treating patients.

Didactic Training

The didactic component of the training program is outlined in Table 12-1. Each meeting would last for 1½ hours. A lecture of 45 minutes would be followed by time for discussion, case examples from the teacher's clinical experience, and role-playing exercises similar in format to those described in the previous section.

This book could serve as a basic text, but it should be supplemented with readings on sexual dysfunction, sex and marital therapy, and other relevant techniques. Table 12-2 lists books we have found especially useful in teaching. Journal articles should be assigned as reading in areas that are new or controversial.

Clinical Supervision

Supervision of ongoing clinical work is the heart of any psychotherapy training, and sex therapy is no exception. We cannot review basic super-

Table 12-1. Curriculum for a Seminar for Sexual Health Care Specialists

Session	Topic[a]
1	The therapist's sexual attitudes
2	Discussing sex with patients
3	Sexual response cycle and the range of normalcy in behavior
4	Intrapsychic causes of sexual dysfunction
5	Relationship causes of sexual dysfunction
6	Medical causes of sexual dysfunction
7	Diagnosis of sexual dysfunction: Schemas and questionnaires
8	Diagnosis of sexual dysfunction: Medical tests
9	The initial assessment interview
10	Taking a sexual history
11	Providing sex education to patients
12	Formats of sex therapy: Couple, group, or individual
13	Giving homework assignments and debriefing
14	Sensate focus sequences
15	Techniques to change sexual attitudes
16	Techniques to enhance caring and intimacy
17	Communication training: Marital and sexual
18	Problem solving and contracting for couples
19	Anger management for couples
20	Techniques to minimize physical handicaps during sexual activity
21	Treatment strategies for premature ejaculation
22	Treatment strategies for erectile dysfunction
23	Treatment strategies for male difficulty reaching orgasm and reduced orgasmic intensity
24	Treatment strategies for women with lifelong inorgasmia
25	Treatment strategies for less severe female orgasm problems
26	Treatment strategies for vaginismus and dyspareunia
27	Treatment strategies for aversion to sex
28	Treatment strategies for global low sexual desire
29	Treatment strategies for situational low sexual desire
30	Combining sex therapy with medical treatment of sexual dysfunction
31	Ethical issues in sex therapy
32	Sexual trauma and paraphilias
33	Sexuality and aging
34	Sexuality and cardiovascular disease
35	Sexuality and diabetes
36	Sexuality and cancer
37	Sexuality and renal disease
38	Sexuality and COPD
39	Sexuality and major psychiatric disorders
40	Sexuality and substance abuse
41	Sexuality and chronic pain
42	Sexuality and infertility

[a]Each topic should include a 45-minute lecture. Afterward, another 45 minutes should be devoted to discussion, case examples, and role playing.

Table 12-2. Bibliography for Seminar for Sexual Health Care Specialists

---

Sex Therapy

Arentewicz, G., & Schmidt, G. (1983). *The treatment of sexual disorders.* New York: Basic Books.

Kaplan, H. S. (1974). *The new sex therapy.* New York: Brunner/Mazel.

Kaplan, H. S. (1979). *Disorders of sexual desire.* New York: Brunner/Mazel.

Kaplan, H. S. (1983)). *The evaluation of sexual disorders.* New York: Brunner/Mazel.

Leiblum, S. R., & Pervin, L. A. (1980). *Principles and practice of sex therapy.* New York: Guilford Press.

LoPiccolo, J., & LoPiccolo, L. (1978). *Handbook of sex therapy.* New York: Plenum Press.

Medical Issues and Erectile Dysfunction

Krane, R. J., Siroky, M. B., & Goldstein, I. (1983). *Male sexual dysfunction.* Boston: Little, Brown & Co.

Segraves, R. T., & Schoenberg, H. W. (1985). *Diagnosis and treatment of erectile disturbances: A guide for clinicians.* New York: Plenum Press.

Wagner, G., & Green, R. (1981). *Impotence: Psychological, physiological, surgical diagnosis and treatment.* New York: Plenum Press.

Self-Help Books for Patients

Barbach, L. (1984). *For yourself: The fulfillment of female sexuality.* Garden City, NY: Anchor Press/Doubleday.

Barbach, L. (1982). *For each other: Sharing sexual intimacy.* Garden City, NY: Anchor Press/Doubleday.

Barbach, L. (1984). *Pleasures: Women write erotica.* Garden City, NY: Doubleday & Co.

Heiman, J., LoPiccolo, L., & LoPiccolo, J. (1976). *Becoming orgasmic: A sexual growth program for women.* Englewood Cliffs, NJ: Prentice-Hall.

Schover, L. R. (1984). *Prime time: Sexual health for men over fifty.* New York: Holt, Rinehart & Winston.

Zilbergeld, B. (1978). *Male sexuality.* New York: Bantam Books.

---

vision skills in this brief chapter; rather, we focus on supervision issues particularly relevant to training the sexuality specialist. A supervision group that meets once weekly is a very effective training format. Students take turns presenting their cases, getting feedback not only from the supervisor (or for a large seminar, perhaps a team of supervisors) but also from their peers. Group supervision, however, is usually too infrequent to serve as the major source of clinical guidance for a student. Each therapist in training also needs to meet weekly with an individual supervisor.

Probably the best way to supervise couple therapy is to videotape each session with the patients' permission. Although videotaping may seem intrusive at first, both therapist and couple usually quickly forget about the camera (which can be fixed to focus on the patients). The videotape affords a chance to examine subtle, nonverbal aspects of the therapy process as well as to analyze the verbal interaction in depth. The therapy process comes alive for the supervisor and supervision group in a way that no narrated account of a session can equal. The complexity of couple therapy makes an "instant replay" especially valuable in understanding lines of communication and in catching unspoken messages. Since videotaping is expensive, audiotaping therapy sessions is a helpful alternative.

Another important goal of the group supervision is to help trainees examine their own sexual attitudes and potential clinical blind spots. In the early months of the seminar, group supervision sessions could be used for experiential learning. For example, pairs of trainees could take each other's sexual histories and then discuss their emotional reactions to the experience in the group. When being taught how to assign the sensate focus exercises or other homework, trainees could actually carry out the exercises with a partner at home and bring some reactions back into the group.

How can the supervisor make a group safe for such experiences? Rules about confidentiality are imperative. Group members should agree not to discuss each other's or the patients' personal lives outside of the group sessions. Trainees should never be pressured to disclose more than is comfortable. Those who have physical disabilities, do not have a committed sexual partner, or have a homosexual orientation must not be made to feel excluded when heterosexual couple issues are in focus. Such individual differences should instead be sources of enlightenment for the group. For example, when an assignment is suggested to try a couple sensate focus exercise, an alternative for any trainee could be to practice sensate focus techniques individually, caressing his or her own body and noticing the sensations evoked. All experiential exercises and self-disclosure should be optional rather than required.

If personal material concerns a very taboo topic, for example, sexual fantasies, trainees may be more able to share and discuss such material when their anonymity is preserved. If the group is not too small, trainees could write their opinion or experience on an index card. Cards can be collected, shuffled, and handed out so that each trainee reads some unknown person's thoughts to the group. Trainees can also explore personal attitudes and feelings without self-disclosure by role playing using case material.

Learning to be a sex therapist also has an impact on the trainee's close relationships. For example, trainees' partners may feel anxious about being involved with a nascent "sex expert," or the supervision process may spotlight deficiencies in communication or sexual function in the trainee's own relationship. Although a supervisor usually has little or no contact with the trainee's sexual partner, personal effects of the new learning should be discussed at intervals and all trainees should be made aware of resources for couple counseling outside of the supervision setting. A special group session or two including partners is another alternative. The focus of sex therapy on intimacy and pleasure rather than on performance should minimize pressure on trainee and partner to live up to an unrealistic standard of sexual or marital perfection.

Many sex therapy seminars pair trainees into male–female cotherapy teams, adding another dimension to the emotional experience. The supervisor may need to mediate between cotherapists who are struggling to dominate one another. The normal insecurities of a clinician who is practicing new skills can escalate into a battle to show patients and supervisor that one cotherapist is more competent than the other. When husband and wife teams work together as cotherapists, power struggles take on an added intensity, particularly when the husband has a more prestigious professional degree than the wife, a common situation (Golden & Golden, 1976).

The exhilaration of working in tandem and dealing with sexually charged material may also eroticize the relationship between cotherapists (Dunn & Dickes, 1977; Zentner & Pouyat, 1978). In fact, one function of the cotherapy team is to model a good relationship for the patient couple. When the enjoyment of teamwork develops into a sexual relationship between cotherapists, consequences may be mixed professionally and personally. If both partners are single and the relationship can be overt, the energy produced from falling in love can be inspiring for patients and coworkers. The ability to share work interests as well as family life has been a dream for many couples in this field. Just as the cotherapists have an image of the patients' relationship in its ideal form, they can seek to transform their own lives to match their picture of intimacy and love. Even in the least compli- cated situation, however, negative fallout is possible. The patient couple may feel that their therapists are more focused on each other than on the therapy. The patients may also feel as if they are competing with the therapist couple to attain the perfect relationship or that the therapists present a picture of happiness that is discouraging because it is so hard to match. Coworkers may be jealous of the cotherapists' absorption in each other.

When the cotherapists' relationship is secret, the dynamics are even more complex. The spouse of one therapist may become suspicious of the affair. Indeed, jealousy on the part of a spouse is common even when cotherapists are simply good friends and colleagues. Such affairs rarely remain undetected for long within the supervision group. Other group members often take sides about whether the affair is acceptable, and some degree of turmoil and resentment is almost inevitable.

We believe that the ethics of cotherapist sexual relationships depend mainly on their impact on the therapy process and on the work group. Cotherapists share power equally when both are trainees. Each individual must examine his or her own values and consider the pros and cons.

We feel strongly, however, that sexual relationships between supervi- sors and trainees are unethical during a formal training program. The supervisor must often evaluate the trainee's performance, creating a conflict of roles if a sexual relationship also exists. Another problem is inherent in the nature of supervision, a process similar to psychotherapy. The supervi- sor elicits transferential feelings because of his or her position of power and guise of wisdom. To engage in a sexual relationship with a trainee is to abuse that transference and to betray a trust. Research has demonstrated that sexual contacts between professors or supervisors and graduate students, at least in clinical psychology, frequently have negative emotional and professional consequences for the trainee (Glazer & Thorpe, 1986; Pope, Levenson, & Schover, 1979). Such affairs can also engender jealousy and suspicions of favoritism in the other students in a supervision group. Those of us who work in a controversial clinical area must take care to be sensitive and ethical role models. Because of the extreme importance of such ethical considerations in the training and practice of sex therapy, we devote the chapter that follows to this subject.

Teaching Supervisory Skills

The supervisor serves as a role model not only in professional conduct, but also in teaching trainees to assume supervisory responsibility. Group supervision provides a good opportunity for trainees to comment on their peers' cases and to learn how to give constructive feedback. Therapists who treat sexual and marital cases have an edge in learning to be good supervisors because they must already be expert in the principles of good communication. As in any close relationship, the supervisor's feedback to a trainee should be framed positively, be specific, be limited to the here and now, and allow for discussion and negotiation. Good listening skills and a high degree of empathy are crucial for supervision, as they are for psychotherapy.

When treatment focuses on the sensitive issues of sexuality, the supervisor must be especially careful to prevent the trainee's sexual biases from intruding on the patient and to keep the supervision free of his or her own sexual attitudes. Being nonjudgmental as a sex therapist requires a constant awareness of one's own sexual beliefs and emotional reactions so that one does not automatically perceive the patient through an idiosyncratic or distorted frame of reference (Schover, 1983).

In addition to supervising the group, and perhaps to assigning advanced trainees to supervise beginners later in the seminar, the seminar leader can provide students with practical experience in building a consultation service. In the model presented in this book, the sexuality specialist increases referrals and improves care for the majority of chronically ill patients by teaching the primary care team to provide sexual information and brief counseling routinely. Toward the end of the seminar year, teams of two or three trainees could be assigned to give a half-day workshop to a group of health professionals working with a special target population of patients. The workshop would include material on incidence and types of sexual dysfunctions in that population, types of assessment and treatment available, and practical demonstrations and role playing of brief education and counseling techniques.

If the sexuality training program is set in a medical school or large hospital, many potential settings for workshops would be available. Otherwise, the seminar leader and students can reach out into the community, approaching smaller hospitals, nursing homes, rehabilitation facilities, or the staff of nonprofit societies that serve patients with particular illnesses (e.g., the American Cancer Society, the Heart Association, Alcoholics Anonymous, etc.). The supervisor's task is a heavy one, however, because trainees need to handle contacts with other professionals with dignity and tact. One insensitive student could damage the training program's reputation in the community and harm future efforts at education and outreach. If only one supervisor is available, it might be wise to limit the number of workshops to allow close supervision, giving more trainees a smaller role in each. However a workshop is structured, experience interacting with other health professionals is crucial to the sexuality specialist working in this rapidly developing interdisciplinary area.

13

Ethical and Professional Issues in Treating Sexual Problems in the Chronically Ill

This final chapter is the product of our experiences in designing sexuality programs for medical patients and in training health care professionals. Issues regarding ethics and professionalism often arise unexpectedly, leaving the clinician confused and anxious. We hope to anticipate the most common dilemmas so that readers can develop preferred ways of handling them and either prevent conflicts or be prepared to contain them quickly and effectively.

THE CLINICIAN'S NEED TO KNOW: ALTRUISM OR VOYEURISM?

As we stressed earlier, the clinician who asks a medical patient about sexuality risks a rebuff. Patients have responded, "I'm here to get medical treatment, not to answer questions about my sex life." A sensitive therapist learns to bring up the topic of sexuality in a nonthreatening way. Even if patient and partner are willing to discuss their sexual function, however, the type of meticulous assessment needed to plan intensive sex therapy is usually not warranted for a medical patient who simply needs basic facts and some reassurance or advice.

Because relationships are so fascinating, clinicians may find themselves asking more than they need to know, especially in the beginning of their work in this area. Patients who are very attractive or who have rare and interesting illnesses often receive the most superfluous attention. The risk is that patients feel the clinician is being voyeuristic rather than therapeutic, or feel engulfed by the therapist. Clinicians can avoid such accusations by asking themselves, "How much do I need to know about this couple's sex life to provide brief counseling and assess the need for intensive therapy?" If the therapist wants to learn about sexual function after a specific medical procedure, the assessment should be presented as a research evaluation rather than in the guise of counseling. Medical patients often enjoy providing information that could help others with the same illness, but their rights to privacy and informed consent must remain paramount.

DEALING WITH STAFF RESISTANCE TO A SEXUALITY PROGRAM

Treating patients with respect and sensitivity is vital, too, because a sexuality program in a medical setting must be, like Caesar's wife, above reproach. Many physicians and other health professionals regard sex as a taboo subject and sex therapists as unethical quacks. Sadly enough, the lack of control over this relatively new area of psychotherapy has allowed many incompetent and even destructive clinicians to call themselves sex therapists, confirming the public's worst fears (LoPiccolo, 1978). Those of us who are highly trained professionals constantly battle these stereotypes. In the United States, a recent proliferation of sex therapy media shows offering callers instant advice has made it even more difficult for the serious clinician to be recognized as a skilled psychotherapist and scientific investigator.

Health professionals in medical settings greet a sexuality program, or even a lecture about treatment of sexual dysfunction, with mixed feelings. Some are fascinated and eager to refer patients. These are often the sensitive clinicians who had been trying to provide brief counseling, but with little training or opportunity for supervision. Another minority are those who scoff at the idea that sexuality could be an important issue for someone faced with a chronic illness. Often these physicians, nurses, or other caretakers are dissatisfied with their own sex lives and have chosen denial as a mechanism for coping with their frustration. Others have rigid religious or moral beliefs and fear that sexual counseling will lure patients from the paths of righteousness.

Some anxious clinicians treat the sexuality program as a joke. A common reaction is to ask, with a laugh, if services are available to the professional staff as well as to the patients. The sexuality specialist must also be prepared for an avalanche of "dirty jokes" and double entendres. We believe that the best response is to keep one's own sense of humor, but also to steer the conversation to case examples that illustrate how sexual counseling can benefit patients and make a real difference in quality of life. Citing normative statistics or research findings also can be helpful. Sometimes the education of staff is inadvertent, as when a physician down the hall received one of our copies of *Archives of Sexual Behavior* by mistake in the mail. He returned it to the sexuality specialist with the comment, "I never realized that there was so much scientific research about sex!"

In the beginning days of a program, even a small incident can give disastrous bad press. When one of us (LRS) was starting a sexuality unit in a cancer center, she showed a videotape about sex therapy for erectile dysfunction to a patient couple to illustrate sensate focus techniques. She warned husband and wife beforehand that explicit sexual activity would be shown. After the tape was over, she spent a few minutes discussing their emotional reactions to it. Believing that a helpful and therapeutic session had taken place, she went on about her day, only to be called in by her department chairman 2 hours later. The couple had gone from her office to their enterostomal therapist and had told her that they were furious with the psychologist who had probed into the details of their sex life and then had shown them a pornographic film. The enterostomal therapist, who later became one of program's chief advocates, had not met the sex therapist yet. Protective of her patients, she went directly to the department chairman, demanding to know what kind of bizarre unit he was sponsoring. Although the staff involved finally understood the circumstances, the patients refused to see the therapist to discuss their reactions. After that incident, we decided not to use explicit educational films in our program.

Building a referral network takes patience. Busy physicians rarely take the time to conduct routine sexual evaluations. Nurses, social workers, physical therapists, and others who are more likely to hear about a patient's sexual problems may not have the authority to ask for a consultation. The sexuality specialist needs to give frequent lectures and workshops. Some referring clinicians want feedback on the patient's progress, but others are simply relieved to have the sexual issue handled by someone else, becoming impatient if the sex therapist wants to discuss the case. Since sexuality is so private, the sex therapist should ask the patient's permission to give feedback to the referring physician, a safeguard that may be alien to the usual cross-specialty sharing in a hospital.

CONFIDENTIALITY IN MEDICAL SETTINGS

Confidentiality is a salient concern for the clinician who provides sexual counseling in medical settings. Not only do professional staff assume that case material can be shared freely, without special permission, but the patient's medical record is read by clerks, nurses, and other personnel.

We recommend that the sexuality specialist obtain permission from the institution to keep private therapy files on each patient. Reports of evaluations in the patient's medical chart should be limited to information fulfilling legal requirements and contributing to good, interdisciplinary care. The patient's diagnosis of sexual dysfunction, possible physiological factors, and psychological variables that play a causal role can be listed. The treatment plan should be briefly described initially, followed by short progress notes for each session. The clinician should not describe specific sexual practices, note extramarital affairs, or give details of a sexual history in the medical chart. It is also wise to assume that the patient may read his or her own chart. Not only is freedom of medical information a legal right in the United States, but charts in most medical settings are easily accessible to determined patients who do not wish to go through official channels. A good rule is not to write a note that you would not wish your patient to read.

Patients also may prefer that a diagnosis of sexual dysfunction not appear on insurance claim forms. The insurance clerk at their workplace or their employer might see the diagnosis. Clinicians should be familiar with billing guidelines of their own institutions and of third-party payers and keep the diagnosis as confidential as is possible.

RESPECTING THE RELATIONSHIP BETWEEN PRIMARY CARE CLINICIAN AND PATIENT

The sexuality specialist often functions as a consultation resource. Since health care professionals receive so little training in sexuality, patients are occasionally referred only after the primary care clinician has provided misinformation about sexual function. The specialist's dilemma is how to set the patient straight without damaging trust in the primary caretaker.

A frequent example in the cancer center was the man whose urologist in the community told him that sexual desire and orgasm were eliminated by operations such as radical cystectomy or prostatectomy. It is also all too common for physicians to tell diabetic men that erectile failure is just a matter of time. Other physicians prescribe unnecessary replacement testosterone or use tranquilizers to "treat" premature ejaculation.

We often begin by telling the patient that medicine has become too complex for any physician to be expert in all areas. We state that knowledge about sexual problems has grown so rapidly in the past several years that few physicians are completely up-to-date, and that although the doctor usually means well and is undoubtedly using his or her best judgment, our own specialized experience has taught us a different way of seeing things. We make it clear that we assume that the primary care doctor could run circles around us in his or her specialty area.

Even this gentle style of contradiction may alienate some referral sources, but we put the patient's best interest above our wish to be congenial colleagues. If a primary care clinician appears receptive, the sexuality specialist can tactfully share a recent journal article or case history containing correct information as part of providing feedback on the referred patient.

RESISTING PRESSURE TO PROVIDE A QUICK FIX

Recent advances in technology have made it possible to restore erections with surgery or penile injections in many patients. So much financial and research support for pharmacological manipulations of sexual desire and arousal currently exists that within the next few years we may well see a true aphrodisiac pill, able to increase seuxal desire or stimulate erections or vaginal lubrication. In many large U.S. cities, newspapers already carry advertisements for potency clinics, promising that medical therapies can cure sexual problems.

Given this atmosphere, patients are angry and disappointed if a clinician recommends against papaverine injections or a penile prosthesis. They threaten to go elsewhere for their care, and sometimes a conscientious physician is tempted to provide the service rather than see the patient mistreated by a less than scrupulous caretaker. The lines blur when a man with a clearly psychogenic problem begs for just one papaverine injection so that he can have a successful experience with his wife. What would be the harm? On the other hand, when one learns that the wife is an alcoholic, does not even know that her husband is seeing a doctor about the sexual problem, and has told her husband that she no longer is interested in sex, the clinician begins to see the possibility that a sudden, 3-hour erection could provoke a marital crisis or, at the least, set the scene for one more dismal sexual failure.

The very patient who says he understands all the risks of surgery or medical treatment and admits the problem is psychogenic but wishes a medical cure anyway, is the one likely to turn around and sue the physician because the penile prosthesis left his penis one inch shorter than in its original erect condition. Giving in to pressure is a disservice to one's patient and oneself.

SEXUAL FREEDOM IN INSTITUTIONS

Clinicians who treat inpatients in hospitals, nursing homes, or rehabilitation programs may be asked to mediate between the institution and patient when issues arise concerning the right to engage in sexual activity.

Sometimes an institutional policy forbids sex between residents, ostensibly to protect them, but more often to avoid offending staff or patients' families. Patients who are severely mentally impaired do need protection from sexual abuse, but limits on consensual sex between patients are hard to defend, especially if contraception and safeguards against sexually transmitted diseases are provided, for example, by teaching patients to use barrier contraceptives and by routine, periodic health screening.

The practice of many residental homes for the elderly of banning all sexual contact, even between spouses, is particularly indefensible (Kassel, 1983). Residents of nursing homes need privacy for masturbation or for partner sexual activity. Some facilities have special rooms that patients can use. Even in a medical hospital, long-term patients need the right to hang a "Do Not Disturb" sign on the door for reasonable periods. Nurses, physicians, and other caretakers should be educated about the human need for touch and the disruption to emotional and physical health that occurs in the absence of intimacy.

The sexuality specialist occasionally has the chance to act as a consultant to change staff's beliefs and practices regarding sexuality for patients.

Ricky was a 32-year-old man with a mental age of 5. He had been institutionalized since early childhood and since puberty had needed frequent sedation and sometimes even physical restraints because of explosive episodes of aggression. Some of the aggression seemed to be evoked by sexual frustration and was directed at female caretakers. Ricky's father continued to visit him periodically. On one such occasion he brought his son an inflatable plastic doll that had breasts and a vagina. He dressed the doll in women's clothes and Ricky was fascinated by it. The psychologist in the institution supported Ricky's father and got the caretakers to agree to give Ricky daily private time with his doll. After that time Ricky's aggressive outbursts decreased greatly, except on a few occasions when other residents or a new caretaker teased him by taking his doll. His need for sedation also declined and he could often be calmed down by a quiet talk.

PREVENTION OF SEXUAL ABUSE BY CLINICIANS

Statistics on sexual relationships between mental health professionals and their patients have been consistent across a number of surveys (Pope, Keith-Spiegel, & Tabachnick, 1986). About 5% to 10% of male therapists and 1% or 2% of women surveyed anonymously admit to having had sex with a patient. Another consistent finding has been a syndrome of traumatization, anger, and distrust in women who were involved as patients with their therapist (Apfel & Simon, 1985; Feldman-Summers & Jones, 1984; Pope *et al.*, 1986). Although our view of such relationships may be negatively biased by the characteristics of women who volunteer to participate in research on this topic or who seek further psychotherapy after an exploitive relationship, the potential for damage to the patient is clear (Pope & Bouhoutsos, 1986). In the United States, both the American Psychological and American Psychiatric Associations have declared sex between therapist and patient to be unethical. Psychotherapy involves a special kind of relationship, but sexual contacts with other health professionals can also be detrimental to the patient if a breach of trust is involved (Burgess, 1981; Feldman-Summers & Jones, 1984). Sexual exploitation of patients by technicians and caretakers in institutions is reported to be an even more common problem than sexual relationships with fully trained professionals (Bell, 1983; Edelwich & Brodsky, 1982).

As Pope and Bouhoutsos (1986) have pointed out, training programs for mental health clinicians, as well as other health care professionals, pay little or no attention to coping with feelings of sexual attraction to patients. Many psychotherapists regard their own sexual arousal as a taboo feeling that should never occur in a session (Schover, 1983). Yet, in a recent survey of psychologists, Pope *et al.* (1986) found that only 5% of men and 24% of women had never felt attracted to a patient. Men were more likely to notice a female patient's appearance, whereas women therapists were impressed by a male patient's professional success.

We agree with Pope and Bouhoutsos (1986) and with Holroyd (1983) that therapists need to learn to use their sexual response to patients in a therapeutic way. Like any emotional response to a patient, sexual feelings may simply be an indicator of the therapist's own state of mind. Perhaps the clinician is lonely or sexually frustrated. Sometimes a patient has qualities that are close to the therapist's ideal in a lover. More often, however, sexual attraction to a patient is a valuable clue to the patient's interactive style. Some patients are sexually seductive when they want attention or nurturance. Sexual feelings expressed early in therapy often fall into this category. In a more positive light, a sexual attraction between patient and therapist can signal a new depth of trust and sharing, especially as the patient improves and becomes more independent and mature (Searles, 1959).

A therapist must remain aware of sexual attraction to a patient, since denying the feelings can lead to ignoring or negatively reinforcing important clinical material, especially when the patient is exploring sexual issues (Schover, 1981, 1983). When therapists are comfortable with their own sexuality and have evolved personal boundaries about socializing with patients and physical touching of patients, sexual attraction becomes no more disturbing than anger toward a patient. Both reactions can be tricky to manage but are a routine aspect of being a clinician. Good clinical supervision is indispensable in this learning process. Pope *et al.* (1986) also suggest that training programs for therapists integrate material on handling sexual issues and feelings into their basic curricula. We would add that health care professionals who are not psychotherapists could also benefit from such instruction.

COPING WITH THE SEDUCTIVE OR
ACTING-OUT PATIENT

One of us (Jensen & Møhl, 1987) often uses a training exercise in which student therapists write down their worst fears about working with patients' sexual issues. We find that men most commonly fear feeling tempted to have sex with a patient, and women fear the male patient who is aggressively angry or seductive. A minority of patients do make sexual advances to therapists, confirming both men's and women's negative fantasies. Situations range from the hospitalized patient deliberately exposing his or her genitals or touching a caretaker inappropriately to the psychotherapy patient who propositions the therapist verbally.

The following guidelines can help the clinician feel prepared to deal with seductive or acting-out patients:

- Remember that sexual advances from patients usually have some hidden goal. Is the patient seeking nurturance, expressing rage, or perhaps testing the limits to see if the therapist can be trusted? Understanding the patient's motivation is helpful in determining your own response.
- Inappropriate sexual behavior may be a symptom of cognitive impairment or psychosis. Hospitalized patients whose acting out is disruptive may be managed with a behavior modification program that extinguishes sexual acting out or limits sexual behavior such as masturbation to certain locations. The patient's needs for affection and touch should be met in alternate ways. In severe cases, neuroleptic medication may be prescribed.
- If a patient has a history of violent sexual aggression, therapy sessions should take place in an office that is not isolated, where the therapist can get immediate help. Having a "panic button" under the desk can increase the therapist's safety and thus enhance her or his ability to focus on treating the patient.
- Reacting with anger to a seductive patient is counterproductive. The angry therapist just gives the message that indeed, the patient has succeeded in sabotaging the therapeutic relationship.
- The therapist can ignore a seductive comment the first time or two it occurs, but continued signs of an eroticized transference reaction need to be discussed with the patient. The focus is on helping the patient examine his or her own feelings and exploring what the therapy process reveals about other close relationships in the patient's life.
- When a patient's sexual feelings are disturbing the therapy process, consult a colleague and get supervision. An objective supervisor can help you decide whether to refer the patient out or to continue, and may be able to suggest good therapeutic strategies. Timely supervision prevents therapist errors such as sexual acting out with patients or unnecessary terminations. If you feel you can no longer work productively in the therapy relationship, you still have an ethical obligation to refer the patient to a therapist who may be more effective. Many patients set themselves up for abandonment by their excessive dependency or obnoxious sexual comments. A skillful therapist tries to interrupt this destructive cycle.

CONCLUDING COMMENTS

This book is intended as a practical guide to understanding, assessing, and treating sexual problems in chronically ill patients. No book is a substitute for direct training and supervision, but we hope readers whose work touches on this new area of care will feel inspired to learn more and to apply our approach to the many medical patients in need of sexual education, brief counseling, or intensive therapy. We will feel satisfied only when sexual health care becomes a standard aspect of medical and psychological care worldwide.

References

Abel, E. L. (1985). *Psychoactive drugs and sex*. New York: Plenum Press.

Abelson, D. (1975). Diagnostic value of the penile pulse and blood pressure: A Doppler study of impotence in diabetics. *Journal of Urology, 113*, 636–639.

Akhtar, S., Crocker, E., Dickey, N., Helfrich, J., & Rheuban, W. J. (1977). Overt sexual behavior among psychiatric inpatients. *Diseases of the Nervous System, 38*, 359–361.

Althof, S. E., Coffman, C. B., & Levine, S. B. (1984). The effects of coronary bypass surgery on female sexual, psychological, and vocational adaptation. *Journal of Sex and Marital Therapy, 10*, 176–184.

Alzate, H. (1985). Vaginal eroticism: A replication study. *Archives of Sexual Behavior, 14*, 529–537.

Amberson, J. I., & Hoon, P. (1985). Hemodynamics of sequential orgasm. *Archives of Sexual Behavior, 14*, 351–360.

Amelar, R. D., & Dubin, L. (1982). Sexual function and fertility in paraplegic males. *Urology, 20*, 62–65.

American Council on Science and Health. (1983). Postmenopausal estrogen therapy (Report). Summit, NJ: Author.

American Psychiatric Association. (1980). *Quick reference to the diagnostic criteria from Diagnostic and Statistical Manual of Mental Disorders (3rd ed.)*. Washington, DC: American Psychiatric Association.

Andersen, B. L. (1983). Primary orgasmic dysfunction: Diagnostic considerations and review of treatment. *Psychological Bulletin, 93*, 105–136.

Andersen, B. L. (1985). Sexual functioning morbidity among cancer survivors: Current status and future directions. *Cancer, 55*, 1835–1842.

Andersen, B. L., & Hacker, N. E. (1983). Psychosexual adjustment after vulvar surgery. *Obstetrics and Gynecology, 62*, 457–462.

Anderson, F., & Bardach, J. L. (1983). Sexuality and neuromuscular disease: A pilot study. *International Rehabilitation Medicine, 5*, 21–26.

Annon, J. S. & Robinson, C. H. (1978). The use of vicarious learning models in treatment of sexual concerns. In J. LoPiccolo & L. LoPiccolo (Eds.), *Handbook of sex therapy* (pp. 35–56). New York: Plenum Press.

Apfel, R. J., & Simon, B. (1985). Patient–therapist sexual contact: II. Problems of subsequent psychotherapy. *Psychotherapy and Psychosomatics, 43*, 63–68.

Apfelbaum, B. (1984). The ego-analytic approach to individual bodywork sex therapy: Five case examples. *Journal of Sex Research, 20*, 1–27.

Appelt, H., & Strauss, B. (1984). Effects of antiandrogen treatment on the sexuality of women with hyperandrogenism. *Psychotherapy and Psychosomatics, 42*, 177–181.

Arentewicz, G., & Schmidt, G. (1983). *The treatment of sexual disorders*. New York: Basic Books.

Arthritis Foundation (1982). *Arthritis: Living and loving: Information about sex* (9190, 9197–9182). Atlanta, GA: Arthritis Foundation.

317

Bachmann, G. A., Leiblum, S. R., Kemmann, E., Colburn, D. W., Swartzman, L., & Shelden, R. (1984). Sexual expression and its determinants in the post-menopausal woman. *Maturitas, 6,* 19–29.

Bachmann, G. A., Leiblum, S. R., Sandler, B., Ainsley, W., Narcessian, R., Shelden, R., & Hymans, H. N. (1985). Correlates of sexual desire in postmenopausal women. *Maturitas, 7,* 211–216.

Backstrom, T., Sanders, D., Leask, R., Davidson, D., Warner, P., & Bancroft, J. (1983). Mood, sexuality, hormones, and the menstrual cycle: II. Hormone levels and their relationship to the premenstrual syndrome. *Psychosomatic Medicine, 45,* 503–507.

Balslev, I., & Harling, H. (1983). Sexual dysfunction following operation for carcinoma of the rectum. *Diseases of the Colon and Rectum, 26,* 785–788.

Bancroft, J. (1984). Hormones and human sexual behavior. *Journal of Sex and Marital Therapy, 10,* 3–21.

Bancroft, J., Sanders, D., Davidson, D., & Warner, P. (1983). Mood, sexuality, hormones, and the menstrual cycle: III. Sexuality and the role of androgens. *Psychosomatic Medicine, 45,* 509–516.

Bancroft, J., & Wu, F. C. W. (1983). Changes in erectile responsiveness during androgen replacement therapy. *Archives of Sexual Behavior, 12,* 59–66.

Bansal, S., Wincze, J. P., Nirenberg, T., Liepman, M. R., & Engle-Friedman, A. (1986, September). *Evolution of sexual function and pituitary-Leydig cell axis in chronic alcoholic males during sobriety.* Paper presented at the annual meeting of the International Academy of Sex Research, Amsterdam, The Netherlands.

Banting, F. G., & Best, C. H. (1922). The internal secretion of the pancreas. *Journal of Laboratory and Clinical Medicine, 7,* 251.

Barbach. L. (1982). *For each other: Sharing sexual intimacy.* New York: Anchor Press/Doubleday.

Barry, J. M., Blank, B. H., & Boileau, M. (1980). Nocturnal penile tumescence monitoring with stamps. *Urology, 15,* 171–172.

Bass, C. (1984). Psychosocial outcome after coronary bypass surgery. *British Journal of Psychiatry, 145,* 526–532.

Battaglia, A. R., Graziano, M. R., & Fonti, M. G. S. (1983). Experimental research into the changes in the way sexuality is experienced by the infertile woman. *Acta Europaea Fertilitatis, 14,* 67–73.

Beaser, R. S., Van der Hoek, C., Jacobson, A. M., Flood, T. M., & Desautels, R. E. (1982). Experience with penile prostheses in the treatment of impotence in diabetic men. *Journal of the American Medical Association, 248,* 943–948.

Beck, J. G., & Barlow, D. H. (1984). Current conceptualizations of sexual dysfunction: A review and an alternative perspective. *Clinical Psychology Review, 4,* 363–378.

Beck, J. G., Sakheim, D. K., & Barlow, D. H. (1983). Operating characteristics of the vaginal photoplethysmograph: Some implications for its use. *Archives of Sexual Behavior, 12,* 43–58.

Bedsworth, J. A., & Molen, M. T. (1982). Psychological stress in spouses of patients with myocardial infarction. *Heart and Lung, 11,* 450–456.

Bell, C. C. (1983). On sex and the psychiatric patient [Letter to the editor]. *American Journal of Psychiatry, 140,* 1269.

Bell, D., Lewis, R., & Kerstein, M. D. (1983). Hyperemic stress test in diagnosis of vasculogenic impotence. *Urology, 22,* 611–613.

Belzer, E. G., Whipple, B., & Moger, W. (1984). On female ejaculation. *Journal of Sex Research, 20,* 403–406.

Benedek, T. G., & Kubinec, J. (1982). The evaluation of impotence by sexual congress and alternatives thereto in divorce proceedings. *Transdisciplinary Studies of the College of Physicians, Philadelphia, 4,* 122–153.

Benkert, O., Witt, W., Adam, W., & Leitz, A. (1979). Effects of testosterone undecanoate on sexual potency and the hypothalamic-pituitary-gonadal axis of impotent males. *Archives of Sexual Behavior, 8*, 471-479.

Benson, G. S., & McConnell, J. (1983). Erectile physiology: Adrenergic innervation of the penis: In vitro studies. In R. J. Krane, M. B. Siroky, & I. Goldstein (Eds.), *Male sexual dysfunction* (pp. 21-26). Boston: Little, Brown & Co.

Berg, R., Mindus, P., Berg, G., & Gustafson, H. (1984). Penile implants in erectile impotence: Outcome and prognostic indicators. *Scandinavian Journal of Urology and Nephrology, 18*, 277-282.

Bergman, B., Damber, J. E., Littbrand, B., Sjögren, K., & Tomic, R. (1984). Sexual function in prostatic cancer patients treated with radiotherapy, orchiectomy, or oestrogens. *British Journal of Urology, 56*, 64-69.

Bergman, B., Nilsson, S., & Petersen, I. (1979). The effect on erection and orgasm of cystectomy, prostatectomy, and vesiculectomy for cancer of the bladder: A clinical and electromyographic study. *British Journal of Urology, 51*, 114-120.

Berkman, A. H., Katz, L. A., & Weissman, R. (1982). Sexuality and the lifestyle of home dialysis patients. *Archives of Physical Medicine and Rehabilitation, 63*, 272-275.

Bernstein, J., Potts, N., & Mattox, J. H. (1985). Assessment of psychological dysfunction associated with infertility. *Journal of Obstetrical, Gynecological, and Neonatal Nursing, 14* (Suppl.), 63-66.

Billet, A., Dagher, F. J., & Queral, L. A. (1982). Surgical correction of vasculogenic impotence in a patient after bilateral renal transplantation. *Surgery, 91*, 108-112.

Blair, J. H., & Simpson, G. M. (1966). Effect of antipsychotic drugs on reproductive functions. *Diseases of the Nervous System, 27*, 645-647.

Blaivas, J. G., Nagler, H., Katz, G., White, R. D., & Barballas, G. A. (1982). The diagnosis and treatment of erectile dysfunction [Abstract 391]. *Journal of Urology, 130*, 175.

Blaivas, J. G., Zayed, A. A. H., & Labib, K. B. (1981). The bulbocavernosus reflex in urology: A prospective study of 299 patients. *Journal of Urology, 126*, 191-199.

Blay, S. L., Ferraz, M. P. T., & Calil, H. M. (1982). Lithium-induced male sexual impairment: Two case reports. *Journal of Clinical Psychiatry, 43*, 497-498.

Blumstein, P., & Schwartz, P. (1983). *American couples: Money, work, sex.* New York: Pocket Books.

Bohlen, J. G. (1982). "Female ejaculation" and urinary stress incontinence. *Journal of Sex Research, 18*, 360-363.

Bohlen, J. G., Held, J. P., Sanderson, M. O., & Ahlgren, A. (1982a). The female orgasm: Pelvic contractions. *Archives of Sexual Behavior, 11*, 367-386.

Bohlen, J. G., Held, J. P., Sanderson, M. O., & Boyer, C. M. (1982b). Development of a woman's multiple orgasm pattern: A research case report. *Journal of Sex Research, 18*, 130-145.

Bohlen, J. G., Held, J. P., Sanderson, M. O., & Patterson, R. P. (1984). Heart rate, rate-pressure product, and oxygen uptake during four sexual activities. *Archives of Internal Medicine, 144*, 1745-1748.

Bouchelouche, P., Bartram P., & Jensen, S. B. (1985). The sexual consequences and problems in marital relations in patients with chronic renal disease. *Ugeskrift for Laeger, 147*, 3347-3350.

Bradley, W. E., Timm, G. W., Gallagher, J. M., & Johnson, B. K. (1985). New method for continuous measurement of noctural penile tumescence and rigidity. *Urology, 26*, 4-9.

Brannen, G. E., Peters, T. G., Hambridge, K. M., Kumpe, D. A., Kempczinski, R., Schroter, G. P. J., & Weil, R. (1980). Impotence after kidney transplantation. *Urology, 15*, 138-146.

Brashear, R. E. (1980). Chronic obstructive pulmonary disease. In D. Simmons (Ed.), *Current pulmonology: Volume 2.* Boston: Houghton-Mifflin.

Bray, G. P., DeFrank, R. S., & Wolfe, T. C. (1981). Sexual functioning in stroke survivors. *Archives of Physical Medicine and Rehabilitation, 62*, 286–288.

Brecher, E. M. (1984). *Love, sex, and aging.* Mount Vernon, NY: Consumers Union.

Brindley, G. S. (1983). Cavernosal alpha-blockade: A new technique for investigating and treating erectile impotence. *British Journal of Psychiatry, 143*, 332–337.

Brindley, G. S., & Gillan, P. (1982). Men and women who do not have orgasms. *British Journal of Psychiatry, 140*, 351–356.

Brooks, M. E., Berezin, J., & Braf, Z. F. (1982). Effect of phenoxybenzamine on penile tumescence in diabetic men. *Urological Research, 10*, 249–251.

Brown, H. N., & Zinberg, N. E. (1982). Difficulties in the integration of psychological and medical practices. *American Journal of Psychiatry, 139*, 1576–1582.

Brownell, K. D., Marlatt, G. A., Lichtenstein, E., & Wilson, G. T. (1986). Understanding and preventing relapse. *American Psychologist, 41*, 765–782.

Brownell, K. D., & Stunkard, A. J. (1981). Couples training, pharmacotherapy, and behavior therapy in the treatment of obesity. *Archives of General Psychiatry, 38*, 1224–1229.

Buckwalter, K. C., Wernimont, T., & Buckwalter, J. A. (1982). Musculoskeletal conditions and sexuality (Part II). *Sexuality and Disability, 5*, 195–207.

Bukberg, J., Penman, D., & Holland, S. C. (1984). Depression in hospitalized cancer patients. *Psychosomatic Medicine, 46*, 199–212.

Burgess, A. W. (1981). Physician sexual misconduct and patients' responses. *American Journal of Psychiatry, 138*, 1335–1342.

Burrows, B. (1976). Pulmonary terms and symbols. *Chest, 67*, 583–593.

Burton, G., & Kaplan, H. M. (1968). Sexual behavior and adjustment of married alcoholics. *Quarterly Journal of Studies on Alcohol, 29*, 603–609.

Buvat, J., Buvat-Herbaut, M., Dehaene, J. L., & Lemaire, A. (1986a). Is intracavernous injection of papaverine a reliable screening test for vascular impotence? *Journal of Urology, 135*, 476–478.

Buvat, J., Lemaire, A., Buvat-Herbaut, M., Fourlinnie, J. C., Racadot, A., & Fossati, P. (1985a). Hyperprolactinemia and sexual function in men. *Hormone Research, 22*, 196–203.

Buvat, J., Lemaire, A., Buvat-Herbaut, M., Guieu, J. D., Bailleul, J. P., & Fossati, P. (1985b). Comparative investigations in 26 impotent and 26 nonimpotent diabetic patients. *Journal of Urology, 133*, 34–38.

Buvat, J., Lemaire, A., Dehaene, J. L., Buvat-Herbaut, M., & Guieu, J. D. (1986b). Venous incompetence: Critical study of the organic basis of high maintenance flow rates during artificial erection test. *Journal of Urology, 135*, 926–928.

Campese, V. M., Procci, W. R., Levitan, D., Romoff, M. S., Goldstein, D. A., & Massry, S. G. (1982). Autonomic nervous system dysfunction and impotence in uremia. *American Journal of Nephrology, 2*, 140–143.

Cancer Facts and Figures. (1986). New York: American Cancer Society.

Caplan, G. (1964). *Principles of preventive psychiatry.* New York: Basic Books.

Carmelli, D., Swan, G. E., & Rosenman, R. H. (1985). The relationship between wives' social and psychologic status and their husband's coronary heart disease: A case–control study from the Western Collaborative Group Study. *American Journal of Epidemiology, 122*, 90–100.

Chambless, D. L., Stein, T., Sultan, F. E., Williams, A. J., Goldstein, A. J., Lineberger, M. H., Lifshitz, J. L., & Kelly, L. (1982). The pubococcygens and female orgasm: A correlational study with normal subjects. *Archives of Sexual Behavior, 11*, 479–490.

Chandra, V., Szklo, M., Goldberg, R., & Tonascia, J. (1983). The impact of marital status on survival after an acute myocardial infarction: A population-based study. *American Journal of Epidemiology, 117*, 320–325.

Chapman, R. M. (1982). Effect of cytotoxic therapy on sexuality and gonadal function. *Seminars in Oncology*, *9*, 84–94.

Charles, D., & Glover, D. D. (1985). Psychosexual problems related to pelvic pain. In M. Farber (Ed.), *Human sexuality: Psychosexual effects of disease* (pp. 159–168). New York: Macmillan.

Chowanec, G. D., & Binik, Y. M. (1982). End stage renal disease (ESRD) and the marital dyad: A literature review and critique. *Social Science and Medicine*, *16*, 1551–1558.

Christensen, D. N. (1983). Postmastectomy couple counseling: An outcome study of a structured treatment protocol. *Journal of Sex and Marital Therapy*, *9*, 266–275.

Clark, J. T., Smith, E. R., & Davidson, J. M. (1984). Enhancement of sexual motivation in male rats by yohimbine. *Science*, *225*, 847–849.

Clulow, C. (1984). Sexual dysfunction and interpersonal stress: The significance of the presenting complaint in seeking and engaging help. *British Journal of Medical Psychology*, *57*, 371–380.

Cluss, P. A., & Fireman, P. (1985). Recent trends in asthma research. *Annals of Behavioral Medicine*, *7*, 11–16.

Coffman, C. B., Levine, S. B., Althof, S. E., & Stern, R. C. (1984). Sexual adaptation among single young adults with cystic fibrosis. *Chest*, *86*, 412–418.

Cole, C. M. (1979). A treatment strategy for postmyocardial sexual dysfunction. *Sexuality and Disability*, *2*, 122–129.

Cole, C. M., Levin, E. M., Whitley, J. O., & Young, S. H. (1979). Brief sexual counseling during cardiac rehabilitation. *Heart and Lung*, *8*, 124–129.

Comarr, A. E., & Vigue, M. (1978). Sexual counseling among male and female patients with spinal cord and/or cauda equina injury. *American Journal of Physical Medicine*, *57*, 215–227.

Condra, M., Morales, A., Owen, J. A., Surridge, D. H., & Fenemore, J. (1986a). Prevalence and significance of tobacco smoking in impotence. *Urology*, *27*, 495–498.

Condra, M., Morales, A., Surridge, D. H., Owen, J. A., Marshall, P., & Fenemore, J. (1986b). The unreliability of nocturnal penile tumescence recording as an outcome measurement in the treatment of organic impotence. *Journal of Urology*, *135*, 280–282.

Cooper, A. J. (1985). Myocardial infarction and advice on sexual activity. *The Practitioner*, *229*, 575–579.

Cooper, A. J. (1986). Progestogens in the treatment of male sex offenders: A review. *Canadian Journal of Psychiatry*, *31*, 73–79.

Cooper, A. J., & Magnus, R. V. (1984). A clinical trial of the beta blocker propranolol in premature ejaculation. *Journal of Psychosomatic Research*, *28*, 331–336.

Corby, N., & Zarit, J. M. (1983). Old and alone: The unmarried in later life. In R. B. Weg (Ed.), *Sexuality in the later years: Roles and behavior* (pp. 131–147). New York: Academic Press.

Coyne, J. C. (1986). Strategic marital therapy for depression. In N. S. Jacobson & A. S. Gurman (Eds.), *Clinical Handbook of Marital Therapy* (pp. 495–512). New York: Guilford Press.

Coyne, J. C., & Holroyd, K. (1982). Stress, coping, and illness: A transactional perspective. In T. Millon, C. Green, & R. Meagher (Eds.), *Handbook of clinical health psychology* (pp. 103–128). New York: Plenum Press.

Critchlow, B. (1986). The powers of John Barleycorn: Beliefs about the effects of alcohol on social behavior. *American Psychologist*, *41*, 751–764.

Crowe, R., Lincoln, J., Blacklay, P. F., Pryor, J. P., Lumley, J. S. P., & Burnstock, G. (1983). Vasoactive intestinal polypeptide-like immunoreactive nerves in diabetic penis. *Diabetes*, *32*, 1075–1077.

Crowther, J. H. (1985). The relationship between depression and marital maladjustment: A descriptive study. *Journal of Nervous and Mental Disease*, *173*, 227–231.

Cullberg, J. (1984). *Psykodynamisk psykiatri.* Copenhagen, Hans Reitzels Forlag.

Cutler, W. B., Garcia, C., Edwards, D. A. (1983). *Menopause: A guide for women and the men who love them.* New York: W. W. Norton & Co.

Davidson, J. M., Camargo, C. A., & Smith, E. R. (1979). Effects of androgen on sexual behavior in hypogonadal men. *Journal of Clinical Endocrinology and Metabolism, 48*, 955–958.

Davidson, J. M., Camargo, C. A., Smith, E. R., & Kwan, M. (1983). Maintenance of sexual function in a castrated man treated with ovarian steroids. *Archives of Sexual Behavior, 12*, 263–274.

De Amicis, L. A., Goldberg, D. C., LoPiccolo, J., Friedman, J., & Davies, L. (1985). Clinical follow-up of couples treated for sexual dysfunction. *Archives of Sexual Behavior, 14*, 467–490.

De La Fuente, J. R., & Rosenbaum, A. H. (1981). Prolactin in psychiatry. *American Journal of Psychiatry, 138*, 1154–1160.

Del Bene, E., Conti, C., Poggioni, M., & Sicuteri, F. (1982). Sexuality and headache. *Advances in Neurology, 33*, 209–214.

Delcour, C., Wespes, E., Schulman, C. C., & Struyven, J. (1984). Investigation of the venous system in impotence of vascular origin. *Urologic Radiology, 6*, 190–193.

DeLeo, D., & Magni, G. (1983). Sexual side effects of antidepressant drugs. *Psychosomatics, 24*, 1076–1082.

Dennerstein, L., & Burrows, G. D. (1982). Hormone replacement therapy and sexuality in women. *Clinics in Endocrinology and Metabolism, 11*, 661–679.

Derogatis, L. R. (1983a). Psychological testing: Diagnosis and diagnostic techniques. In J. K. Meyer, C. W. Schmidt, & T. N. Wise (Eds.), *Clinical management of sexual disorders* (2nd ed.) (pp. 76–85). Baltimore, MD: Williams & Wilkins.

Derogatis, L. R. (1983b). *Psychosocial Adjustment to Illness Scale (PAIS & PAIS-SR): Administration, scoring and procedures manual—I.* Baltimore, MD: Clinical Psychometric Research.

Derogatis, L. R., & King, K. M. (1981). The coital coronary: A reassessment of the concept. *Archives of Sexual Behavior, 10*, 325–335.

Derogatis, L. R., & Melisaratos, N. (1983). The Brief Symptom Inventory: An introductory report. *Psychological Medicine, 13*, 595–605.

Derogatis, L. R., Meyer, J. K., & King, K. M. (1981). Psychopathology in individuals with sexual dysfunction. *American Journal of Psychiatry, 138*, 757–763.

Derogatis, L. R., Morrow, G. R., Fetting, J., Penman, D., Piasetsky, S., Schmale, A. M., Henrichs, M., & Carnicke, L. M. (1983). The prevalence of psychiatric disorders among cancer patients. *Journal of the American Medical Association, 249*, 751–757.

de Tejada, I. S., Goldstein, I., Heeren, T., & Krane, R. J. (1985). Association of vascular risk factors with penile brachial pressure index [Abstract 852]. *Journal of Urology, 133*, 327A.

Devins, G. M., Binik, Y. M., Hollomby, D. J., Barré, P. E., & Guttman, R. D. (1981). Helplessness and depression in end-stage renal disease. *Journal of Abnormal Psychology, 90*, 531–545.

De Vries, K., Degani, S., Eibschitz, I., Oettinger, M., Zilberman, A., & Sharf, M. (1984). The influence of the postcoital test on the sexual function of infertile women. *Journal of Psychosomatic Obstetrics and Gynaecology, 3*, 101–106.

Dewar, M. L., Blundell, P. E., Lidstone, D., Herba, M. J., & Chiu, R. C. (1985). Effects of abdominal aneurysmectomy, aortoiliac bypass grafting and angioplasty on male sexual potency: A prospective study. *Canadian Journal of Surgery, 28*, 154–159.

Dhabuwala, C. B., Ghayad, P., Smith, J. B., & Pierce, J. M. (1983). Penile calibration for nocturnal penile tumescence studies. *Urology, 22*, 614–616.

Dhabuwala, C. B., Kumar, A., & Pierce, J. M. (1986). Myocardial infarction and its influence on male sexual function. *Archives of Sexual Behavior, 15*, 499–504.

Dirks, J. F., Brown, E. L., & Robinson, S. K. (1982). The Battery of Asthma Illness Behavior: II. Independence from airways hyperactivity. *Journal of Asthma, 19*, 79–83.

Doherty, W. J., & Baird, M. A. (1984). *Family therapy and family medicine.* New York: Guilford Press.

Drago, F. (1984). Prolactin and sexual behavior: A review. *Neuroscience and Biobehavioral Reviews, 8*, 433–439.

Dunn, M. E., & Dickes, R. (1977). Erotic issues in cotherapy. *Journal of Sex and Marital Therapy, 3*, 205–211.

D'Zurilla, T. J., & Goldfried, M. R. (1971). Problem solving and behavior modification. *Journal of Abnormal Psychology, 78*, 107–126.

Ebbehøj, J., & Wagner, G. (1979). Insufficient penile erection due to abnormal drainage of cavernous bodies. *Urology, 13*, 507–510.

Edelwich, J., & Brodsky, A. (1982). *Sexual dilemmas for the helping professional.* New York: Brunner/Mazel.

Edwards, C. L., Loeffler, M., & Rutledge, F. N. (1981). Vaginal reconstruction. In A. C. von Eschenbach & D. B. Rodrieguez (Eds.), *Sexual rehabilitation of the urologic cancer patient* (pp. 250–265). Boston: G. K. Hall.

Ek, A., Bradley, W. E., & Krane, R. J. (1983). Nocturnal penile rigidity measured by the snap-gauge band. *Journal of Urology, 129*, 964–966.

Flist, J., Jarman, W. D., & Edson, M. (1984). Evaluating medical treatment of impotence. *Urology, 23*, 374–375.

Ellenberg, M. (1971). Impotence and diabetes mellitus: The neurological factor. *Annals of Internal Medicine, 75*, 213–219.

Ellenberg, M. (1977). Sexual aspects of the female diabetic. *Mount Sinai Journal of Medicine, 44*, 495–500.

Ellis, W. J., & Grayhack, J. T. (1963). Sexual function in aging males after orchiectomy and estrogen therapy. *Journal of Urology, 89*, 895–899.

Elst, P., Sybesma, T., van der Stadt, R. J., Prins, A. P. A., Muller, W. H., & den Butter, A. (1984). Sexual problems in rheumatoid arthritis and ankylosing spondylitis. *Arthritis and Rheumatism, 27*, 217–220.

Engel, G. L. (1977). The need for a new medical model: A challenge for biomedicine. *Science, 196*, 129–136.

Engel, G. L. (1980). The clinical application of the biopsychosocial model. *American Journal of Psychiatry, 137*, 535–544.

Erikson, E. (1963). *Childhood and Society.* New York: Norton.

Ermolenko, V. M., Kukhtevich, A. V., Dedov, I. I., Bunatian, A. F., Melnichenko, G. A., & Gitel, E. P. (1986). Parlodel treatment of uremic hypogonadism in men. *Nephron, 42*, 19–22.

Ertekin, C., Akyurekli, O., Gurses, A. N., & Turgut, H. (1985). The value of somatosensory-evoked potentials and bulbocavernosus reflex in patients with impotence. *Acta Neurologica Scandinavica, 71*, 48–53.

Ertekin, C., & Reel, F. (1976). Bulbocavernosus reflex in normal men and in patients with neurogenic bladder and/or impotence. *Journal of the Neurological Sciences, 28*, 1–15.

Fagan, P. J., Schmidt, C. W., Rick, J. A., Damewood, M. D., Halle, E., & Wise, T. N. (1986). Sexual functioning and psychologic evaluation of in vitro fertilization couples. *Fertility and Sterility, 46*, 668–672.

Fahrner, E. M. (1987). Sexual dysfunction of male alcohol addicts: Prevalence and treatment. *Archives of Sexual Behavior, 16*, 247–257.

Fairburn, C. G., Wu, F. C. W., McCulloch, D. K., Borsay, D. Q., Ewing, D. J., Clarke, B. F., & Bancroft, J. H. J. (1982). The clinical features of diabetic impotence: A preliminary study. *British Journal of Psychiatry, 140*, 447–452.

Fava, G. A. (1984). More data on hyperprolactinemia. [Letter to the editor]. *American Journal of Psychiatry, 141*, 1131–1132.

Feldman-Summers, S., & Jones, G. (1984). Psychological impacts of sexual contact between therapists or other health care practitioners and their clients. *Journal of Consulting and Clinical Psychology, 52*, 1054–1061.

Felstein, I. (1977). Respiratory problems in sexual medicine. *British Journal of Sexual Medicine, 78*, 24–25.

Ferguson, K., & Figley, B. (1979). Sexuality and rheumatic disease: A prospective study. *Sexuality and Disability, 2*, 130–138.

Ficher, M., Zuckerman, M., Fishkin, R. E., Goldman, A., Neeb, M., Fink, P. J., Cohen, S. N., Jacobs, J. A., & Weisberg, M. (1984). Do endocrines play an etiological role in diabetic and nondiabetic sexual dysfunctions? *Journal of Andrology, 5*, 8–16.

Fisher, C., Cohen, H. D., Schiavi, R. C., Davis, D., Furman, B., Ward, K., Edwards, A., & Cunningham, J. (1983). Patterns of female sexual arousal during sleep and waking: Vaginal thermoconductance studies. *Archives of Sexual Behavior, 12*, 97–122.

Fishman, I. J., Scott, F. B., Light, J. K. (1984). Experience with inflatable penile prosthesis. *Urology, 23*, 86–92.

Flanigan, D. P., Schuler, J. J., Kiefer, T., Schwartz, J. A., & Lim, L. T. (1982). Elimination of iatrogenic impotence and improvement of sexual function after aortoiliac revascularization. *Archives of Surgery, 117*, 544–549.

Flechner, S. M., Novick, A. C., Braun, W. E., Popowniak, K. L., & Steinmuller, D. (1983). Functional capacity and rehabilitation of recipients with a functioning renal allograft for ten years or more. *Transplantation, 35*, 572–576.

Fletcher, E. C., & Martin, R. J. (1982). Sexual dysfunction and erectile impotence in chronic obstructive pulmonary disease. *Chest, 81*, 413–421.

Flind, A. C. (1984). Cavernosal alpha-blockade: A Warning. *British Journal of Psychiatry, 144*, 329–330.

Flor, H., Turk, D. C., & Scholz, O. B. (1987). Impact of chronic pain on the spouse: Marital, emotional and physical consequences. *Journal of Psychosomatic Research, 31*, 63–71.

Fordney, D. S. (1978). Dyspareunia and vaginismus. *Clinical Obstetrics and Gynecology, 21*, 205–221.

Forsberg, L., Olsson, A. M., & Neglen, P. (1982). Erectile function before and after aorto-iliac reconstruction: A comparison between measurements of Doppler acceleration ratio, blood pressure and angiography. *Journal of Urology, 127*, 379–382.

Forstein, M. (1984). The psychosocial impact of the Acquired Immune Deficiency Syndrome. *Seminars in Oncology, 11*, 77–82.

Frank, E., Anderson, C., & Rubinstein, D. (1978). Frequency of sexual dysfunction in normal couples. *New England Journal of Medicine, 299*, 111–115.

Frank, E., & Boller, F. (1982). *Sexual dysfunction in neurological disorders*. New York: Raven Press.

Frantz, A. G., Wardlaw, S. L., Ragavan, V. V., Thoron, L., Wehrenberg, W. B., & Ferin, M. (1982). Opioid regulation of pituitary secretion. In A. F. DeNicola & J. A. Blaquier (Eds.), *Physiopathology of hypophysial disturbances and diseases of reproduction* (pp. 153–177). New York: Alan R. Liss.

Friedman, S., & Harrison, G. (1984). Sexual histories, attitudes, and behavior of schizophrenic and "normal" women. *Archives of Sexual Behavior, 13*, 555–568.

Fugl-Meyer, A. R., Sjögren, K., & Johansson, K. (1984). A vaginal temperature registration system. *Archives of Sexual Behavior, 13*, 247–260.

Garcea, N., Caruso, A., Campo, S., & Siccardi, P. (1982). Retrograde ejaculation: A more convenient method for artificial insemination. *European Journal of Obstetrics, Gynecology, and Reproductive Biology, 14,* 175–178.

Garde, K., & Lunde, I. (1982). *Voksne kvinder.* Copenhagen, Denmark: Lindhardt & Ringhoff.

Gartrell, N. (1986). Increased libido in women receiving trazodone. *American Journal of Psychiatry, 143,* 781–782.

Gay Men's Health Crisis (1985). An ounce of prevention: STD AIDS risk reduction guidelines for healthier sex as recommended by New York Physicians for Human Rights. New York: GMHC.

Gee, W. F., McRoberts, J. W., Raney, J. O., & Ansell, J. S. (1974). The impotent patient: Surgical treatment with penile prosthesis and psychiatric evaluation. *Journal of Urology, 111,* 41–43.

George, L. K., & Weiler, S. J. (1981). Sexuality in middle and late life: The effects of age, cohort, and gender. *Archives of General Psychiatry, 38,* 919–923.

Germaine, L. M., & Freedman, R. R. (1984). Behavioral treatment of menopausal hot flashes: Evaluation by objective methods. *Journal of Consulting and Clinical Psychology, 52,* 1072–1079.

Giambra, L. M., & Martin, C. E. (1977). Sexual daydreams and quantitative aspects of sexual activity: Some relations for males across adulthood. *Archives of Sexual Behavior, 6,* 497–505.

Girgis, S. M., El-Haggar, S., & El-Hermouzy, S. (1982). A double-blind trial of clomipramine in premature ejaculation. *Andrologia, 14,* 364–368.

Glass, C. A., Fielding, D. M., Evans, C., & Ashcroft, J. B. (1987). Factors related to sexual functioning in male patients undergoing hemodialysis and with kidney transplants. *Archives of Sexual Behavior, 16,* 189–208.

Glazer, R. D., & Thorpe, J. S. (1986). Unethical intimacy: A survey of sexual contact and advances between psychology educators and female graduate students. *American Psychologist, 41,* 43–51.

Godec, C. J. (1985). Comparative evaluation of impotence with vibration and nocturnal monitoring. *Urology, 25,* 135–138.

Goldberg, D. C., Whipple, B., Fishkin, R. E., Waxman, H., Fink, P. J., & Weisberg, M. (1983). The Grafenberg Spot and female ejaculation: A review of initial hypotheses. *Journal of Sex and Marital Therapy, 9,* 27–37.

Golden, J. S., & Golden, M. A. (1976). You know who and what's her name: The woman's role in sex therapy. *Journal of Sex and Marital Therapy, 2,* 6–16.

Goldman, J. A., Schechter, A., & Eckerling, B. (1970). Carbohydrate metabolism in infertile and impotent men. *Fertility and Sterility, 21,* 397–401.

Goldstein, I. (1983). Neurologic impotence. In R. J. Krane, M. B. Siroky, & I. Goldstein (Eds.), *Male sexual dysfunction* (pp. 193–201). Boston: Little, Brown & Co.

Goldstein, I., Feldman, M. I., Deckers, P. J., Babayan, R. K., & Krane, R. J. (1984). Radiation-associated impotence: A clinical study of its mechanism. *Journal of the American Medical Association, 251,* 903–910.

Goldstein, I., Mortara, R. W., & Krane, R. J. (1985). Penile revascularization: Three years' experience [Abstract 304]. *Journal of Urology, 133,* 189A.

Goldstein, I., Siroky, M. B., Nath, R. L., McMillian, T. N., Menzoian, J. O., & Krane, R. J. (1982a). Vasculogenic impotence: Role of the pelvic steal test. *Journal of Urology, 128,* 300–306.

Goldstein, I., Siroky, M. B., Sax, D. S., & Krane, R. J. (1982b). Neurourologic abnormalities in multiple sclerosis. *Journal of Urology, 128,* 541–545.

Goldwasser, B., Carson, C. C., Braun, S. D., & McCann, R. L. (1985). Impotence due to the pelvic steal syndrome: Treatment by iliac transluminal angioplasty. *Journal of Urology, 133,* 860–861.

Goldwasser, B., Madgar, I., Jonas, P., Lunenfeld, B., & Many, M. (1983). Imipramine for the treatment of sterility in patients following retroperitoneal node dissection. *Andrologia, 15*, 588–591.

Goodstein, R. K. (1983). Overview: Cerebrovascular accident and the hospitalized elderly—A multidimensional clinical problem. *American Journal of Psychiatry, 140*, 141–147.

Gould, R. J., Murphy, K. M. M., Reynolds, I. J., & Snyder, S. H. (1984). Calcium channel blockade: Possible explanation for thioridazine's peripheral side effects. *American Journal of Psychiatry, 141*, 352–357.

Gove, W. R., Hughes, M., & Style, C. B. (1983). Does marriage have positive effects on the psychological well-being of an individual? *Journal of Health and Social Behavior, 24*, 122–131.

Graber, B., & Kline-Graber, P. (1979). Female orgasm: Role of the pubococcygeous muscle. *Journal of Clinical Psychiatry, 40*, 348–351.

Green, C. J. (1982). Psychological assessment in medical settings. In T. Millon, C. Green, & R. Meagher (Eds.), *Handbook of clinical health psychology* (pp. 339–375). New York: Plenum Press.

Gross, M. D. (1982). Reversal by bethanechol of sexual dysfunction caused by anticholinergic antidepressants. *American Journal of Psychiatry, 139*, 1193–1194.

Grunstein, H., Clifton-Bligh, P., Colagiuri, S., Rushworth, R., Robertson, S., Wilkinson, M., & Posen, S. (1984). Clinical disorders in patients with hyperprolactinemia. *The Medical Journal of Australia, 5*, 64–69.

Gu, J., Polak, J. M., Probert, L., Islam, K. N., Marangos, P. J., Mina, S., Adrian, T. E., McGregor, G. P., O'Shaughnessy, D. J., & Bloom, S. R. (1983). Peptidergic innervation of the human genital tract. *Journal of Urology, 130*, 386–391.

Haeberle, E. J. (1983). *The birth of sexology: A brief history in documents.* Bloomington, IN: The Kinsey Institute.

Hager, T. (1983). Pacemaker studied for impotence. *Journal of the American Medical Association, 250*, 583.

Haldeman, S., Bradley, W. E., Bhatia, N. N., & Johnson, B. K. (1982). Pudendal evoked responses. *Archives of Neurology, 39*, 280–283.

Hale, W. D. Cochran, C. D., & Hedgepeth, B. E. (1984). Norms for the elderly on the Brief Symptom Inventory. *Journal of Consulting and Clinical Psychology, 52*, 321–322.

Halpert, R., Fruchter, R. G., Sedlis, A., Butt, K., Boyce, J. G., & Sillman, F. H. (1986). Human papilloma virus and lower genital neoplasia in renal transplant patients. *Obstetrics and Gynecology, 68*, 251–258.

Hanson, E. I. (1982). Effects of chronic lung disease on life in general and on sexuality: Perceptions of adult patients. *Heart and Lung, 11*, 435–441.

Harman, S. M., & Tsitouras, P. D. (1980). Reproductive hormones in aging men. I. Measurement of sex steroids, basal luteinizing hormone, and Leydig cell response to human chorionic gonadotropin. *Journal of Clinical Endocrinology and Metabolism, 51*, 35–40.

Harrison, W., Stewart, J., Ehrhardt, A., Rabkin, J., McGrath, P., Liebowitz, M., & Quitkin, F. M. (1985). A controlled study of the effects of antidepressants on sexual function. *Psychopharmacology Bulletin, 21*, 85–88.

Hartman, W. A., & Fithian, M. A. (1972). *Treatment of sexual dysfunction: A bio-psycho-social approach.* Long Beach, CA: Center for Marital and Sexual Studies.

Hartman, W. A., & Fithian, M. A. (1984). *Any man can: The multiple orgasmic technique for every loving man.* New York: St. Martin.

Harvey, M., & Beckman, L. J. (1986). Alcohol consumption, female sexual behavior and contraceptive use. *Journal of Studies on Alcohol, 47*, 327–332.

Hawatmeh, I. S., Houttuin, E., Gregory, J. G., & Purcell, M. H. (1983). Vascular surgery for the treatment of the impotent male. In R. J. Krane, M. B. Siroky, & I. Goldstein (Eds.), *Male sexual dysfunction* (pp. 291–300). Boston: Little, Brown & Co.

Hawton, K. (1984). Sexual adjustment of men who have had strokes. *Journal of Psychosomatic Research, 28,* 243–249.

Haynes, S. G., Eaker, E. D., & Feinleib, M. (1983). Spouse behavior and coronary heart disease in men: Prospective results from the Framingham Heart Study: I. Concordance of risk factors and the relationship of psychosocial status to coronary incidence. *American Journal of Epidemiology, 118,* 1–22.

Heim, N. (1981). Sexual behavior of castrated sex offenders. *Archives of Sexual Behavior, 10,* 11–19.

Heiman, J. R., & LoPiccolo, J. (1983). Clinical outcome of sex therapy: Effects of daily vs. weekly treatment. *Archives of General Psychiatry, 40,* 443–449.

Heiman, J. R., LoPiccolo, L., & LoPiccolo, J. (1976). *Becoming orgasmic: A sexual growth program for women.* Englewood Cliffs, NJ: Prentice-Hall, Inc.

Heinrich, R. L., Schag, C. C., & Ganz, P. (1984). Living with cancer: The Cancer Inventory of Problem Situations. *Journal of Clinical Psychology, 40,* 972–980.

Hejl, B. L. (1984). Toward a psychosomatic understanding. *Nordisk Sexologi, 2,* 9–19.

Hellerstein, H. K., & Friedman, E. H. (1970). Sexual activity and the postcoronary patient. *Archives of Internal Medicine, 125,* 987–999.

Henson, D. E., Rubin, H. B., & Henson, C. (1982). Labial and vaginal blood volume responses to visual and tactile stimuli. *Archives of Sexual Behavior, 11,* 23–32.

Herd, A. J. (1984). Cardiovascular disease and hypertension. In W. D. Gentry (Ed.), *Handbook of behavioral medicine* (pp. 222–281). New York: Guilford Press.

Herstein, A., Hill, R. H., & Walters, K. (1977). Adult sexuality and juvenile rheumatoid arthritis. *Journal of Rheumatology, 4,* 35–39.

Hertoft, P. (1983). *Det er måske en galskab. Om sexualreform bevaegelsen.* Copenhagen, Denmark: Gyldendal.

Higgins, G. E. (1978). Aspects of sexual response in adults with spinal cord injury: A review of the literature. In J. LoPiccolo & L. LoPiccolo (Eds.), *Handbook of Sex Therapy* (pp. 387–410). New York: Plenum Press.

Hilsted, J., & Jensen, S. B. (1979). A simple test for autonomic neuropathy in juvenile diabetics. *Acta Medica Scandinavica, 205,* 385–387.

Hite, S. (1976). *The Hite Report.* New York: Dell Publishing Co.

Hite, S. (1981). *The Hite Report on Male Sexuality.* New York: Ballantine Books.

Hoch, Z. (1983). The G Spot [Letter to the editor]. *Journal of Sex and Marital Therapy, 9,* 166–167.

Holroyd, J. D. (1983). Erotic contact as an instance of sex-biased therapy. In J. Murray & P. R. Abramson (Eds.), *Bias in psychotherapy* (pp. 285–308). New York: Praeger.

Hoon, P. W. (1984). Physiologic assessment of sexual response in women: The unfulfilled promise. *Clinical Obstetrics and Gynecology, 27,* 767–780.

Horowitz, M. J. (1982). Psychological processes induced by illness, injury, and loss. In T. Millon, C. Green, & R. Meagher (Eds.), *Handbook of clinical health psychology* (pp. 53–67). New York: Plenum Press.

Horwith, M., & Imperato-McGinley, J. (1983). The medical evaluation of disorders of sexual desire in males and females. In H. S. Kaplan (Ed.) *The evaluation of sexual disorders: Psychological and medical aspects* (pp. 183–196). New York: Brunner/Mazel.

House, W. C., & Pendleton, L. (1986). Sexual dysfunction in diabetes: A survey of physicians' responses to patients' problems. *Postgraduate Medicine, 79,* 227–235.

Huckins, C. (1983). Adult spermatogenesis: Characteristics, kinetics, and control. In L. I. Lipschultz, & S. S. Howards (Eds.), *Infertility in the male* (pp. 249–264). New York: Churchill Livingstone.

Hunt, M. (1974). *Sexual behavior in the 1970's.* Chicago: Playboy Press.

Infante, M. C. (1981). Sexual dysfunction in the patient with chronic back pain. *Sexuality and Disability, 4,* 173–178.

International Association for the Study of Pain, Subcommittee on Taxonomy (1979). Pain terms: A list with definitions and notes on usage. *Pain, 6*, 249–252.

Jackson, G. (1981). Sexual intercourse and angina pectoris. *International Rehabilitation Medicine, 3*, 92–94.

Jacobson, N. S., & Margolin, G. (1979). *Marital therapy: Strategies based on social learning and behavior exchange principles.* New York: Brunner/Mazel.

Jenkins, C. D., Zyzanski, S. J., & Rosenman, R. H. (1971). Progress towards validation of a computer-scored test for the Type-A coronary prone behavior pattern. *Psychosomatic Medicine, 33*, 193–202.

Jensen, S. B. (1979a). Sexual customs and dysfunction in alcoholics: Part I. *British Journal of Sexual Medicine, 53*, 29–32.

Jensen, S. B. (1979b). Sexual customs and dysfunction in alcoholics: Part II. *British Journal of Sexual Medicine, 54*, 30–34.

Jensen, S. B. (1981a). Diabetic sexual dysfunction: A comparative study of 160 insulin-treated diabetic men and women and age-matched control group. *Archives of Sexual Behavior, 10*, 493–497.

Jensen, S. B. (1981b). Sexual dysfunction in male diabetics and alcoholics; A comparative study. *Sexuality and Disability, 4*, 215–219.

Jensen, S. B. (1982). Klinisk sexologi i almen praksis. *Ugeskrift for Laeger, 144*, 2484–2489.

Jensen, S. B. (1983). Sexologisk workshop. *Nordisk Sexologi, 1*, 86–87.

Jensen, S. B. (1984a). [Editorial]. *Nordic Sexology, 2*, 107–108.

Jensen, S. B. (1984b). Sexual dysfunction in younger married alcoholics: A comparative study. *Acta Psychiatrica Scandinavica, 69*, 543–559.

Jensen, S. B. (1985a). Emotional aspects in diabetes mellitus: A study of somatopsychologic reactions in 51 couples in which one partner has insulin-treated diabetes. *Journal of Psychosomatic Research, 29*, 353–359.

Jensen, S. B. (1985b). Sexual relationships in couples with a diabetic partner. *Journal of Sex and Marital Therapy, 11*, 259–270.

Jensen, S. B. (1986). Sexual dysfunction and diabetes mellitus: A six-year follow-up study. *Archives of Sexual Behavior, 15*, 271–284.

Jensen, S. B., Colstrup, H., Wagner, G., Nystrup, J., & Hertoft, P. (1983). Erective dysfunctions: Assessment of a screening program of investigation with particular attention to the significance of urodynamic and hormonal factors. *Ugeskrift for Laeger, 145*, 158–162.

Jensen, S. B., & Gluud, C. (1985). Sexual dysfunction in men with alcoholic liver cirrhosis: A comparative study. *Liver, 5*, 94–100.

Jensen, S. B., Hagen, C., Frøland, A., & Pedersen, P. B. (1979). Sexual function and pituitary gonadal axis in insulin-treated diabetic man. *Acta Medica Scandinavica, 624* (Suppl.), 65–68.

Jensen, S. B., & Hejl, B. L. (Eds.) (1987). *Par i behandling.* Copenhagen: Munksgaards Forlag.

Jensen, S. B., & Hertoft, P. (1984). Multiaxial diagnosis in sexual dysfunctions. *Ugeskrift for Laeger, 146*, 2854–2857.

Jensen, S. B., Meidahl, B., & Sjögren, K. (1984). Sexologiske data belyst ved brug af standardsporgeskemaer. *Nordisk Sexologi, 2*, 133–142.

Jensen, S. B., & Møhl, B. (in press). Vi er ikke af trae [We are not made of wood]. In S. B. Jensen & B. L. Hejl (Eds.), *Par i behandling* (pp. 240–256). Copenhagen: Munksgaards Forlag.

Jensen, S. B., Olsen, P. S., Rønne, H. R. (1980). Seksuel dysfunktion i almen praksis. *Ugeskrift for Laeger, 142*, 401–404.

Jensen, S. B., Sjögren, K., & Meidahl, B. (1984). Sexologiske data hos 117 konsekutive personer henvist til sexologisk klinik. *Ugeskrift for Laeger, 146*, 489–493.

Jevtich, M. J. (1983). Vascular noninvasive diagnostic techniques. In R. J. Krane, M. B. Siroky, & I. Goldstein (Eds.), *Male sexual dysfunction* (pp. 139–164). Boston: Little, Brown & Co.

Jevtich, M. J., Edson, M., Jarman, W. D., & Herrera, H. H. (1982). Vascular factor in erectile failure among diabetics. *Urology, 19*, 163–168.

Jevtich, M. J., Kass, M., & Khawand, N. (1985). Changes in the corpora cavernosa of impotent diabetics: Comparing histological and clinical findings. *Journal d'Urologie, 91*, 281–285.

Jevtich, M. J., & Maxwell, D. D. (1983). Invasive vascular procedures. In R. J. Krane, M. B. Siroky, & I. Goldstein (Eds.), *Male sexual dysfunction* (pp. 165–183). Boston: Little, Brown & Co.

Johns, D. R. (1986). Benign sexual headache within a family. *Archives of Neurology, 43*, 1158–1160.

Jonas, D., Linzbach, P., & Weber, W. (1979). The use of midodrin in the treatment of ejaculation disorders following retroperitoneal lymphadenectomy. *European Urology, 5*, 184–187.

Jones, S. D. (1984). Ejaculatory inhibition with trazodone. *Journal of Clinical Psychopharmacology, 4*, 279–281.

Judd, L. L., Risch, S. C., Parker, D. C., Janowsky, D. S., Segal, D. S., & Huey, L. Y. (1982). Blunted prolactin response: A neuroendocrine abnormality manifested by depressed patients. *Archives of General Psychiatry, 39*, 1413–1416.

Kahn, E., & Fisher, C. (1969). REM sleep and sexuality in the aged. *Journal of Geriatric Psychiatry, 2*, 181–199.

Kaplan, H. S. (1974). *The new sex therapy.* New York: Brunner/Mazel.

Kaplan, H. S. (1979). *Disorders of sexual desire.* New York: Brunner/Mazel.

Kaplan, H. S. (1983). *The evaluation of sexual disorders.* New York: Brunner/Mazel.

Kaplan, H. S. (1987). *The real truth about women and AIDS: How to eliminate the risks without giving up love and sex.* New York: Fireside Books, Simon & Schuster.

Kaplan, R. M., Reis, A., & Atkins, C. J. (1985). Behavioral issues in the management of chronic obstructive pulmonary disease. *Annals of Behavioral Medicine, 7*, 5–10.

Kaplan, W., & Kimball, C. (1982). The risks and course of coronary artery disease. A biopsychosocial explanation. In T. Millon, C. Green, & R. Meagher (Eds.), *Handbook of clinical health psychology* (pp. 69–90). New York: Plenum Press.

Karacan, I., & Moore, C. A. (1982). Nocturnal penile tumescence: An objective diagnostic aid for erectile dysfunction. In A. H. Bennett (Ed.), *Management of male impotence* (pp. 62–72). Baltimore: Williams & Wilkins.

Karacan, I., Williams, R. L., Thornby, J. I., & Salis, P. J. (1975). Sleep-related penile tumescence as a function of age. *American Journal of Psychiatry, 132*, 932–937.

Kass, I., Updegraff, K., & Muffly, R. B. (1972). Sex in chronic obstructive pulmonary disease. *Medical Aspects of Human Sexuality, 63*, 33–42.

Kassel, V. (1983). Long-term care institutions. In R. B. Weg (Ed.), *Sexuality in the later years: Roles and behavior* (pp. 167–184). New York: Academic Press.

Kaufman, J. J. (1982). Penile prosthetic surgery under local anesthesia. *Journal of Urology, 128*, 1190–1191.

Kedia, K. R. (1983a). Ejaculation and emission: Normal physiology, dysfunction, and therapy. In R. J. Krane, M. B. Siroky, & I. Goldstein (Eds.), *Male sexual dysfunction* (pp. 37–54). Boston: Little, Brown & Co.

Kedia, K. R. (1983b). Penile plethysmography useful in diagnosis of vasculogenic impotence. *Urology, 22*, 235–239.

Kelami, A. (1985). A new description: Urethral manipulation Syndrome [Abstract 1061]. *Journal of Urology, 133*, 379A.

Kellner, R., Buckman, M. T., Fava, G. A., & Pathak, D. (1984). Hyperprolactinemia, distress, and hostility. *American Journal of Psychiatry, 141*, 759–763.

Kempczinski, R. F. (1979). Role of the vascular diagnostic laboratory in the evaluation of male impotence. *American Journal of Surgery, 138*, 278–282.

Kerstein, M. D., Gould, S. A., French-Sherry, E., & Pirman, C. (1982). Diagnostic value of penile blood pressure. *American Surgeon, 48*, 271–272.

Keye, W. R. (1984). Psychosexual responses to infertility. *Clinical Obstetrics and Gynecology, 27*, 760–766.

Kinchla, J., & Weiss, T. (1985). Psychologic and social outcomes following coronary artery bypass surgery. *Journal of Cardiopulmonary Rehabilitation, 5*, 274–283.

King, B. D., Pitchon, R., Stern, E. H., Schweitzer, P., Schneider, R. R., & Weiner, I. (1983). Impotence during therapy with verapamil. *Archives of Internal Medicine, 143*, 1248–1249.

Kinsey, A. C., Pomeroy, W. B., & Martin, C. E. (1948). *Sexual behavior in the human male*. Philadelphia: W. B. Saunders.

Kinsey, A. C., Pomeroy, W. B., Martin, C. E., & Gebhard, P. H. (1953). *Sexual behavior in the human female*. Philadelphia: W. B. Saunders.

Kolodny, R. C. (1971). Sexual dysfunction in diabetic females. *Diabetes, 20*, 557–559.

Kolodny, R. C., Kahn, C. B., Goldstein, H. H., & Barnett, D. M. (1974). Sexual dysfunction in diabetic men. *Diabetes, 23*, 306–309.

Kolodny, R. C., Masters, W. H., & Johnson, V. E. (1979). *Textbook of sexual medicine*. Boston: Little, Brown & Co.

Kornfeld, D. S., Heller, S. S., Frank, K. A., Wilson, S. N., & Malm, J. R. (1982). Psychological and behavioral responses after coronary artery bypass surgery. *Circulation, 66* (Suppl. 3), 24–28.

Krant, M. J., & Johnston, L. (1978). Family members' perceptions of communications in late stage cancer. *International Journal of Psychiatry in Medicine, 8*, 203–216.

Krantz, D. S., & Glass, D. C. (1984). Personality, behavior patterns, and physical illness: Conceptual and methodological issues. In W. D. Gentry (Ed.), *Handbook of behavioral medicine* (pp. 38–86). New York: Guilford Press.

Kristensen, J. K. (1973). Side effects in disulfiram treatment. *Ugeskrift for Laeger, 135*, 1457–1459.

Kristensen, J. K., Rønsted, P., & Vaag, U. (1984). Side effects after disulfiram. *Acta Psychiatrica Scandinavica, 69*, 265–273.

Ladas, A. K., Whipple, B., & Perry, J. D. (1982). *The G Spot*. New York: Holt, Rinehart & Winston.

Lang, A. R. (1985). The social psychology of drinking and human sexuality. *Journal of Drug Issues, 2*, 273–289.

Larsen, E., & Hejgaard, N. (1984). Sexual dysfunction after spinal cord or cauda equina lesions. *Paraplegia, 22*, 66–74.

Larsen, E. H., Gasser, T., & Bruskewitz, R. C. (1987). Fibrosis of corpus cavernosum after intracavernous injection of phentolamine/papaverine. *Journal of Urology, 137*, 292–293.

Lazarus, R. S. (1966). *Psychological stress and the coping process*. New York: McGraw-Hill.

Lazarus, R. S., & Folkman, S. (1984). Coping and adaptation. In W. D. Gentry (Ed.), *Handbook of behavioral medicine* (pp. 282–325). New York: Guilford Press.

Lee, K., Hardt, F., Møller, L., Haubek, A., & Jensen, E. (1979). Alcohol induced brain damage and liver damage in young alcoholics. *Lancet, 8231*, 759–761.

Lehman, T. P., & Jacobs, J. A. (1983). Etiology of diabetic impotence. *Journal of Urology, 129*, 291–294.

Leiblum, S. R., Bachmann, G., Kemmann, E., Colburn, D., & Swartzman, L. (1983). Vaginal atrophy in the postmenopausal woman: The importance of sexual activity and hormones. *Journal of the American Medical Association, 249*, 2195–2198.

Leiblum, S. R., & Pervin, L. A. (1980). *Principles and practice of sex therapy*. New York: Guilford Press.

Lemere, F., & Smith, J. W. (1973). Alcohol-induced sexual impotence. *American Journal of Psychiatry, 130*, 212–213.

Lepor, H., Gregerman, M., Crosby, R., Mostofi, F. K., & Walsh, P. C. (1985). Precise localization of the autonomic nerves from the pelvic plexus to the corpora cavernosa: A detailed anatomical study of the adult male penis. *Journal of Urology, 133*, 207–212.

Leriche, A., & Morel, A. (1948). The syndrome of thrombotic obliteration of the aortic bifurcation. *Annals of Surgery, 127*, 193–208.

Lesko, L. M., Stotland, N. L., & Segraves, R. T. (1982). Three cases of female anorgasmia associated with MAOIs. *American Journal of Psychiatry, 139*, 1353–1354.

Lester, E., Grant, A. J. & Woodroffe, F. J. (1980). Impotence in diabetic and nondiabetic outpatients. *British Medical Journal, 281*, 354–355.

Levin, R. J. (1984, September). *Pelvic contractions, duration and intensity of orgasm and the ejaculate volume: A longitudinal human study.* Paper presented at the meeting of the International Academy of Sex Research, Cambridge, England.

Levin, R. J., & Wagner, G. (1985). Orgasm in women in the laboratory: Quantitative studies in duration, intensity, latency, and vaginal blood flow. *Archives of Sexual Behavior, 14*, 439–449.

Levy, N. B. (1983). Sexual dysfunctions of hemodialysis patients. *Clinical and Experimental Dialysis and Apheresis, 7*, 275–288.

Levy, N. B. (1986). Renal transplantation and the new medical era. *Advances in Psychosomatic Medicine, 15*, 167–179.

Levy, S. M. (1985). *Behavior and cancer.* San Francisco: Jossey-Bass.

Lilius, H. G., Valtonen, E. J., & Wikström, J. (1976). Sexual problems in patients suffering from multiple sclerosis. *Journal of Chronic Diseases, 29*, 643–647.

Lin, J. T., & Bradley, W. E. (1985). Penile neuropathy in insulin dependent diabetes mellitus. *Journal of Urology, 133*, 213–215.

Lindemann, E. (1944). Symptomatology and management of acute grief. *American Journal of Psychiatry, 101*, 1–11.

Lindenberg, S., Hjardem, I., Kelbaek, H., Munkgaard, S., & Jensen, S. B. (1980). Beat-to-beat variation in chronic alcoholics. *Ugeskrift for Laeger, 143*, 1325–1326.

Link, P. W., & Darling, C. A. (1986). Couples undergoing treatment for infertility: Dimensions of life satisfaction. *Journal of Sex and Marital Therapy, 12*, 46–59.

Lipschultz, L. I., Cunningham, G., & Howards, S. S. (1983). Differential diagnosis of male infertility. In L. I. Lipschultz, & S. S. Howards (Eds.), *Infertility in the male* (pp. 249–264). New York: Churchill Livingstone.

Lipschultz, L. I., McConnell, J., & Benson, G. S. (1981). Current concepts of the mechanisms of ejaculation: Normal and abnormal studies. *Journal of Reproductive Medicine, 26*, 449–507.

Lipson, L. G. (1984). Treatment of hypertension in diabetic men: Problems with sexual dysfunction. *American Journal of Cardiology, 53*, 46–50.

LoPiccolo, J. (1978). The professionalization of sex therapy: Issues and problems. In J. LoPiccolo & L. LoPiccolo (Eds.), *Handbook of sex therapy* (pp. 511–525). New York: Plenum Press.

LoPiccolo, J. (Consultant). (1984). *Treating vaginismus* [Film]. New York: Multi-Focus, Inc.

LoPiccolo, J., & Heiman, J. R. (1978). The role of cultural values in the prevention and treatment of sexual problems. In C. B. Qualls, J. P. Wincze, & D. H. Barlow (Eds.), *The prevention of sexual disorders: Issues and approaches* (pp. 43–74). New York: Plenum Press.

LoPiccolo, J., Heiman, J. R., Hogan, D. R., & Roberts, C. W. (1985). Effectiveness of single therapists vs. co-therapy teams in sex therapy. *Journal of Consulting and Clinical Psychology, 53*, 287–294.

LoPiccolo, J. & LoPiccolo, L. (Eds.). (1978). *Handbook of sex therapy.* New York: Plenum Press.

LoPiccolo, J., & Miller, V. H. (1978). A program for enhancing the sexual relationship of normal couples. In J. LoPiccolo & L. LoPiccolo (Eds.), *Handbook of Sex Therapy* (pp. 451–458). New York: Plenum Press.

LoPiccolo, J., & Steger, J. C. (1978). The Sexual Interaction Inventory: A new instrument for assessment of sexual dysfunction. In J. LoPiccolo & L. LoPiccolo (Eds.), *Handbook of sex therapy* (pp. 113–122). New York: Plenum Press.

LoPiccolo, L. & Heiman, J. R. (Writers & Producers) (1976). *Becoming orgasmic: A sexual growth program for women* [Film]. New York: Multi-Focus Films.

LoPiccolo, L., Heiman, J. R., & LoPiccolo J. (1976). *Becoming orgasmic: A sexual growth program for women.* Englewood Cliffs, NJ: Prentice-Hall.

Lorimy, F., Loo, H., & Deniker, P. (1977). Effets cliniques des traitements prolongés par les sels de lithium sur le sommeil, l'appetit, et la sexualité. *L'Encèphale, 3*, 227–239.

Lue, T. F., Hricak, H., Marich, K. W., & Tanagho, E. A. (1985a). Evaluation of arteriogenic impotence with intracorporeal injection of papaverine and the duplex ultrasound scanner. *Seminars in Urology, 3*, 43–48.

Lue, T. F., Hricak, H., Schmidt, R. A., & Tanagho, E. A. (1986). Functional evaluation of penile veins by cavernosography in papaverine-induced erection. *Journal of Urology, 135*, 479–482.

Lue, T. F., Schmidt, R. A., & Tanagho, E. A. (1985b). Electrostimulation of penile erection. *Urology International, 40*, 60–64.

Lue, T. F., Zeineh, S. J., Schmidt, R. A., & Tanagho, E. A. (1984). Neuroanatomy of penile erection: Its relevance to iatrogenic impotence. *Journal of Urology, 131*, 273–280.

Lundberg, P. O. (1981). Sexual dysfunction in female patients with multiple sclerosis. *International Rehabilitation Medicine, 3*, 32–34.

Lundberg, P. O., Hulter, B., & Wide, L. (1985, September). *Sexual libido in women with hypothalamo-pituitary disorders.* Paper presented at the annual meeting of the International Academy of Sex Research, Seattle, WA.

Maatman, T. J., & Montague, D. K. (1985). Is routine hormonal screening of impotent men worthwhile [Abstract 302]? *Journal of Urology, 133*, 189A.

Mahajan, S. K., Prasad, A. S., & McDonald, F. D. (1984). Sexual dysfunction in uremic males: Improvement following oral zinc supplementation. *Controversies in Nephrology, 38*, 103–111.

Malatesta, V. J., Pollack, R. H., Crotty, T. D., & Peacock, L. J. (1982). Acute alcohol intoxication and female orgasmic response. *Journal of Sex Research, 18*, 1–17.

Malatesta, V. J., Pollack, R. H., Wilbanks, W. A., & Adams, H. E. (1979). Alcohol effects of the orgasmic-ejaculatory response in human males. *Journal of Sex Research, 15*, 101–107.

Mann, S., Craig, M. W. M., Gould, B. A., Melville, D. I., & Raftery, E. B. (1982). Coital blood pressure in hypertensives: Cephalgia, syncope, and effects of beta-blockade. *British Heart Journal, 47*, 84–89.

Marshall, P., McGrath, P., & Schillinger, J. (1983). Importance of electromyographic data in interpreting nocturnal penile tumescence. *Urology, 22*, 153–156.

Maruta, T., Osborne, D., Swanson, D. W., & Halling, J. M. (1981). Chronic pain patients and spouses: Marital and sexual adjustment. *Mayo Clinic Proceedings, 56*, 307–310.

Martin, C. E. (1981). Factors affecting sexual functioning in 60–79-year-old married males. *Archives of Sexual Behavior, 10*, 399–420.

Masters, W. H., & Johnson, V. E. (1966). *Human sexual response.* Boston: Little, Brown & Co.

Masters, W. H., & Johnson, V. E. (1970). *Human sexual inadequacy.* Boston: Little, Brown & Co.

Masters, W. H., & Johnson, V. E. (1981). Sex and the aging process. *Journal of the American Geriatrics Society, 9*, 385–390.

Mastrogiacomo, I., De Besi, L., Serafini, E., Zussa, S., Zucchetta, P., Romagholi, G. F., Saporiti, E., Dean, P., Ronco, C., & Adami, A. (1984). Hyperprolactinemia and sexual disturbances among uremic women on hemodialysis. *Nephron, 37*, 195–199.

Mathew, R. J., & Weinman, M. L. (1982). Sexual dysfunctions in depression. *Archives of Sexual Behavior, 11*, 323–328.

Mazor, M. D. (1984). Emotional reactions to infertility. In M. D. Mazor & H. F. Simons (Eds.), *Infertility: Medical, emotional, and social considerations* (pp. 23–35). New York: Human Sciences Press.

McCoy, N., Cutler, W., & Davidson, J. (1985). Relationships among sexual behavior, hot flashes, and hormone levels in perimenopausal women. *Archives of Sexual Behavior, 14*, 385–394.

McCulloch, D. K., Hosking, D. J., Tobert, A. (1986). A pragmatic approach to sexual dysfunction in diabetic men: Psychosexual counselling. *Diabetic Medicine, 3*, 485–489.

McCulloch, D. K., Young, R. J., Prescott, R. J., Campbell, I. W., & Clarke, B. F. (1984). The natural history of impotence in diabetic men. *Diabetologia, 26*, 437–440.

McIntosh, T. K., & Barfield, R. J. (1984a). Brain monoaminergic control of male reproductive behavior: I. Serotonin and the post-ejaculatory refractory period. *Behavioral Brain Research, 12*, 255–265.

McIntosh, T. K., & Barfield, R. J. (1984b). Brain monoaminergic control of male reproductive behavior: II. Dopamine and the post-ejaculatory refractory period. *Behavioral Brain Research, 12*, 267–273.

McIntosh, T. K., & Barfield R. J. (1984c). Brain monoaminergic control of male reproductive behavior: III. Norepinephrine and the post-ejaculatory refractory period. *Behavioral Brain Research, 12*, 275–281.

Melman, A. (1983). Catecholamine levels in penile corpora. In R. J. Kranc, M. B. Siroky, & I. Goldstein (Eds.), *Male sexual dysfunction* (pp. 27–32). Boston: Little, Brown & Co.

Melman, A., & Frye, S. (1983). Use of the evoked sacral potential in evaluation of erectile impotence. *Neurourology and Urodynamics, 2*, 295–300.

Melman, A., Kaplan, D., & Redfield, J. (1984). Evaluation of the first 70 patients in the center for male sexual dysfunction of Beth Israel Medical Center. *Journal of Urology, 131*, 53–55.

Melman, A., & Maayani, S. (1985, September). *Alpha-1-adrenergic receptor mediated contraction of diabetic human erectile tissue in vitro*. Paper presented at the annual meeting of the International Academy of Sex Research, Seattle, WA.

Mendelson, J. H., Ellingboe, J., Keuhnle, J. C., & Mello, N. K. (1979). Effects of naltrexone on mood and neuroendocrine function in males. *Psychoneuroendocrinology, 3*, 231–236.

Merikangas, K. R. (1982). Assortative mating for psychiatric disorders and psychological traits. *Archives of General Psychiatry, 39*, 1173–1180.

Merikangas, K. R., Prusoff, B. A., Kupfer, D. J., & Frank, E. (1985). Marital adjustment in major depression. *Journal of Affective Disorders, 9*, 5–11.

Merrill, D. C. (1984). Mentor inflatable penile prosthesis: Clinical experience in 52 patients. *British Journal of Urology, 56*, 512–515.

Metz, P. (1983). Erectile function in men with occlusive arterial disease in the legs. *Danish Medical Bulletin, 30*, 185–189.

Metz, P., Christensen, J., Mathiesen, F. R., & Ostri, P. (1983a). Ultrasonic Doppler pulse wave analysis vs. penile blood pressure measurement in the evaluation of arteriogenic impotence. *VASA, 12*, 363–366.

Metz, P., Ebbehøj, J., Uhrenholdt, A., & Wagner, G. (1983b). Peyronie's disease and erectile failure. *Journal of Urology, 130*, 1103–1104.

Metz, P., Frimodt-Møller, & Mathiesen, F. R. (1983c). Erectile function before and after reconstructive arterial surgery in men with occlusive arterial leg disease. *Scandinavian Journal of Thoracic and Cardiovascular Surgery, 17*, 45–50.

Metz, P., & Mathiesen, F. R. (1979). External iliac "steal syndrome" leading to a defect in penile erection and impotence. *Vascular Surgery, 13*, 70–72.

Meyer-Bahlburg, H. F. L., & Ehrhardt, A. A. (1983). *Sexual Behavior Assessment Schedule— Adult (SEBAS-A)*. New York: New York State Psychiatric Institute.

Miccoli, R., Gianpietro, O., Tognarelli, M., Basile Fasolo, C., Menchini Fabris, G. F., Lenzi, S., Rossi, B., & Navalesi, R. (1985). Prevalence of sexual dysfunctions in non-insulin dependent (type II) diabetic males. *Acta Europaea Fertilitatis, 16*, 241–244.

Michal, V. (1982). Arterial disease as a cause of impotence. *Clinics in Endocrinology and Metabolism, 11*, 725–748.

Michal, V., Kramar, R., & Pospichal, J. (1978). External iliac "steal syndrome." *Journal of Cardiovascular Surgery, 19*, 255–257.

Michal, V., Kramar, R., Pospichal, J., & Hejhal, L. (1977). Arterial epigastricocavernosus anastomosis for the treatment of sexual impotence. *World Journal of Surgery, 1*, 515–520.

Michalski, S. M. (1986). Case history of a homosexual male on CAPD. *American Nephrology Nursing Association Journal, 13*, 70–71.

Miller, W. R., & Hester, R. K. (1986). Inpatient alcoholic treatment: Who benefits? *American Psychologist, 41*, 794–805.

Mills, K. H., & Kilmann, P. R. (1982). Group treatment of sexual dysfunctions: A methodological review of the outcome literature. *Journal of Sex and Marital Therapy, 8*, 259–296.

Mimoun, M. S. (1984). Sexualité et douleurs chroniques urologiques sans causes cliniquement décelables chez l'homme. *Annales d'Urologie, 18*, 331–336.

Minderhoud, J. M., Leemhuis, J. G., Kremer, J., Laban, E., & Smits, P. M. L. (1984). Sexual disturbances arising from multiple sclerosis. *Acta Neurologica Scandinavica, 70*, 299–306.

Minuchin, S., Rosman, B. L., & Baker, L. (1978). *Psychosomatic families*. Cambridge, MA: Harvard University Press.

Mirin, S. M., Meyer, R. E., Mendelson, J. H., & Ellingboe, J. (1980). Opiate use and sexual function. *American Journal of Psychiatry, 137*, 909–915.

Mitchell, J. E., & Popkin, M. K. (1982). Antipsychotic drug therapy and sexual dysfunction in men. *American Journal of Psychiatry, 139*, 633–637.

Mitchell, J. E., & Popkin, M. K. (1983). The pathophysiology of sexual dysfunction associated with antipsychotic drug therapy in males: A review. *Archives of Sexual Behavior, 12*, 173–183.

Mittal, B. (1985). A study of penile circulation before and after radiation in patients with prostate cancer and its effect on impotence. *International Journal of Radiation Oncology, Biology, and Physics, 11*, 1121–1125.

Møller-Nielsen, C., Lundhus, E., Møller-Madsen, B., Norgaard, J. P., Simonsen, O. H., Hansen, S. L., & Birkler, N. (1985). Sexual life following "minimal" and "total" transurethral prostatic resection. *Urology International, 40*, 3–4.

Montenero, P., & Donatone, E. (1962). Diabète et activité sexuelle chez l'homme. *Le Diabète, 10*, 327–335.

Mooney, T., Cole, T., & Chilgren, R. (1975). *Sexual options for paraplegics and quadriplegics*. Boston: Little, Brown & Co.

Moos, R. H. (1982). Coping with acute health crises. In T. Millon, C. Green, & R. Meagher (Eds.), *Handbook of clinical health psychology* (pp. 129–151). New York: Plenum Press.

Morales, A., Surridge, D. H., Marshall, P. G., & Fenemore, J. (1982). Nonhormonal pharmacological treatment of organic impotence. *Journal of Urology, 128*, 45–47.

Morin, S. F., Charles, K. A., & Malyon, K. A. (1984). The psychological impact of AIDS on gay men. *American Psychologist, 39*, 1288–1293.

Morokoff, P. (1978). Determinants of female orgasm. In J. LoPiccolo & L. LoPiccolo (Eds.), *Handbook of sex therapy* (pp. 147–166). New York: Plenum Press.

Morrell, M. J., Dixen, J. M., Carter, S., & Davidson, J. M. (1984). The influence of age and cycling status on sexual arousability in women. *American Journal of Obstetrics and Gynecology, 148*, 66–71.

Moses, R. G., & Colagiuri, S. (1985). Diabetes mellitus and intercourse. *Diabetes Care, 8*, 623–624.

Moss, H. B., & Procci, W. R. (1982). Sexual dysfunction associated with oral antihypertensive medication: A critical survey of the literature. *General Hospital Psychiatry, 4*, 121–129.

Moth, I., Andreasson, B., Jensen, S. B., & Bock, J. E. (1983). Sexual function and somatopsychic reactions after vulvectomy. *Danish Medical Bulletin, 30*, 27–30.

Muir, J. W., Besser, G. M., Edwards, C. R. W., Rees, L. H., Cattell, W. R., Ackrill, P., & Baker, L. R. I. (1983). Bromocriptine improves reduced libido and potency in men receiving maintenance hemodialysis. *Clinical Nephrology, 20*, 308–314.

Nahoum, C. R. D., & Freire, F. R. (1985). Nonhormonal mechanism of sexual inadequacy in patients with varicocele. *Urology, 25*, 49–52.

Neff, M. S., Eiser, A. R., Slifkin, R. F., Baum, M., Baez, A., Gupta, S., & Amarga, E. (1983). Patients surviving 10 years of hemodialysis. *American Journal of Medicine, 74*, 996–1004.

Neri, A., Aygen, M., Zukerman, Z., & Bahary, C. (1980). Subjective assessment of sexual dysfunction of patients on long-term administration of digoxin. *Archives of Sexual Behavior, 9*, 343–347.

Nestoros, J. N., Lehmann, H. E., & Ban, T. A. (1981). Sexual behavior of the male schizophrenic: The impact of illness and medications. *Archives of Sexual Behavior, 10*, 421–442.

Newman, A. S., & Bertelson, A. D. (1986). Sexual dysfunction in diabetic women. *Journal of Behavioral Medicine, 9*, 261–270.

Newman, H. F., & Marcus, H. (1985). Erectile dysfunction in diabetes and hypertension. *Urology, 26*, 135–137.

Newman, H. F., & Reiss, H. (1984). Artificial perfusion in impotence. *Urology, 24*, 469–471.

Newman, H. F., Reiss, H., & Northup, J. D. (1982). Physical basis of emission, ejaculation, and orgasm in the male. *Urology, 19*, 341–350.

Ngiem, D. D., Corry, R. J., Mendez, G. P., & Lee, H. M. (1982). Pelvic hemodynamics and male sexual impotence after renal transplantation. *Annals of Surgery, 48*, 532–535.

Ngiem, D. D., Corry, R. J., Mendez, G. P., & Lee, H. M. (1983). Factors influencing male sexual impotence after renal transplantation. *Urology, 21*, 49–52.

Nichols, K. A., & Springford, V. (1984). The psycho-social stressors associated with survival by dialysis. *Behaviour Research and Therapy, 22*, 563–574.

Nickel, J. C., Morales, A., Condra, M., Fenemore, J., & Surridge, D. H. (1984). Endocrine dysfunction in impotence: Incidence, significance, and cost-effective screening. *Journal of Urology, 132*, 40–43.

Nielsen, I. L., Fog, E., Larsen, G. K., Madsen, J., Garde, K., & Kelstrup, J. (1986a). A presentation of the sexual behavior, experience, knowledge, and attitudes of 70-year-old women. *Ugeskrift for Laeger, 148*, 2863–2866.

Nielsen, I. L., Larsen, G. K., Fog, E., Madsen, J., Garde, K., & Kelstrup, J. (1986b). A presentation of the sexual behavior, experience, knowledge, and attitudes of 22-year-old women. *Ugeskrift for Laeger, 148*, 2867–2869.

Nowlin, N. S., Brick, J. E., Weaver, P. J., Wilson, D. A., Judd, H. L., Lu, J. K. H., & Carlson, H. E. (1986). Impotence in scleroderma. *Annals of Internal Medicine, 104*, 794–798.

O'Carroll, R., & Bancroft, J. (1984). Testosterone therapy for low sexual interest and erectile dysfunction in men: A controlled study. *British Journal of Psychiatry, 145*, 146–151.

O'Carroll, R., Shapiro, C., & Bancroft, J. (1985). Androgens, behaviour and nocturnal erection in hypogonadal men: The effects of varying the replacement dose. *Clinical Endocrinology, 23*, 527–538.

O'Donnell, P., Leach, G., & Raz, S. (1983). Surgical treatment of Peyronie's disease. In R. J. Krane, M. B. Siroky, & I. Goldstein (Eds.), *Male sexual dysfunction* (pp. 225–242). Boston: Little, Brown & Co.

Orenstein, D. M., & Wachnowsky, D. B. (1985). Behavioral aspects of cystic fibrosis. *Annals of Behavioral Medicine, 7*, 17–20.

Ottesen, B. (1983). Vasoactive polypeptide as a neurotransmitter in the female genital tract. *American Journal of Obstetrics and Gynecology, 147*, 208–224.

Owen, J. A., Nakatsu, S. L., Condra, M., Fenemore, J., Surridge, D. H., & Morales, A. (1985). The pharmacokinetics of yohimbine in man [Abstract 594]. *Journal of Urology, 133*, 262A.

Paff, B. A. (1985). Sexual dysfunction in gay men requesting treatment. *Journal of Sex and Marital Therapy, 11*, 3–18.

Papadopoulos, C., Beaumont, C., Shelley, S. I., & Larrimore, P. (1983). Myocardial infarction and sexual activity of the female patient. *Archives of Internal Medicine, 143*, 1528–1530.

Papadopoulos, C., Shelley, S. I., Piccolo, M., Beaumont, C., & Barnett, L. (1986). Sexual activity after coronary bypass surgery. *Chest, 90*, 681–685.

Peele, S. (1984). The cultural context of alcoholism: Can we control the effects of alcohol? *American Psychologist, 39*, 1337–1351.

Perelman, M. A. (1980). Treatment of premature ejaculation. In S. R. Leiblum & L. A. Pervin (Eds.), *Principles and practice of sex therapy* (pp. 199–234). New York: Guilford Press.

Persky, H., Dreisbach, L., Miller, W. R., O'Brien, C. P., Khan, M. A., Lief, H. I., Charney, N., & Strauss, D. (1982). The relation of plasma androgen levels to sexual behaviors and attitudes of women. *Psychosomatic Medicine, 44*, 305–319.

Peterson, H. R., Best, J. D., Berger, R., Reenan, A., Porte, D., Halter, J. B., & Pfeifer, M. A. (1985). Attitudes of diabetic men after implantation of a semi-rigid penile prosthesis. *Diabetes Care, 8*, 156–160.

Peterson, J. S., Hartsock, N., & Lawson, G. (1984). Sexual dissatisfaction of female alcoholics. *Psychological Reports, 55*, 744–746.

Pierini, A. A., & Nusimovich, B. (1981). Male diabetic sexual impotence: Effects of dopaminergic agents. *Archives of Andrology, 6*, 347–350.

Pinderhughes, C. A., Grace, E. B., & Reyna, L. J. (1972). Psychiatric disorders and sexual functioning. *American Journal of Psychiatry, 128*, 1276–1283.

Pogach, L. M., & Vaitukaitis, J. L. (1983). Endocrine disorders associated with erectile dysfunction. In R. J. Krane, M. B. Siroky, & I. Goldstein (Eds.), *Male sexual dysfunction* (pp. 63–76). Boston: Little, Brown & Co.

Poland, M. L., & Evans, T. N. (1985). Psychologic aspects of vaginal agenesis. *Journal of Reproductive Medicine, 30*, 340–344.

Pope, K. S., & Bouhoutsos, J. C. (1986). *Sexual intimacy between therapists and patients.* New York: Praeger Publishers.

Pope, K. S., Keith-Spiegel, P., & Tabachnick, B. G. (1986). Sexual attraction to clients: The human therapist and the (sometimes) inhuman training system. *American Psychologist, 41*, 147–158.

Pope, K. S., Levenson, H., & Schover, L. R. (1979). Sexual intimacy in psychology training: Results and implications of a national survey. *American Psychologist, 34*, 682–689.

Prigatano, G. P., Wright, E., Levin, D. C., & Hawryluk, G. (1983). Neuropsychological test performance in mildly hypoxemic patients with chronic obstructive pulmonary disease. *Journal of Consulting and Clinical Psychology, 51*, 108–116.

Procci, W. R. (1983). The study of sexual dysfunction in uremic males: Problems for patients and investigators. *Clinical and Experimental Dialysis and Apheresis, 7*, 289–302.

Procci, W. R., & Martin, D. J. (1985). Effect of maintenance hemodialysis on male sexual performance. *Journal of Nervous and Mental Disease, 173,* 366–372.

Psychology Today (1970, July). Sex. *Psychology Today,* 30–52.

Purifoy, F. E., Koopmans, L. H., & Mayes, D. M. (1981). Age differences in serum androgen levels in normal adult males. *Human Biology, 53,* 499–511.

Quadland, M. C. (1985). Compulsive sexual behavior: Definition of a problem and an approach to treatment. *Journal of Sex and Marital Therapy, 11,* 121–132.

Raboch, J. (1984). The sexual development and life of female schizophrenic patients. *Archives of Sexual Behavior, 13,* 341–350.

Raboch, J. (1986). Sexual development and life of female psychiatric patients. *Archives of Sexual Behavior, 15,* 231–254.

Raboch, J., Kobilkova, J., Raboch, J., & Starka, L. (1985). Sexual life of women with the Stein-Leventhal syndrome. *Archives of Sexual Behavior, 14,* 263–270.

Raboch, J., Smolik, P., & Soucek, V. (1983). Lithium and male sexuality. *Ceskoslovenska Psychiatrie, 79,* 19–21.

Ramirez, G., Butcher, D. E., Newton, J. L., Brueggemeyer, C. D., Moon, J., & Gomez-Sanchez, C. (1985). Bromocriptine and the hypothalamic hypophyseal function in patients with chronic renal failure on chronic dialysis. *American Journal of Kidney Diseases, 6,* 111–118.

Ramshaw, J. E., & Stanley, G. (1984). Psychological adjustment to coronary artery surgery. *British Journal of Clinical Psychology, 23,* 101–108.

Remes, K., Kuoppasalmi, K., & Adlercreutz, H. (1979). Effect of long-term physical training on plasma testosterone, androstenedione, luteinizing hormone and sex-hormone-binding globulin capacity. *Scandinavian Journal of Clinical and Laboratory Investigation, 39,* 743–749.

Renshaw, D. (1982). *Incest.* Boston: Little, Brown & Co.

Richards, J. S. (1980). Sex and arthritis. *Sexuality and Disability, 3,* 97–104.

Rieker, P. P., Edbril, S. D., & Garnick, M. (1985). Curative testis cancer therapy: Social and emotional consequences. *Journal of Clinical Oncology, 3,* 1117–1126.

Riley, A. J., & Riley, E. (1982). Partial ejaculatory incompetence: The therapeutic effect of midodrine, an orally active selective alpha-adrenoceptor agonist. *European Urology, 8,* 155–160.

Robinson, P. K. (1983). The sociological perspective. In R. B. Weg (Ed.), *Sexuality in the later years: Roles and behavior* (pp. 82–104). New York: Academic Press.

Rocco, A., Falaschi, P., Pompei, P., D'Urso, R., & Frajese, G. (1983). Reproductive parameters in prolactinaemic men. *Archives of Androgy, 10,* 179–183.

Rodger, R. S. C., Brook, A. C., Muirhead, N., & Kerr, D. N. S. (1984). Zinc metabolism does not influence sexual function in chronic renal insufficiency. *Controversies in Nephrology, 38,* 112–115.

Rodger, R. S. C., Fletcher, K., Dewar, J. H., Genner, D., McHugh, M., Wilkinson, R., Ward, M. K., & Kerr, D. N. S. (1985a). Prevalence and pathogenesis of impotence in one hundred uremic men. *Uremia Investigation, 8,* 89–96.

Rodger, R. S. C., Morrison, L., Dewar, J. H., Wilkinson, R., Ward, M. K., & Kerr, D. N. S. (1985b). Loss of pulsatile luteinising hormone secretion in men with chronic renal failure. *British Medical Journal, 291,* 1598–1600.

Rogers, G. S., Van de Castle, R. L., Evans, W. S., & Critelli, J. W. (1985). Vaginal pulse amplitude response patterns during erotic conditions and sleep. *Archives of Sexual Behavior, 14,* 327–342.

Rollo, J. (1798). *An account of two cases of diabetes mellitus with remarks as they arose during the progress of the case.* London: C. Dilly.

Roose, S. P., Glassman, A. H., Walsh, B. T., & Cullen, K. (1982). Reversible loss of nocturnal penile tumescence during depression: A preliminary report. *Neuropsychobiology, 8,* 284–288.

Roughan, P. A., & Kunst, L. (1981). Do pelvic floor exercises really improve orgasmic potential? *Journal of Sex and Marital Therapy, 7*, 223–229.

Roviaro, S., Holmes, D. S., & Holmstein, R. D. (1984). Influence of a cardiac rehabilitation program on the cardiovascular, psychological, and social functioning of cardiac patients. *Journal of Behavioral Medicine, 7*, 61–80.

Roy, R. (1985). Chronic pain and marital difficulties. *Health and Social Work, 10*, 199–207.

Royal College of Psychiatrists (1979). *Alcohol and alcoholism.* London: Tavistock Publications.

Rubin, A., & Babbott, D. (1958). Impotence and diabetes mellitus. *Journal of the American Medical Association, 168*, 498–500.

Rubinow, D. R., & Roy-Byrne, P. (1984). Premenstrual syndromes: Overview from a methodologic perspective. *American Journal of Psychiatry, 141*, 163–172.

Ruilope, L., Garcia-Robles, R., Paya, C., de Villa, L. R., Miranda, B., Morales, J. M., Parada, J., Sancho, J., & Rodicio, J. L. (1985). Influence of Lisuride, a dopaminergic agonist, on the sexual function of male patients with chronic renal failure. *American Journal of Kidney Disease, 5*, 182–185.

Rush, A. J. (1982). *Short-term psychotherapies for depression: Behavioral, interpersonal, cognitive, and psychodynamic approaches.* New York: Guilford Press.

Ruzbarsky, V., & Michal, V. (1977). Morphologic changes in the arterial bed of the penis with aging: Relationship to the pathogenesis of impotence. *Investigative Urology, 15*, 194–199.

Sager, C. J. (1976). *Marriage contracts and couple therapy: Hidden forces in intimate relationships.* New York: Brunner/Mazel.

Salmimies, P., Kockott, G., Pirke, K. M., Vogt, H. J., & Schill, W. B. (1982). Effects of testosterone replacement on sexual behavior in hypogonadal men. *Archives of Sexual Behavior, 11*, 345–354.

Sanders, D., & Bancroft, J. (1982). Hormones and the sexuality of women: The menstrual cycle. *Clinics in Endocrinology & Metabolism, 11*, 639–659.

Sanders, D., Warner, P., Backstrom, T., & Bancroft, J. (1983). Mood, sexuality, hormones and the menstrual cycle. I. Changes in mood and physical state: Description of subjects and method. *Psychosomatic Medicine, 45*, 487–501.

Sanders, J. D., & Sprenkle, D. H. (1980). Sexual therapy for the post coronary patient. *Journal of Sex and Marital Therapy, 6*, 174–186.

Sarason, I. G., Johnson, J. H., & Siegel, J. M. (1978). Assessing the impact of life changes: Development of the Life Experiences Survey. *Journal of Consulting and Clinical Psychology, 46*, 932–946.

Sarrel, L. J., & Sarrel, P. M. (1984). *Sexual turning points.* New York: Macmillan.

Sarrel, P. M. (1984). Biological considerations of sexual function during the climacteric. *SIECUS Report, 13*(2), pp. 6–7.

Sarrel, P. M., & DeCherney, A. H. (1985). Psychotherapeutic intervention for treatment of couples with secondary infertility. *Fertility & Sterility, 43*, 897–900.

Sarrel, P. M., Steege, J. F., Maltzer, M., & Bolinsky, D. (1983). Pain during sex response due to occlusion of the Bartholin gland duct. *Obstetrics and Gynecology, 62*, 261–264.

Schain, W. S., Jacobs, E., & Wellisch, D. K. (1984). Psychosocial issues in breast reconstruction: Intrapsychic, interpersonal, and practical concerns. *Clinics in Plastic Surgery, 11*, 237–251.

Schain, W. S., Wellisch, D. K., Pasnau, R. O., & Landsverk, J. (1985). The sooner the better: A study of psychological factors in women undergoing immediate versus delayed breast reconstruction. *American Journal of Psychiatry, 142*, 40–46.

Schein, M., Levine, S., Zyzanski, S., Medalie, J., Dickman, R., & Alemango, S. (1986, March). *Frequency of sexual problems in a family medicine practice.* Paper presented at the annual meeting of the Society for Sex Therapy and Research, Philadelphia, PA.

Schiavi, R. C., Fisher, C., Quadland, M., & Glover, A. (1985). Nocturnal penile tumescent evaluation of erectile function in insulin-dependent diabetic men. *Diabetologia, 28*, 90–94.

Schiavi, R. C., Fisher, C., White, D. Beers, P., & Szechter, R. (1984). Pituitary-gonadal function during sleep in men with erectile impotence and normal controls. *Psychosomatic Medicine, 46*, 239–254.

Schinfeld, J. S. (1985). Psychosexual dysfunction and infertility. In M. Farber (Ed.), *Human sexuality: Psychosexual effects of disease* (pp. 141–153). New York: MacMillan.

Schipper, H., Clinch, J., McMurray, A., & Levitt, M. (1984). Measuring the quality of life of cancer patients: The Functional Living Index—Cancer: Development and validation. *Journal of Clinical Oncology, 2*, 472–783.

Schlebusch, L., & Levin, A. (1983). A psychological profile of women selected for augmentation mammaplasty. *South African Medical Journal, 64*, 481–483.

Schover, L. R. (1981). Male and female therapists' responses to male and female client sexual material: An analogue study. *Archives of Sexual Behavior, 10*, 477–491.

Schover, L. R. (1983). Psychotherapists' responses to client sexuality: A source of bias in treatment? In J. Murray & P. R. Abramson (Eds.), *Bias in psychotherapy* (pp. 256–284). New York: Praeger.

Schover, L. R. (1984). *Prime time: Sexual health for men over fifty.* New York: Holt, Rinehart & Winston.

Schover, L. R. (1986a). Sex and the cancer patient. In B. A. Stoll (Ed.), *Coping with cancer stress* (pp. 71–80). Dordrecht, The Netherlands: Martinus Nijhoff.

Schover, L. R. (1986b). Sexual problems. In L. Teri, & P. M. Lewinsohn (Eds.), *Geropsychological assessment and treatment* (pp. 145–188). New York: Springer.

Schover, L. R. (1986c). Sexual rehabilitation of the ostomy patient. In D. B. Smith & D. E. Johnson (Eds.), *Ostomy care and the cancer patient: Surgical and clinical considerations* (pp. 103–120). Orlando, FL: Grune & Stratton, Inc.

Schover, L. R. (1987). Sexuality and fertility in urologic cancer patients. *Cancer, 60* (Suppl.), 553–558.

Schover, L. R., & von Eschenbach, A. C. (1984). Sexual and marital counseling with men treated for testicular cancer. *Journal of Sex and Marital Therapy, 10*, 29–40.

Schover, L. R., & von Eschenbach, A. C. (1985a). Sex therapy and the penile prosthesis: A synthesis. *Journal of Sex and Marital Therapy, 11*, 57–66.

Schover, L. R., & von Eschenbach, A. C. (1985b). Sexual and marital relationships after treatment for nonseminomatous testicular cancer. *Urology, 25*, 251–255.

Schover, L. R., & von Eschenbach, A. C. (1985c). Sexual function and female radical cystectomy: A case series. *Journal of Urology, 134*, 465–468.

Schover, L. R., von Eschenbach, A. C., Smith, D. B., & Gonzalez, J. (1984). Sexual rehabilitation of urologic cancer patients: A practical approach. *CA: A Cancer Journal for Clinicians, 34*, 3–11.

Schover, L. R., Evans, R. B., & von Eschenbach, A. C. (1986a). Sexual rehabilitation and male radical cystectomy. *Journal of Urology, 136*, 1015–1017.

Schover, L. R., Evans, R. B., & von Eschenbach, A. C. (1987). Sexual rehabilitation in a cancer center: Diagnosis and outcome in 384 cases. *Archives of Sexual Behavior, 16*, 445–461.

Schover, L. R., & Fife, M. (1985). Sexual counseling and radical pelvic or genital cancer surgery. *Journal of Psychosocial Oncology, 3*, 21–41.

Schover, L. R., Fife, M., & Gershenson, D. (1985, September). *Sexual and marital relationships in cervical cancer patients.* Paper presented at the International Academy of Sex Research Annual Meeting, Seattle, WA.

Schover, L. R., Friedman, J. M., Weiler, S. J., Heiman, J. R., & LoPiccolo, J. (1982). Multiaxial problem-oriented system for sexual dysfunctions. *Archives of General Psychiatry, 39*, 614–619.

Schover, L. R., Gonzales, M., & von Eschenbach, A. C. (1986b). Sexual and marital relationships after radiotherapy for seminoma. *Urology, 27,* 117–123.

Schover, L. R., & LoPiccolo, J. (1982). Treatment effectiveness for dysfunctions of sexual desire. *Journal of Sex and Marital Therapy, 8,* 179–197.

Schreiner-Engel, P., Schiavi, R. C., Smith, H., & White, D. (1981). Sexual arousability and the menstrual cycle. *Psychosomatic Medicine, 43,* 199–214.

Schreiner-Engel, P., Schiavi, R. C., Vietorisz, D., Eichel, J. D. S., & Smith, H. (1985). Diabetes and female sexuality: A comparative study of women in relationships. *Journal of Sex and Marital Therapy, 11,* 165–175.

Schreiner-Engel, P., Schiavi, R. C., Vietorisz, D., & Smith, H. (1987). The differential impact of diabetes type on female sexuality. *Journal of Psychosomatic Research, 31,* 23–33.

Schwartz, M. F., Bauman, J. E., & Masters, W. H. (1982). Hyperprolactinemia and sexual disorders in men. *Biological Psychiatry, 17,* 861–876.

Searles, H. F. (1959). Oedipal love in the countertransference. *International Journal of Psychoanalysis, 40,* 180–190.

Segraves, R. T. (1982a). Male sexual dysfunction and psychoactive drug use. *Postgraduate Medicine, 71,* 227–233.

Segraves, R. T. (1982b). *Marital therapy: A combined psychodynamic-behavioral approach.* New York: Plenum Press.

Segraves, R. T., Madsen, R., Carter, C. S., & Davis, J. M. (1985). Erectile dysfunction associated with pharmacological agents. In R. T. Segraves & H. W. Schoenberg (Eds.), *Diagnosis and treatment of erectile disturbances* (pp. 23–64). New York: Plenum Press.

Segraves, R. T., Schoenberg, H. W., & Ivanoff, J. (1983). Serum testosterone and prolactin levels in erectile dysfunction. *Journal of Sex and Marital Therapy, 9,* 19–26.

Selzer, M. L., Vinokur, A., & Van Rooijen, L. (1975). A self-administered Short Michigan Alcoholism Screening Test (SMAST). *Journal of Studies on Alcohol, 36,* 117–126.

Semmens, J. P., & Semmens, E. C. (1984). Sexual function and the menopause. *Clinical Obstetrics and Gynecology, 27,* 717–723.

Semmens, J. P., Rouse, I., Beilin, L. F., & Masarei, J. R. L. (1983). Relationship of plasma HDL-cholesterol to testosterone, estradiol, and sex-hormone-binding globulin levels in men and women. *Metabolism, 32,* 428–432.

Semmens, J. P., Tsai, C. C., Semmens, E. C., & Loadholt, C. B. (1985). Effects of estrogen therapy on vaginal physiology during menopause. *Obstetrics & Gynecology, 66,* 15–18.

Semmens, J. P., & Wagner, G. (1982). Estrogen deprivation and vaginal function in postmenopausal women. *Journal of the American Medical Association, 248,* 445–448.

Semmlow, J. L., & Lubowsky, J. (1983). Sexual instrumentation. *IEEE Transactions on Biomedical Engineering, 6,* 309–319.

Semple, P. D., Beastall, G. H., Brown, T. M., Stirling, K. W., Mills, R. J., & Watson, W. S. (1984). Sex hormone suppression and sexual impotence in hypoxic pulmonary fibrosis. *Thorax, 39,* 46–51.

Semple, P. D., Beastall, G. H., & Hume, R. (1980). Male sexual dysfunction, low serum testosterone and respiratory hypoxia. *British Journal of Sexual Medicine, 62,* 48–53.

Sharlip, I. D. (1981). Penile arteriography in impotence after pelvic trauma. *Journal of Urology, 126,* 477–481.

Shaw, W. W., & Zorgniotti, A. W. (1984). Surgical techniques in penile revascularization. *Urology, 23,* 76–78.

Shen, W. W. (1982). Female orgasmic inhibition by amoxapine [Letter to the editor]. *American Journal of Psychiatry, 139,* 1220–1221.

Shen, W. W., & Sata, L. S. (1983). Inhibited female orgasm resulting from psychotropic drugs: A clinical review. *Journal of Reproductive Medicine, 28,* 497–499.

Sherwin, B. B. (1985). Changes in sexual behavior as a function of plasma sex steroid levels in post-menopausal women. *Maturitas, 7,* 225–233.

Sherwin, B. B., Gelfand, M. M., & Brender, W. (1985). Androgen enhances sexual motivation in females: A prospective, crossover study of sex steroid administration in the surgical menopause. *Psychosomatic Medicine, 47,* 339–351.

Shilon, M., Paz, G. F., & Homonnai, Z. T. (1984). The use of phenoxybenzamine treatment in premature ejaculation. *Fertility and Sterility, 42,* 659–661.

Shontz, F. C. (1982). Adaption to chronic illness and disability. In T. Millon, C. Green, & R. Meagher (Eds.), *Handbook of clinical psychology* (pp. 153–171). New York: Plenum Press.

Sidi, A., Cameron, J. S., Duffy, L. M., & Lange, P. H. (1986). Intracavernous drug-induced erections in the management of male erectile dysfunction: Experience with 100 patients. *Journal of Urology, 135,* 704–706.

Sikorski, J. M. (1985). Knowledge, concerns, and questions of wives of convalescent coronary artery bypass graft surgery patients. *Journal of Cardiac Rehabilitation, 5,* 74–85.

Siroky, M. B., Sax, D. S., & Krane, R. J. (1979). Sacral signal tracing: The electrophysiology of the bulbocavernosus reflex. *Journal of Urology, 122,* 661–664.

Sjögren, K. (1983). Sexuality after stroke with hemiplegia. II. With special regard to partnership adjustment and to fulfillment. *Scandinavian Journal of Rehabilitation Medicine, 15,* 63–69.

Sjögren, K., & Fugl-Meyer, A. R. (1981). Chronic back pain and sexuality. *International Rehabilitation Medicine, 3,* 19–25.

Sjögren, K., & Fugl-Meyer, A. R. (1982). Adjustment to life after stroke with special reference to sexual intercourse and leisure. *Journal of Psychosomatic Research, 26,* 409–417.

Sjögren, K., & Fugl Meyer, A. R. (1983). Some factors influencing quality of sexual life after myocardial infarction. *International Rehabilitation Medicine, 5,* 197–201.

Slag, M. F., Morley, J. E., Elson, M. K., Trence, D. L., Nelson, C. J., Nelson, A. E. Kinlaw, W. B., Beyer, S., Nuttall, F. Q., & Shafer, R. B. (1983). Impotence in medical clinic outpatients. *Journal of the American Medical Association, 249,* 1736–1740.

Small, M. P. (1983). The Small-Carrion penile implant. In R. J. Krane, M. B. Siroky, & I. Goldstein (Eds.), *Male sexual dysfunction* (pp. 253–265). Boston: Little, Brown & Co.

So, E. P., Ho, P. C., Bodenstab, W., & Parsons, C. L. (1982). Erectile impotence associated with transurethral prostatectomy. *Urology, 19,* 259–262.

Sovner, R. (1983). Anorgasmia associated with imipramine but not desimipramine: Case report. *Clinical Psychiatry, 44,* 345–346.

Spanier, G. B. (1976). Measuring dyadic adjustment: New scales for assessing the quality of marriage and similar dyads. *Journal of Marriage and the Family, 38,* 15–28.

Spark, R. F., White, R. A., & Connolly, P. B. (1980). Impotence is not always psychogenic. *Journal of the American Medical Association, 243,* 750–755.

Sprenger, K. B. G., Schmitz, J., Hetzel, D., Bundschu, D., & Franz, H. E., (1984). Zinc and sexual dysfunction. *Controversies in Nephrology, 38,* 119–125.

Staff. (1985, Second Quarter). Impotence support groups: A win-win situtation. *Colleagues in Urology,* p. 5.

Stauffer, D., & Depalma, R. G. (1983). A comparison of penile-brachial index (PBI) and penile pulse volume recordings for diagnosis of vasculogenic impotence. *Bruit, 7,* 29–32.

Steger, J. C., & Fordyce, W. E. (1982). Behavioral health care in the management of chronic pain. In T. Millon, C. Green, & R. Meagher (Eds.), *Handbook of clinical health psychology* (pp. 467–498). New York: Plenum Press.

Stein, R. A. (1980). Sexual counseling and coronary heart disease. In S. R. Leiblum & L. A. Pervin (Eds.), *Principles and practice of sex therapy* (pp. 301–319). New York: Guilford Press.

Steinglass, P., Tislenko, L., & Reiss, D. (1985). Stability/instability in the alcoholic marriage: The interrelationships between course of alcoholism, family process, and marital outcome. *Family Process, 24,* 365–383.

Stellman, R. E., Goodwin, J. M., Robinson, J., Dansak, D., & Hilgers, R. D. (1984). Psychological effects of vulvectomy. *Psychosomatics, 25,* 779–783.

Stevens, L. A., McGrath, M. H., Druss, R. G., Kister, S. J., Gump, F. E., & Forde, K. A. (1984). The psychological impact of immediate breast reconstruction for women with early breast cancer. *Plastic and Reconstructive Surgery, 73,* 619–626.

Stroebe, M. S., & Stroebe, W. (1983). Who suffers more? Sex differences in health risks of the widowed. *Psychological Bulletin, 93,* 279–301.

Stuart, R. B. (1976). *Helping couples change.* New York: Guilford Press.

Szasz, G. (1983). Sexual incidents in an extended care unit for aged men. *Journal of the American Geriatrics Society, 31,* 407–411.

Szasz, G., Paty, D., Lawton-Speert, S., & Eisen, K. (1984). A sexual functioning scale in multiple sclerosis. *Acta Neurologica Scandinavica, 101,* 37–43.

Task Force on Concerns of Physically Disabled Women (1980). *Toward intimacy.* New York: Human Sciences Press.

Taylor, C. B., Bandura, A., Ewart, C. K., Miller, N. H., & DeBusk, R. F. (1985). Exercise testing to enhance wives' confidence in their husbands' cardiac capability soon after clinically uncomplicated myocardial infarction. *American Journal of Cardiology, 55,* 635–638.

Tepper, S. L., Jagirdar, J., Heath, D., & Geller, S. A. (1984). Homology between the female paraurethral (Skene's) glands and the prostate. *Archives of Pathology and Laboratory Medicine, 108,* 423–425.

Thase, M. E., Reynolds, C. F., Glanz, L. M., Jennings, R., Sewitch, D. E., Kupfer, D. J., & Frank, E. (1986, March). *Nocturnal penile tumescence in depressed men.* Paper presented at the annual meeting of the Society of Sex Therapy and Research, Philadelphia, PA.

Thornton, C. E. (1981). Sexuality counseling of women with spinal cord injuries. In D. G. Bullard & S. E. Knight (Eds.), *Sexuality and physical disability: Personal perspectives* (pp. 156–168). St. Louis, MO: C. V. Mosby & Co.

Thurer, S. L. (1982). The long-term sexual response to coronary bypass surgery: Some preliminary findings. *Sexuality and Disability, 5,* 208–212.

Toledo-Pereyra, L. H., Schneider, A., Baskin, S., McNichol, L., Thavarajah, K., Lin, W. J., & Whitten, J. (1985). Rehabilitation after dialysis and kidney transplantation. *Bol. Asociacion Medicin de Puerto Rico, 77,* 227–230.

Torrens, M. J. (1983). Neurologic and neurosurgical disorders associated with impotence. In R. J. Krane, M. B. Siroky, & I. Goldstein (Eds.), *Male sexual dysfunction* (pp. 55–62). Boston: Little, Brown & Co.

Trudel, G., & Saint-Laurent, S. (1983). A comparison between the effects of Kegel's exercises and a combination of sexual awareness relaxation and breathing on situational orgasmic dysfunction in women. *Journal of Sex and Marital Therapy, 9,* 204–209.

Tsitouras, P. D., Martin, C. E., & Harman, S. M. (1982). Relationship of serum testosterone to sexual activity in healthy elderly men. *Journal of Gerontology, 37,* 288–293.

Turk, D. C., Meichenbaum, D., & Genest, M. (1983). *Pain and behavioral medicine: A cognitive-behavioral perspective.* New York: Guilford Press.

Tyrer, G., Steel, J. M., Ewing, D. J., Bancroft, J., Warner, P., & Clarke, B. F. (1983). Sexual responsiveness in diabetic women. *Diabetologia, 3,* 166–171.

Valleroy, M. L., & Kraft, G. H. (1984). Sexual dysfunction in multiple sclerosis. *Archives of Physical Medicine and Rehabilitation, 65,* 125–128.

Van Hasselt, V. B., Morrison, R. L., & Bellack, A. S. (1985). Alcohol use in wife abusers and their spouses. *Addictive Behaviors, 10,* 127–135.

Van Thiel, D. H., & Gavaler, J. S. (1986). Hypothalamic-pituitary-gonadal function in liver disease with particular attention to the endocrine effects of chronic alcohol abuse. *Progress in Liver Diseases, 8*, 273-282.

Velcek, D. (1980). Penile flow index utilizing a Doppler wave analysis to identify penile vascular insufficiency. *Journal of Urology, 123*, 669-673.

Verbrugge, L. M. (1979). Marital status and health. *Journal of Marriage and the Family, 42*, 267-285.

Verhulst, J., & Schneidman, B. (1981). Schizophrenia and sexual functioning. *Hospital and Community Psychiatry, 32*, 259-262.

Vermeulen, A., Ando, S., & Verdonck, L. (1982). Prolactinomas, testosterone-binding globulin, and androgen metabolism. *Journal of Clinical Endocrinology and Metabolism, 54*, 409-412.

Vigersky, R. S. (1983). Pituitary-testicular axis. In L. I. Lipschultz, & S. S. Howards (Eds.), *Infertility in the male* (pp. 19-42). New York: Churchill Livingstone.

Virag, R., Bouilly, P., & Frydman, D. (1985a). Is impotence an arterial disorder: A study of arterial risk factors in 440 impotent men. *The Lancet, 8422*, 181-184.

Virag, R., Frydman, D., Legman, M., & Virag, H. (1984). Intracavernous injection of papaverine as diagnostic and therapeutic method in erectile failure. *Angiology, 35*, 79-87.

Virag, R., Virag, H., & Lajujie, J. (1985b). A new device for measuring penile rigidity. *Urology, 25*, 80-81.

Virag, R., Zwang, G., Dermange, H., & Legman, M. (1981). Vascologenic impotence: A review of 92 cases with 54 surgical operations. *Vascular Surgery, 15*, 9-17.

Vircburger, M. I., Prelevic, G. M., Peric, L. A., Knezevic, J., & Djukanovic, L. (1985). Testosterone levels after bromocriptine treatment in patients undergoing long-term hemodialysis. *Journal of Andrology, 6*, 113-116.

Wabrek, A. J. (1985). Bulbocavernosus reflex testing in 100 consecutive cases of erectile dysfunction. *Urology, 25*, 495-498.

Wabrek, A. J., & Burchell, R. C. (1980). Male sexual dysfunction associated with coronary heart disease. *Archives of Sexual Behavior, 9*, 69-75.

Wabrek, A. J., Shelley, M. M., Horowitz, L. M., Bastarache, M. M., & Giuca, J. E. (1983). Noninvasive penile arterial evaluation in 120 males with erectile dysfunction. *Urology, 22*, 230-234.

Wagner, G. (1982). Vascular mechanisms involved in erection and erectile disorders. *Clinics in Endocrinology and Metabolism, 11*, 717-723.

Wagner, G. (1985). Penile erection provoked by vibration. *Nordisk Sexologi, 3*, 113-118.

Wagner, G., & Green, R. (1981). *Impotence: Physiological, psychological, surgical diagnosis and treatment.* New York: Plenum Press.

Wagner, G., Hllsted, J., & Jensen, S. B. (1981). Diabetes mellitus and erectile failure. In G. Wagner & R. Green (Eds.), *Impotence: Physiological, psychological, and surgical diagnosis and treatment* (pp. 51-61). New York: Plenum Press.

Wagner, G., & Levin, R. (1978). Oxygen tension of the vaginal surface during sexual stimulation in the human. *Fertility and Sterility, 30*, 50-53.

Walker, H. E. (1983). Psychiatric aspects of infertility. In R. de Vere White (Eds.), *Aspects of male infertility* (pp. 250-260). Baltimore: Williams & Wilkins.

Walsh, P. C., & Mostwin, J. L. (1984). Radical prostatectomy and cystoprostatectomy with preservation of potency: Results using a new nerve-sparing technique. *British Journal of Urology, 56*, 694-697.

Waltzer, W. C. (1981). Sexual and reproductive function in men treated with hemodialysis and renal transplantation. *Journal of Urology, 126*, 713-716.

Waring, E. M., & Patton, D. (1984). Marital intimacy and depression. *British Journal of Psychiatry, 145*, 641-644.

Wasow, M. (1980). Sexuality and the institutionalized mentally ill. *Sexuality and Disability, 3,* 3–16.

Wasow, M., & Loeb, M. B. (1977). Sexuality in nursing homes. In R. L. Solnick (Ed.), *Sexuality and aging.* Los Angeles: University of Southern California Press.

Wein, A. J., Van Arsdalen, K., & Levin, R. M. (1983). Adrenergic corporal receptors. In R. J. Krane, M. B. Siroky, & I. Goldstein (Eds.), *Male sexual dysfunction* (pp. 33–36). Boston: Little, Brown & Co.

Weizman, R., Weizman, A., Levi, J., Gura, V., Zevin, D., Maoz, B., Wijsenbeek, H., & Ben David, M. (1983). Sexual dysfunction associated with hyperprolactinemia in males and females undergoing hemodialysis. *Psychosomatic Medicine, 45,* 259–269.

Whipple, B., & Komisaruk, B. R. (1985). Elevation of pain threshold by vaginal stimulation in women. *Pain, 21,* 357–367.

White, C. B. (1982). Sexual interest, attitudes, knowledge, and sexual history in relation to sexual behavior in the institutionalized aged. *Archives of Sexual Behavior, 11,* 11–23.

Wiklund, I., Sanne, H., Elmfeldt, D., Vedin, A., & Wilhelmsson, C. (1984). Emotional reaction, health preoccupation and sexual activity two months after a myocardial infarction. *Scandinavian Journal of Rehabilitation Medicine, 16,* 47–56.

Williams, W. (1985). Anaesthetic ejaculation. *Journal of Sex and Marital Therapy, 11,* 19–29.

Willis, E. A., Ottesen, B., Wagner, G., Sundler, F., & Fahrenkrug, J. (1983). Vasoactive intestinal polypeptide (VIP) as a putative neurotransmitter in penile erection. *Life Sciences, 33,* 383–391.

Willscher, M. K. (1983). Peyronie's disease. In R. J. Krane, M. B. Siroky, & I. Goldstein (Eds.), *Male sexual dysfunction* (pp. 87–100). Boston: Little, Brown & Co.

Wilson, G. T., Niaura, R. S., & Adler, J. L. (1985). Alcohol, selective attention and sexual arousal in men. *Journal of Studies on Alcohol, 46,* 107–115.

Wincze, J. P., Bansal, S., & Malamud, M. (1986). Effects of medroxyprogesterone acetate on subjective arousal, arousal to erotic stimulation, and nocturnal penile tumescence in male sex offenders. *Archives of Sexual Behavior, 15,* 293–306.

Winn, R. L., & Newton, N. (1982). Sexuality in aging: A study of 106 cultures. *Archives of Sexual Behavior, 11,* 283–298.

Winters, S. J., Sherins, R. J., & Troen, P. (1984). The gonadotropin-suppressive activity of androgen is increased in elderly men. *Metabolism, 33,* 1052–1059.

Winther, G., Jensen, S. B., & Hertoft, P. (1984). The significance of some selected factors for sexological advice and therapy: A review of 397 persons referred on account of sexual dysfunction during the period of 1974–1979. *Ugeskrift for Laeger, 146,* 493–497.

Wise, T. N. (1983). Sexual disorders in medical and surgical conditions. In J. K. Meyer, C. W. Schmidt, Jr., & T. N. Wise (Eds.), *Clinical management of sexual disorders* (pp. 317–332). Baltimore: Williams & Wilkins.

Wise, T. N. (1985). Coping with a transvestite mate. *Journal of Sex and Marital Therapy, 11,* 293–300.

Wise, T. N., Rabins, P. V., & Gahnsley, J. (1984). The older patient with a sexual dysfunction. *Journal of Sex and Marital Therapy, 10,* 117–121.

Witkin, M. H., & Kaplan, H. S. (1983). Sex therapy and penectomy. *Journal of Sex and Marital Therapy, 8,* 209–221.

Woolf, P. D., Hamill, R. W., McDonald, J. V., Lee, L. A., & Kelly, M. (1985). Transient hypogonadotropic hypogonadism caused by critical illness. *Journal of Clinical Endocrinology and Metabolism, 60,* 444–450.

World Health Organization (1975). Education and treatment in human sexuality: The training of health professionals. Geneva, Switzerland: World Health Organization Technical Reports, Series 572.

Yalla, S. V. (1982). Sexual dysfunction in the paraplegic and quadriplegic. In A. H. Bennett (Ed.), *Management of male impotence* (pp. 182–191). Baltimore: Williams & Wilkins.

Young, R. J., & Ismail, A. H. (1978). Ability of biochemical and personality variables in discriminating between high and low physical fitness levels. *Journal of Psychosomatic Research, 22,* 193–199.

Zeidler, A., Gelfand, R., Tamagna, E., Marrs, R., Chopp, R., & Kletzky, O. (1982). Pituitary gonadal function in diabetic male patients with and without impotence. *Andrologia, 14,* 62–68.

Zentner, E. B., & Pouyat, S. P. (1978). The erotic factor as a complication in the dual-sex therapy team's effective functioning. *Journal of Sex and Marital Therapy, 4,* 114–121.

Zilbergeld, B. (1978). *Male sexuality.* New York: Bantam Books.

Zilbergeld, B. (1980). Alternatives to couples counseling for sex problems: Group and individual therapy. *Journal of Sex and Marital Therapy, 6,* 3–18.

Zilbergeld, B., & Kilmann, P. R. (1984). The scope and effectiveness of sex therapy. *Psychotherapy: Theory, Research and Practice, 21,* 319–326.

Zorgniotti, A. W. (1984). Practical diagnostic screening for impotence. *Urology, 23,* 98–102.

Zorgniotti, A. W., & Lefleur, R. S. (1985). Auto-injection of the corpus cavernosum with a vasoactive drug combination for vasculogenic impotence. *Journal of Urology, 133,* 39–41.

Zucker, R. A., & Gomberg, E. S. L. (1986). Etiology of alcoholism reconsidered: The case for a biopsychosocial process. *American Psychologist, 41,* 783–793.

Zuckerman, M., Neeb, M., Ficher, M., Fishkin, R. E., Goldman, A., Fink, P. J., Cohen, S. N., Jacobs, J. A., & Weisberg, M. (1985). Nocturnal penile tumescence and penile responses in the waking state in diabetic and nondiabetic sexual dysfunctionals. *Archives of Sexual Behavior, 14,* 109–130.

Index